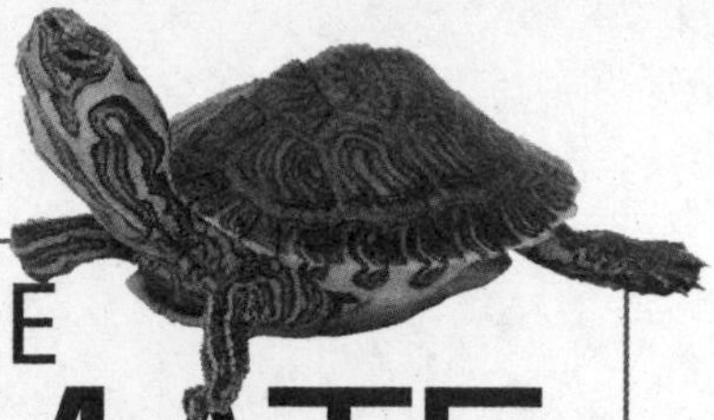

THE ULTIMATE WOMEN'S GUIDE TO BEATING DISEASE

...and living a happy, active life

2019

FROM THE EDITORS OF BOTTOM LINE HEALTH

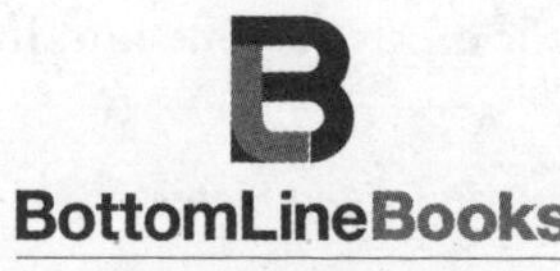

BottomLineInc.com

The Ultimate Women's Guide to Beating Disease and Living a Happy, Active Life

Cover art: In many ancient traditions, the turtle is a symbol of good health, endurance and long life, since turtles can live to one hundred years or more. In many Native American tribes, the turtle is the symbol for Mother Earth.

10 9 8 7 6 5 4 3 2 1

ISBN 0-88723-808-4

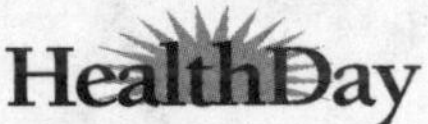

A selection of articles in this book were written by reporters for HealthDay, an award-winning international daily consumer health news service, headquartered in Norwalk, Connecticut.

Bottom Line Books® publishes the advice of expert authorities in many fields. These opinions may at times conflict as there are often different approaches to solving problems. The use of a book is not a substitute for legal, accounting, investment, health or any other professional services. Consult competent professionals for answers to your specific questions.

Offers, prices, rates, addresses, telephone numbers and websites listed in this book are accurate at the time of publication, but they are subject to frequent change.

Bottom Line Books® is a registered trademark of Bottom Line Inc.
3 Landmark Square, Suite 201, Stamford, CT 06901

BottomLineInc.com

Bottom Line Books is an imprint of Bottom Line Inc., publisher of print periodicals, e-letters and books. We are dedicated to bringing you the best information from the most knowledgeable sources in the world. Our goal is to help you gain greater wealth, better health, more wisdom, extra time and increased happiness.

Printed in the United States of America

CONTENTS

10 • PAIN AND AUTOIMMUNE DISEASE

11 • EMOTIONAL HEALING

12 • FOOD AND FITNESS

PREFACE

We are proud to bring to you *The Ultimate Women's Guide to Beating Disease and Living a Happy, Active Life 2019.* This essential volume features trustworthy and actionable life-saving information from the best health experts in the world—information that will help women beat the conditions that are most deadly to them.* In the following chapters, you'll find the latest discoveries, best treatments and scientifically proven remedies to keep you living a long, happy and active life.

Whether it's heart care, the latest on stroke, breast cancer prevention and treatment, breakthrough treatments for hot flashes or cutting-edge nutritional advice, the editors of *Bottom Line Health* talk to the experts—from top women's health doctors to research scientists to leading alternative care practitioners—who are creating the true innovations in health care.

Over the past four decades, we have built a network of literally thousands of leading physicians in both alternative and conventional medicine. They are affiliated with the premier medical and research institutions throughout the world. We read the important medical journals and follow the latest research that is reported at medical conferences. And we regularly talk to our advisors in major teaching hospitals, private practices and government health agencies for their insider perspective.

*"Leading Causes of Death in Females," Centers for Disease Control and Prevention (*http://www.cdc.gov/women/lcod/2014/index.htm*).

In this 2019 edition, we've gone beyond diseases and have included seven chapters of life-enhancing health information on pain, depression, fitness, diet, quality medical care, sexuality and aging...all of which are essential to living a happy, active life. And it's all backed by breaking studies and top health experts. Also note that respiratory diseases, according to the Centers for Disease Control and Prevention, are now considered one of the top three causes of death in women of all ages (same percentage as stroke).

The Ultimate Women's Guide to Beating Disease and Living a Happy, Active Life 2019 is a result of our ongoing research and connection with these experts, and is a distillation of their latest findings and advice. We trust that you will glean new, helpful and affordable information about the health topics that concern you most...and find vital topics of interest to family and friends as well.

As a reader of a Bottom Line book, please be assured that you are receiving well-researched information from a trusted source. But, please use prudence in health matters. Always speak to your physician before taking vitamins, supplements or over-the-counter medication...stopping a medication...changing your diet...or beginning an exercise program. If you experience side effects from any regimen, contact your doctor immediately.

Be well,
The Editors, *Bottom Line Health*
Stamford, Connecticut

Chapter 1

HEART HEALTH FOR WOMEN

Many Women Miss Out on Lifesaving CPR

America's sense of propriety could cost women their lives when their heart suddenly stops, a new study suggests.

Simply put, women suffering from cardiac arrest in a public setting are less likely to get lifesaving CPR from a passerby than men are, researchers reported.

"When it comes to life and death, we need to reassure the public that we're not worrying about what seems socially inappropriate or taboo," said senior study author Benjamin Abella, MD. He is director of the University of Pennsylvania's Center for Resuscitation Science.

"The situation requires action, and it requires people to not hesitate. A life is on the line," Dr. Abella added.

About the Study

But the study showed people do hesitate, especially when the victim is a woman. About 45% of men who suffered cardiac arrest in a public setting received CPR from a bystander, compared with only 39% of women, the researchers found.

The investigators suspect bystanders might be worried about touching a strange woman's chest in public, even if it is to save a life.

The reason the researchers believe that is because people acted very differently when a woman collapsed at home, where she had an equal chance of receiving CPR.

The study involved data gathered by the Resuscitation Outcomes Consortium, a network of US and Canadian hospitals studying cardiac arrest.

About Cardiac Arrest

Cardiac arrest can kill a person within minutes if CPR isn't performed, according to the American Heart Association (AHA).

More than 350,000 cardiac arrests occur outside of a hospital each year. Nine out of 10 of these victims die, but speedy CPR can double or triple the chance of survival, the AHA noted.

Benjamin Abella, MD, director, and Audrey Blewer, MPH, assistant director, University of Pennsylvania's Center for Resuscitation Science, Philadelphia.

Clifton Callaway, MD, PhD, executive vice chair, emergency medicine, University of Pittsburgh Medical Center.

American Heart Association's annual meeting, Anaheim, California.

Study Findings

The researchers reviewed more than 19,000 cases of cardiac arrest that occurred outside of a hospital between 2011 and 2015.

Men in public settings were 23% more likely than women to receive bystander CPR, and they also had 23% better odds of survival, according to the report.

But, "when we looked in the home, there was no difference in terms of response by gender," said study author Audrey Blewer, MPH, an assistant director for educational programs at UPenn's Center for Resuscitation Science.

The study was presented at the AHA's annual meeting, in Anaheim, California.

Expert Commentary

The difference between men and women is "unexpected," said Clifton Callaway, MD, PhD, executive vice chair of emergency medicine at the University of Pittsburgh Medical Center.

"I really would have thought if somebody is on the ground, and not responsive, that people would be equally likely to help a man or woman," said Dr. Callaway, an AHA spokesman.

Bystanders already have a difficult time responding to a sudden collapse in public, Dr. Abella explained. They're shocked by the collapse, and often are afraid of hurting someone by attempting CPR.

"We think these data show yet one more barrier that may be playing a role in low bystander CPR response," Dr. Abella said.

The researchers found that, in all cases, bystanders administered CPR only 37% of the time.

"The most striking thing to me is how few people get CPR overall," Dr. Callaway said. "Those numbers are something we really need to turn around. Two-thirds of people don't get a bystander to do CPR when their heart has stopped. This is something we've known for decades."

What to Do

Witnesses should immediately call 911 and then start hands-only CPR on the person—one hand over the other on the middle of the chest, pushing hard and fast, at about 100 to 120 beats a minute. The disco song "Staying Alive" provides a good beat for CPR, Dr. Abella added.

CPR can be performed through any sort of clothing, Blewer said. Don't worry about any undergarments—just start pressing on the middle of the chest.

Passersby worried about providing CPR should keep in mind that all 50 states have Good Samaritan laws on the books that will protect them against legal action, Dr. Abella noted.

"That's something I think people are not as aware of as they should be," Dr. Abella said.

For more on how to perform CPR, visit the American Heart Association at CPR.heart.org. Under "Programs" choose "Hands-Only CPR."

5 Surprising Ways to Prevent a Heart Attack

Barry A. Franklin, PhD, director of preventive cardiology and cardiac rehabilitation at William Beaumont Hospital, Royal Oak, Michigan. Dr. Franklin has served as president of the American Association of Cardiovascular and Pulmonary Rehabilitation and the American College of Sports Medicine. He is also coeditor of *The Heart-Healthy Handbook*, available at HealthyLearning.com.

There are hopeful signs that Americans are increasingly embracing a heart-healthy lifestyle. The percentage of smokers has plunged to approximately 15% over the last decade. Many people are eating better and doing a better job of controlling high blood pressure and elevated cholesterol.

But despite these gains, cardiovascular disease still accounts for one out of three deaths in the US. Much of the blame goes to the obvious culprits that fuel heart disease—cigarette smoking, elevated blood cholesterol, high blood pressure, obesity, diabetes and a lack of exercise, to name a few. But others might surprise you.

Small Changes Count

Research shows that our daily habits account for 40% to 50% of all deaths caused by cardiovascular disease. The good news is that even small lifestyle choices may offer big benefits. *Five little things you can do to reduce heart attack risk...*

***SECRET #1:* Avoid secondhand smoke.** Most people associate secondhand smoke with lung disease—but the danger to the heart is worse than you may realize.

Here's why: Exposure to cigarette smoke—from smoking yourself or from secondhand smoke—increases arterial inflammation and impairs the ability of arteries to dilate and constrict normally. It also makes blood more likely to coagulate, the major cause of heart attacks.

If you live with an indoor smoker or spend time in other smoke-filled environments, your risk for a heart attack is 30% higher than in someone without this exposure. Cities (and countries) that have adopted public-smoking bans have reported reductions in heart attacks of 20% to 40%—with most of the reductions occurring in nonsmokers.

***SECRET #2:* Know your family genes.** If you have inherited gene variants known to increase the risk for heart disease, your risk of developing coronary disease and having a cardiac event is higher than you probably think. In an important new study, researchers from Massachusetts General Hospital followed more than 55,000 participants for up to 20 years, analyzing genetic variants and lifestyle data.

Conclusion: People with a genetic predisposition for heart disease had nearly double the risk of developing it themselves.

But bad genes don't have to be destiny. The same study found that people who made positive changes in two or three out of four common areas known to negatively impact heart health—smoking, obesity, lack of regular exercise and an unhealthful diet—were able to reduce their cardiovascular risks by nearly 50%.

***SECRET #3:* Get a flu shot.** The flu can be deadly, yet fewer than half of at-risk Americans (including those with chronic health conditions, such as cardiovascular and/or lung disease) get an annual vaccination.

Why it matters: The fever, dehydration and pneumonia that often accompany the flu can be devastating for people who have cardiovascular disease. The flu can worsen preexisting conditions such as heart failure or diabetes or trigger an asthma attack or heart attack in some people.

A 2013 *JAMA* study that looked at more than 6,700 patients (mean age, 67 years) found that those who got a flu vaccination were 36% less likely to suffer cardiovascular events (such as heart attacks) during the following year than those who weren't vaccinated. When researchers looked only at patients who had recent cardiac events, they found that vaccination cut the risk by 55%.

Recommended: An annual flu shot for everyone age 50 or older...and for anyone who has been diagnosed with cardiovascular disease. Adults age 65 and older should discuss the pros and cons of the high-dose flu vaccine with their physicians—it's reported to be about 24% more effective than standard vaccines but may have greater side effects.

***SECRET #4:* Don't stop taking a beta-blocker drug abruptly.** Used for treating high blood pressure, irregular heartbeats, rapid heart rates and many other conditions, beta-blockers are among the most commonly prescribed drugs in the US.

Drugs in this class—*propranolol* (such as Inderal), *atenolol* (Tenormin) and many others—are generally safe but may cause side effects including fatigue, light-headedness and even impotence. As a result, patients sometimes decide on their own to stop taking these drugs.

The danger: If these drugs are suddenly stopped, the patient can have a dangerous upsurge in adrenaline activity, which can cause a faster heart rate, heavy sweating, spikes in blood pressure and an increased risk for heart attack and stroke. People who want to stop taking a beta-blocker are advised to slowly decrease the dose over 10 to 14 days.

Important: If you believe that you need to stop taking any prescribed medication, be sure to first check with your doctor. If side effects are a problem, you can probably switch to another drug or a dose that's easier to tolerate.

Secret #5: **Lower your resting pulse.** When you increase your heart rate during aerobic exercise, you're helping to prevent a heart attack or stroke—this signifies that you're getting the cardiovascular benefits of moderate-to-vigorous exercise. Paradoxically, a slower resting heart rate is also protective.

Here's why: In general, a slower resting rate means a longer life—probably because a slower heart rate exerts less stress on blood vessel walls. Studies have shown that healthy men and women with lower resting heart rates (less than 60 beats per minute) have fewer cardiac events and a lower risk of dying from cardiovascular disease than those with faster rates (greater than 80 beats per minute).

A study of heart patients taking beta-blockers found that each 10-beat reduction in resting heart rate reduced the risk for cardiac death by 30%. For example, if someone with a resting heart rate of 80 beats per minute is given a beta-blocker to slow the rate to 60, the risk for cardiac death will drop by 60%.

Recommended: A resting heart rate of 50 to 70, depending on your cardiac history and typical physical activity level. Regular exercise...quitting smoking...maintaining a healthy weight...and avoiding high doses of caffeine can slow the resting heart rate.

Also important: Your recovery heart rate, the time that it takes your pulse to approach its resting rate after exercise. The fitter you get, the more quickly your heartbeat will return to a resting rate.

Breast Cancer Treatment Can Be Tough on the Heart

Laxmi Mehta, MD, associate professor, medicine, and section director, Women's Cardiovascular Health, Ohio State University Medical Center, Columbus.
Richard Steingart, MD, chief, cardiology service, Memorial Sloan Kettering Cancer Center, New York City.
Circulation.

Certain breast cancer treatments may take a toll on the heart, but women can take steps to minimize the risks, according to a new report from the American Heart Association.

"The intent is not to scare women away from any breast cancer treatments," stressed Laxmi Mehta, MD, the lead author of the report and director of the women's cardiovascular health program at Ohio State University.

Rather, she said, the most important question women should ask when making treatment decisions is, "What is the best treatment for my breast cancer?"

"Then it becomes, 'What are the side effects?' " Dr. Mehta said. "If there is a risk of [heart effects], you can ask, 'How will I be monitored?' "

Background

The good news is that more and more women are beating breast cancer, according to Dr. Mehta.

Still, they will need to pay attention to their risk for heart disease—the No. 1 cause of death for American women, according to the US Centers for Disease Control and Prevention.

In fact, the AHA says, breast cancer survivors—especially those older than 65—are more likely to die of heart disease than a cancer comeback.

The AHA report, published in the journal *Circulation*, gives an overview of the issue as well as some advice for women.

Heart Effects of Cancer Drugs

Because the heart risks associated with certain cancer treatments are well-recognized, those types of discussions should already be happening, according to Richard Steingart, MD, chief of cardiology service at Memorial Sloan Kettering Cancer Center in New York City.

From the start, women should have their cardiovascular health evaluated, Dr. Steingart said. Then, they and their doctors should try to get any heart disease risk factors under the best control possible.

When it comes to chemotherapy, any effects on the heart typically show up in the short term and can be detected during treatment, he said.

For example, drugs called anthracyclines—such as *doxorubicin*—can damage heart muscle cells, sometimes leading to chronic heart failure. In heart failure, the muscle can't pump blood efficiently enough, leading to symptoms such as breathlessness and fatigue.

Heart failure is also a possibility with drugs that target the HER2 gene, such as *trastuzumab* (Herceptin)—though it's largely reversible, according to the AHA report.

Women on those medications will have their heart function monitored during treatment. When signs of trouble are detected, Dr. Steingart said, the "rule of thumb" is to continue treatment, if possible.

Standard heart medications such as beta-blockers and ACE inhibitors may improve heart function in women who develop side effects during treatment, according to the AHA report.

In some cases, women might need a break from their cancer treatment to see whether any heart effects reverse, whereas others might need their treatment plan changed, the report noted.

Dr. Steingart stressed that for any one woman, the risk for serious heart effects is generally low. It also varies, depending on a woman's risk factors for heart disease—such as age, high blood pressure and smoking.

If a woman already has heart disease when she's diagnosed with breast cancer, Dr. Steingart said, her cardiologist should be consulted when treatment is being planned.

Some heart effects, such as those from chest radiation, may not show up until years later.

Migraines Are Associated with Greater Heart Risk

Women who get migraines are 50% more likely to develop major cardiovascular disease than those who do not suffer from the headaches. Migraines probably do not cause heart disease—more likely, the underlying factors that lead to migraines also lead to increased cardiovascular risk. Migraine sufferers should be aware of the association and be especially attentive to signs of a possible heart attack or stroke.

Study of more than 115,000 women ages 25 to 42 over two decades, led by researchers at Harvard T.H. Chan School of Public Health, Boston, published in *The BMJ*.

Expert Advice

According to Dr. Mehta, women should pay attention to any potential heart disease symptoms such as breathlessness and chest pain—and then make sure they tell their doctor about their cancer treatment history.

Those types of symptoms may or may not be concerning on their own, she said. But if you tell your doctor you had chest radiation years ago, that would raise a red flag.

For all women, a healthy lifestyle is vital during and after breast cancer treatment, both Dr. Mehta and Dr. Steingart emphasized.

"You don't want to worsen your risk factors for heart disease," Dr. Mehta said. "So remember that a healthy lifestyle is imperative."

Plus, Dr. Steingart noted, lifestyle choices may help women get through their cancer treatment.

"We believe that if you keep up a healthy lifestyle—stay active, eat a healthy diet—your cancer treatment will be easier to tolerate," he said.

The Susan G. Komen Breast Cancer Foundation has more on the effects of breast cancer treatment at ww5.Komen.org. Search "side effects of breast cancer treatment."

Are Women's Hearts More Vulnerable to Stress?

Viola Vaccarino, MD, PhD, professor, epidemiology and medicine, Rollins School of Public Health, Emory University, Atlanta.

Nieca Goldberg, MD, medical director, Center for Women's Health, NYU Langone Medical Center, New York City.

Arteriosclerosis, Thrombosis and Vascular Biology.

Mental stress can take a toll on blood vessels—and women with heart disease may be especially vulnerable, a new study suggests.

Blood Vessel Constriction

Past research has found that compared with their male counterparts, women with heart disease are more likely to suffer "myocardial ischemia" in response to mental stress.

That refers to a reduction in blood flow to the heart, and it can raise the risk of potentially fatal heart complications.

In the new study, researchers uncovered a reason for the phenomenon: When under psychological stress, women are more prone than men to having their blood vessels constrict.

Experts said the findings underscore some realities.

Physical Versus Mental Stress

Traditionally, doctors have focused on how well the heart and blood vessels respond to physical stress, said Nieca Goldberg, MD, a spokesperson for the American Heart Association who was not involved in the study.

"But we can't ignore the issue of mental stress in treating heart disease," she said.

And that awareness may be especially important for women, said Dr. Goldberg, who is also medical director of NYU Langone's Center for Women's Health in New York City.

There is no single solution for dealing with stress, Dr. Goldberg said. For some people, she noted, a daily walk or an app that teaches relaxation techniques might be enough. Others might need a referral to a mental health professional.

"Everybody's stressors are different," Dr. Goldberg said. "So we as doctors need to work with patients individually."

Study Details

The study involved 678 people with coronary artery disease. That means "plaques" build up in larger arteries, sometimes causing symptoms like chest pain and breathlessness. It can also lead to a heart attack if a plaque ruptures and completely blocks an artery.

Each patient went through a mental stress test—public speaking—and researchers used heart imaging to see whether it triggered myocardial ischemia.

Overall, around 15% of all study patients had stress-induced ischemia—with men and women affected at a similar rate. But the underlying causes differed between the sexes.

In women, it was mainly caused by constriction in small blood vessels, said senior researcher Viola Vaccarino, MD, PhD. She's a professor at Emory University's Rollins School of Public Health in Atlanta.

When men developed ischemia, it was mainly because mental stress triggered a rise in blood pressure and heart rate—which boosted the heart's workload.

It's already known, Dr. Vaccarino said, that women are more likely than men to have "microvascular dysfunction." That refers to problems in the small blood vessels that feed the heart. Those arteries are not clogged up with plaques, but they have damage that can impair blood flow.

"Basically, the small vessels do not relax," Dr. Vaccarino explained.

According to Dr. Goldberg, that higher rate of microvascular dysfunction might help explain why women are more prone to blood vessel constriction when stressed.

The findings were published in *Arteriosclerosis, Thrombosis and Vascular Biology*.

What to Do

What should heart disease patients do? First, Dr. Vaccarino said, many people with stress-related ischemia wouldn't know it. "In most cases, it's asymptomatic—or 'silent,'" she said.

But, she added, people can consider the stressors in their lives, and how well they typically respond. "Stress is universal," Dr. Vaccarino noted. "It's the way we deal with it that matters."

She agreed that simple techniques like guided relaxation or meditation can be a good place to start. Regular exercise, like a daily walk, is another—and not only because it can help a stressed-out person feel better, Dr. Vaccarino noted.

"Physical exercise actually makes the blood vessels dilate. It's the opposite effect of what we see with mental stress," she said.

"The main message is, we need to find healthy ways to cope with stress," Dr. Vaccarino said. And that may be particularly important for women, she added.

"Typically, women often don't put themselves first," she said. "But they need to take breaks every day, find ways to relax."

It's not clear whether stress can cause similar blood vessel constriction in women without heart disease, Dr. Vaccarino noted.

Follow-up Study Planned

And the researchers do not know whether the short-term stress reactions in these study participants could actually raise their risk of heart attack or other complications. The investigators plan to look at that in future studies.

The American Heart Association has more on stress and heart disease at GoRedForWomen.org. Search "stress and heart disease."

For Women, Blocked Arteries Not the Only Trigger for Heart Attacks

Noel Bairey Merz, MD, director, Barbra Streisand Women's Heart Center, Smidt Heart Institute Cedars-Sinai Medical Center, Los Angeles.

Janet Wei, MD, co-director, stress echocardiography laboratory, Cedars-Sinai Heart Institute, Los Angeles.

Cedars-Sinai Medical Center, news release.

Women don't need to have blocked arteries to experience a heart attack, a recent study points out.

Blocked arteries are a main cause of heart attack in men, according to researchers from Cedars-Sinai Medical Center in Los Angeles.

They found, though, that about 8% of women who have chest pain but no blocked arteries actually have scars on their heart that indicate they had a heart attack.

Women who complain of chest pain often are told they haven't had a heart attack if their arteries aren't blocked, the researchers said.

Study Details

Their study included 340 women who reported chest pain but did not have blocked heart arteries.

An imaging procedure—called cardiac magnetic resonance—revealed that 26 of the women (8%) had scars on their heart that indicated prior damage to the heart muscle.

Of those 26 women, about a third were never diagnosed with a heart attack, even though their cardiac scans revealed heart muscle damage.

A year later, 179 of the women had another heart scan. At that point, two women were found to have new heart scarring. In that year, both of the women had been hospitalized for chest pain but were not diagnosed with a heart attack, the study reported.

The study was published in the journal *Circulation*.

Implications

"This study proves that women need to be taken seriously when they complain of chest pain, even if they don't have the typical symptoms we see in men," said first author Janet Wei, MD.

"Too often, these women are told they don't have a heart problem and they are sent home, instead of receiving appropriate medical care," she said.

"Many women go to the hospital with chest pain, but they often aren't tested for a heart attack because doctors felt they were low-risk," said study co-author Noel Bairey Merz, MD. Dr. Merz is director of the Barbra Streisand Women's Heart Center in the Smidt Heart Institute at Cedars-Sinai

"They are considered low-risk because their heart disease symptoms are different than the symptoms men experience," she said.

The American Heart Association outlines heart attack symptoms in women at Heart.org. Search "heart attack symptoms in women."

Tests That Tell Your Real Risk for Heart Disease

James de Lemos, MD, a professor of internal medicine in the division of cardiology at UT Southwestern Medical Center, Dallas. He is the current medical director of the Dallas Heart Study.

Everyone's familiar with the traditional risk factors for heart disease. There's elevated cholesterol...high blood pressure...and diabetes.

What you might not realize is that these measures aren't very effective at predicting who will have a heart attack. More than half of cardiovascular "events," including heart attacks, occur in patients who would not be considered at high risk based on the usual risk factors. Another shortcoming is that these factors address only one particular type of heart disease (due to atherosclerosis, or plaque buildup in the arteries) even though there are other, equally serious heart threats.

A better approach: A simple, relatively inexpensive panel of tests that can identify your risk for a broader range of heart issues, including death from heart disease, as well as heart attack, stroke, heart failure (an inability of the heart to pump blood efficiently) and atrial fibrillation, or AF (an irregular heartbeat that increases risk not only for heart-related death but also for stroke). The panel of tests can even estimate future risks in patients with none of the usual risk factors.

Why it works: Each of the tests detects abnormal processes that affect the heart. But their real strength lies in their collective value. When the tests are combined, they provide an accurate assessment of your risk of developing heart disease within the next 10 years. These tests improve upon the performance of the Heart Disease Risk Calculator, CVRiskCalculator.com, created by the American College of Cardiology and the American Heart Association. (If you know your blood pressure and cholesterol numbers, you can do this online test yourself.)

What's Been Missed

If you worry about heart disease (or already have it), you've probably been told to keep your cholesterol down, stop smoking, manage your blood pressure, etc. It's good advice for everyone, but the benefits mainly involve atherosclerotic cardiovascular disease.

Many people have taken this advice, which is why the prevalence of clot-related heart attacks (as well as stroke) has declined in recent years. But there's been an increase in the rates of heart failure and AF, conditions that are time-consuming and expensive to treat—and are often fatal. The traditional cardiovascular risk factors don't affect your odds of getting AF or heart failure.

The five-test panel can give a better view of cardiovascular risks than the currently used methods. It's particularly useful for people who appear to be in good health and don't have any of the usual risk factors—but who want to ensure that their hearts stay as healthy as possible.

A Broader View

Each of the five tests below reflects a different aspect of heart health. Used individually, the tests are only modestly useful. Their real predictive strength is additive. You might want to do a baseline battery of these tests in your mid-40s and then again on a schedule your doctor suggests. *The five heart tests to have…*

- **A 12-lead EKG.** An electrocardiogram (EKG) measures voltage (the electrical activity created by each heartbeat) using electrodes placed on the chest. Someone with an abnormally enlarged heart will show high voltage. An enlarged heart isn't always dangerous—it often occurs in highly trained athletes in excellent health. But in average adults, an enlarged heart can increase the risk for heart failure, blood clots and cardiac arrest. It can also indicate if someone has had a silent heart attack (one that occurs without noticeable symptoms).
- **Coronary calcium scan.** This low-radiation CT scan looks for calcium deposits in the arteries—a sign of cholesterol plaque buildup and future heart risk.
- **C-reactive protein (CRP) blood test.** Elevated CRP (above 3 mg/L) indicates inflammation in your body and can be a marker for increased risk for coronary artery disease.
- **NT-proBNP blood test.** BNP (B-type natriuretic peptide) is a hormone produced by the heart. It's a protective hormone, so levels rise when the heart is under stress. Levels higher than 100 pg/mL indicate that there might be stress or strain within the chambers of the heart—a sign that heart failure is developing or getting worse.
- **High-sensitivity troponin T blood test.** Troponin T is a protein that's released when the heart muscle is damaged. Hospitals test for it to diagnose heart attacks. The newer, higher-sensitivity test can detect the smallest amounts of damage to the heart muscle caused by high blood pressure, infection or even a heart attack that's so minor that a patient never experiences symptoms.

What the Research Shows

With the exception of the high-sensitivity troponin T test (which only recently received FDA approval), none of these tests are new. Cardiologists have used them individually for years. But they've only recently been tested together as a tool for predicting cardiovascular risks.

Important recent finding: Researchers looked at nearly 9,000 participants from the Dallas Heart Study and the Multi-Ethnic Study of Atherosclerosis for a study that appeared in the journal *Circulation*. The participants, who were followed for more than 10 years, were screened to be sure they had no cardiovascular disease, and all were given the five-test panel at the beginning of the study.

Results: Patients with one abnormal test result (approximately 30%) were about three to four times more likely to be diagnosed with one of the heart conditions described earlier. The risk was sixfold higher in those with two abnormal tests…12 times higher in those with three abnormal tests…and more than 20 times higher in the 5% with four or five abnormal tests. Even after accounting for traditional risk factors such as high blood pressure and weight, people with high scores had five to six times the risk for future heart incidents than those with scores of zero.

Should You Get Tested?

One out of every four deaths in the US is caused by heart disease. Coronary artery disease, commonly linked to smoking, high cholesterol and genetics, is the most prevalent form, but heart failure, AF and other cardiovascular diseases affect millions of Americans.

The five-test panel is the first approach that permits a global view of risk. Previously, there have not been good predictive strategies. Patients who are given the five tests—which will be used along with the traditional tests for cholesterol, blood pressure, etc.—

will have the clearest sense of their future risks. Identifying the risk for heart failure is particularly important because this condition will eventually affect about 25% of Americans…it carries the highest cardiovascular mortality rate…and it isn't predicted by the "standard" risk factors.

For now, we mainly recommend the panel for individuals without obvious risk factors who want to do everything possible to protect their hearts…those with a family history of heart disease…or those interested in the most accurate information about future risk, for example. If you already know you're at risk, the extra information may not be as useful, since your doctor would recommend the same healthful strategies—weight loss, a healthier diet, lower blood pressure and cholesterol, etc.—in either case.

In the future: The panel could be used to target existing treatments and to encourage at-risk patients to make lifestyle changes.

Example: The diabetes drug *empagliflozin* (Jardiance) can reduce heart failure by 35%, but it's expensive. The cost could be justified for diabetics who learn that their heart-failure risk is high. Similarly, heart patients with abnormal test results might be more motivated to get serious about weight loss, fitness, healthy eating and other lifestyle changes.

The panel isn't expensive. You can expect to pay about $50 to $100 for the calcium scan…$25 to $50 for each blood test…and $50 to $100 for an EKG. The entire panel might be offered for about $400. Insurance companies may cover the costs—but check first.

Marijuana May Cause a Heart Problem

In a recent study, pot users were more likely to suffer from stress cardiomyopathy. The rare condition, which usually affects older women, is a sudden temporary weakening of the heart muscle that reduces its pumping ability and can feel like a heart attack.

Analysis of a federal health database of more than 33,000 people by researchers at St. Luke's University Health Network, Bethlehem, Pennsylvania, presented at the annual meeting of the American Heart Association in New Orleans.

"Silent" Heart Attack: Are You at Risk?

Gregory Thomas, MD, a cardiologist, medical director for the MemorialCare Heart & Vascular Institute at Long Beach Memorial Medical Center in California, and clinical professor at the University of California, Irvine.

Most of us think we know what a heart attack looks and feels like. Pain or discomfort in the chest…shortness of breath…a cold sweat…and perhaps even a sense of impending doom. But not so fast. Heart attack symptoms can vary widely from person to person—and may not be noticeable at all.

The reality: Of the 735,000 heart attacks that strike Americans every year, nearly half are silent—that is, there are no obvious symptoms. In fact, people who have had a silent heart attack don't even know they've had one! These heart attacks don't occur only in older adults—they are quite common in middle-aged adults, research shows.

Don't be fooled: Many people assume that a silent heart attack is less harmful than a "real" heart attack, but that's not true. In fact, some studies indicate that a person who has had a silent heart attack has a higher risk of dying from heart disease than a person who has had a recognized heart attack—perhaps because he/she doesn't receive appropriate medical care.

Are You at Risk?

Some risk factors for a silent heart attack are obvious, such as high blood pressure, smoking and being overweight. But many other risks are hidden and largely unrecognized by doctors and patients alike.

If you have one or more of the risk factors below, make an appointment with an internist or a cardiologist and discuss getting an electrocardiogram (see the next page for details) to determine whether you have damage to the heart due to a silent heart attack you may have unknowingly suffered.

If your doctor discovers that you have had a silent heart attack, your treatment—such as medications, a heart-healthy diet and regular exercise—should be the same as that received by a person who has had a recognized heart attack. Your primary care physician can provide much of the care, but if you have had a heart attack, you should be seeing a cardiologist at least yearly. *Important risks for silent heart attack...*

• **Low sensitivity to pain.** Because pain is a major symptom of most heart attacks, it stands to reason that silent heart attacks are more likely in people who are less sensitive to pain—and recent research confirms this theory.

Recent finding: In a study of nearly 5,000 people, published in the *Journal of the American Heart Association*, researchers found that women with lower pain sensitivity were more likely to have had a silent heart attack than those who were more sensitive to pain. According to this study, people who can keep a hand in icy water for up to two minutes have a lower sensitivity to pain.

• **Peripheral neuropathy.** About 20 million Americans—many of them with type 2 diabetes—have peripheral neuropathy, nerve damage that causes symptoms such as numbness, tingling and burning pain, usually in the feet or hands. Having diabetes and peripheral neuropathy more than doubles the likelihood of having a silent heart attack—probably because sensitivity to sensation has been reduced.

• **Elevated blood sugar.** A fasting blood sugar (glucose) test is typically ordered to detect elevated glucose levels and diabetes. You fast overnight for at least eight hours, and your blood is drawn in the morning and sent to a laboratory, where your glucose level is measured. If it's 126 mg/dL or higher, you have diabetes. But if your glucose level is 100 mg/dL or higher, you're 60% more likely to have had a silent heart attack than someone whose glucose level was normal (less than 100 mg/dL). Chronically high levels of glucose (even if they haven't yet reached the point of diabetes) damage arteries, increasing risk for heart attack and stroke. Elevated glucose is common. The average adult in the US has a blood sugar level of 106 mg/dL.

• **Sluggish kidneys.** Two findings on routine laboratory tests that measure kidney function have been linked to a higher risk of having had a silent heart attack...

• Albuminuria. This indicates that there are elevated levels of a protein in your urine that can signal kidney disease. Albuminuria is detected by a combination of two tests—a microalbuminuria test and a creatinine test.

• Low glomerular filtration rate (GFR). This shows your kidneys are struggling to do their main job—filtering impurities out of your blood.

Scientific evidence: A study of nearly 19,000 people by researchers from the University of Alabama at Birmingham found that people with the highest levels of albuminuria (greater than 300 mg/g) were 2.5 times more likely to have had a silent heart attack than those with the lowest levels.

They also found that those with the lowest estimated GFR levels (less than 30) were three times more likely to have had a silent heart attack than those with the highest levels. (Normal GFR varies by age but ranges from 60 to 120.)

• **Fatigue, swollen legs and/or breathing problems.** All three can be symptoms of a weakened heart muscle—including one damaged by a heart attack. If you experience these symptoms but you haven't had a detectable heart attack, you may have had a silent heart attack. Especially if one or more of these symptoms come on suddenly or unexpectedly, see a doctor promptly for an evaluation.

Smart Strategy

Detecting a silent heart attack is easy to do with an electrocardiogram (EKG or ECG). This five- to 10-minute test measures the electrical activity of your heart. If the EKG detects abnormal "Q-waves"—a lack of electrical activity in areas of the heart—your heart muscle has been damaged by a heart attack.

If you've had a silent heart attack, you should promptly treat your heart disease. In my decades as a cardiologist, I've seen over and over again that treating cardiovascular disease with cholesterol-lowering medications, increasing daily exercise and improving diet dramatically decreases the risk for a second heart attack and premature death.

If you have had a silent heart attack, a second one is also more likely to be silent or have atypical symptoms, such as neck, jaw or back pain, nausea, dizziness and/or fatigue. Be on guard for unusual symptoms and a sense that you're feeling "not quite right." Also, be sure to see your physician for regular checkups.

Crash Diets Might Derail Your Heart Health

Jennifer Rayner, MD, clinical research fellow, University of Oxford, United Kingdom.

Gregg Fonarow, MD, codirector, Preventative Cardiology Program, University of California, Los Angeles.

European Society of Cardiology meeting, Barcelona, Spain.

Everyone wants a beach-ready body, and many are willing to starve themselves to achieve it quickly. But new research suggests that fat lost on crash diets may clog the heart and reduce its function.

The good news is that this effect appears temporary. And for healthy people, there probably aren't any ill effects, said the study's lead author Jennifer Rayner, MD.

However, the study researchers are concerned that the fat migration could pose a problem for people who already have heart issues.

For someone who's obese, Dr. Rayner said, "the health benefits of losing weight are huge. But at the moment, we need to do some more research to make sure that these diets are safe in people with heart disease." She is a clinical research fellow at the University of Oxford in England.

Very-low-calorie diets (approximately 600 to 800 calories a day) are an effective method of weight loss and a way to quickly reduce liver fat and reverse diabetes, the researchers said.

The Study

In the current study, the investigators asked 21 obese people to consume meal replacements—special milkshakes or soups—designed to provide 800 or fewer calories daily for eight weeks.

Participants' average age was 52. Their average body mass index (BMI) was 37. BMI is an estimate of a person's fitness level based on a height and weight ratio. A normal BMI is 19.9 to 24.9, while overweight is 25 to 29.9. A BMI of 30 and over is considered obese, according to the US National Heart, Lung, and Blood Institute. For someone who is 5 feet 9 inches tall, a BMI of 30 is over 203 pounds.

All of the study volunteers had MRIs at the study's start, and again after one week and eight weeks on the diet.

After one week, total body fat, abdominal fat and liver fat dropped by 6%, 11% and 42%, respectively. Total cholesterol and triglycerides (another type of blood fat) fell. Insulin resistance and blood sugar levels improved. Blood pressure also improved.

Surprising Decline in Heart Health

Generally, when such measures improve, heart health is expected to get better, too. But that wasn't the case here. After a week on the diet, heart fat went up by 44%. And the researchers noted a decrease in heart function.

Dr. Rayner's team theorized that the sudden drop in calories causes fat to be released from different parts of the body into the blood. It's then taken up by the heart muscle.

But the negative changes didn't last. By eight weeks, heart function and heart fat were better than normal. Body fat, cholesterol and all of the other metabolic measures also continued to improve.

The study was presented at the European Society of Cardiology meeting in Barcelona, Spain.

Expert Commentary

Gregg Fonarow, MD, is codirector of preventative cardiology at the University of California, Los Angeles.

"This study demonstrated there was transient impairment in cardiac function with severe calorie restriction, and there was evidence of increased heart fat content," Dr. Fonarow said.

But the study didn't show why this occurred, he added.

Dr. Fonarow agreed with Dr. Rayner that healthy people probably don't have anything to worry about. But people with heart troubles should talk to their doctor before undertaking any significant diet changes.

Dr. Rayner added that it's unclear if less-severe diets would have similar effects.

Learn more about healthy weight loss from the National Institute of Diabetes and Digestive and Kidney Diseases at NIDDK.nih.gov. Search "safe weight loss."

Heart-Stopping Sex

Heart-stopping sex happens but is very rare. In a study of 4,557 cases of sudden cardiac arrest over a 13-year period, only 34 cases were linked to sex—about one in 100 cardiac arrests in men and about one in 1,000 cases in women.

Sumeet Chugh, MD, associate director, Cedars-Sinai Heart Institute, Los Angeles, and senior author of a study published in *Journal of the American College of Cardiology.*

For Peripheral Artery Disease, Walking Beats Surgery for Pain Relief

Study "Supervised Exercise, Stent Revascularization, or Medical Therapy for Claudication Due to Aortoiliac Peripheral Artery Disease" by researchers at Rhode Island Hospital, Providence, Beth Israel Deaconess Medical Center, Boston, University of Colorado School of Medicine, Aurora, et al., published in *Journal of the American College of Cardiology.*

Walking is miraculous medicine. For a common cardiovascular condition, it can help you avoid surgery. But you'll need some true grit to make it work.

The condition is peripheral artery disease (PAD), a buildup of plaque in the arteries that feed the legs and arms and the rest of the body. It affects one in 20 people over age 55, is more common in women and frequently hurts—in particular, it can be marked by debilitating leg pain.

If you have it, your doctor will likely suggest that you get some exercise and will prescribe medications. If that doesn't help, the go-to treatment usually is revascularization—surgery to insert stents into blocked arteries. It can be effective, but surgery always has risks, entails recuperation and is expensive.

Walking is healthier. The problem, of course, is that if it hurts to walk, you won't want to do it. But the more you walk, the longer you will be able to walk without pain, according to a recent clinical trial of PAD patients with moderate-to-severe leg pain (claudication).

In addition to standard medical treatment, patients had one of three protocols—revascularization...a supervised exercise program...or no additional treatment (placebo). The exercise program consisted of treadmill-walking sessions three times a week for six months—followed by a year-long maintenance phase in which participants were encouraged through telephone calls to continue exercising.

Results: At the end of the 18-month study, those who got regular care could walk for only a mere 12 seconds, on average, without pain. Those who had stenting could last 3.2 minutes. But the exercisers could walk for five minutes, on average, without pain.

Walking, of course, also improves overall health and quality of life. When you have PAD, it's not easy…but it's worth the effort.

Sluggish Circulation?

Neel P. Chokshi, MD, MBA, assistant professor of clinical medicine at Perelman School of Medicine, University of Pennsylvania in Philadelphia, and medical director of the university's Sports Cardiology and Fitness Program. His research has been published in *American Journal of Cardiology* and other professional journals.

If your calves cramp while walking or climbing stairs—especially if the pain eases when you stop—it's a red flag that you may have peripheral artery disease (PAD). With PAD, your arteries are narrowed due to plaque buildup, which prevents the muscles in your extremities (usually your legs) from getting enough blood flow to keep up with the increased oxygen demand when you are active.

It's no small matter—if PAD goes untreated, the condition can lead to infection, loss of the function of the limb and, in severe cases of blockage, amputation.

Here's the irony of treating PAD: People who have this circulatory problem, with its telltale pain while walking, are often prescribed (you guessed it!) walking to relieve their pain. Even though it hurts, walking—when done according to certain guidelines (see below)—does actually improve the symptoms of PAD and slow its progression. In fact, exercise works as well as any medication or surgery, according to research published in *Circulation* (see also previous article).

Walk This Way

What's so great about walking? When you repeatedly put one foot in front of the other, it brings more oxygen to your muscles, which improves your circulation and eases the pain of PAD. The exact reasons why walking helps aren't known, but it's well-established that the more you walk, the farther you'll be able to walk…and with less pain.

Important: If you suspect that you have PAD but haven't been diagnosed, it's important to see your doctor for an evaluation. This will include an ankle-brachial exam, which compares the blood pressure in your arms to that in your feet, to show how well your blood is flowing, and possibly other tests such as an ultrasound. You may also have other related factors, such as high blood pressure, that need to be addressed.

To get the best results from your walking program…

- **Stretch.** Before getting started, your calf muscles need a good stretch to increase blood flow to the area.

What works best: Stand in front of a low step (a curb works fine, too). Place the toes of one foot on the step and drop your heel just enough to feel a stretch in your calf. Don't overdo it…stop at the point of tightness. Hold it for 10 to 15 seconds, then switch feet.

To warm up your thigh muscles, stand on one leg and raise the other foot behind you by bending the knee. Do not pull up on your foot…just rest that ankle in your hand and hold that position long enough to feel a slight stretch in your thigh (usually 10 to 15 seconds). Switch legs and repeat. (If you can't reach your ankle, try standing with a wall behind you and place that foot against the wall to hold it up.)

- **Walk.** Find a flat, safe surface for your walks (neighborhood streets, a local track, a shopping mall or a treadmill).

What works best: Start by walking for five minutes at a pace that causes some pain. On a pain scale from one to five, where one is mild pain and five is severe pain, aim to walk at a three or four.

- **Rest.** After walking for five minutes with moderate pain, stop and rest until the pain goes away.

Helpful: If you like to walk in an area where there aren't any benches for your rest period, treat yourself to a cane with a folding seat attachment. It's not too heavy to carry and gives you a place to sit during your rest stops.

• **Repeat.** Once the pain has dissipated, try to walk for another five minutes. If you find that it's impossible to do the additional five minutes without severe pain, try slowing down your pace to achieve a few extra minutes.

• **Stay focused on your goal.** Try to walk at least three—ideally, five—times a week. During the first two months, build up slowly to a total of 35 minutes of walking during each session, not counting the rest breaks. After you can manage that, keep adding a few minutes each week until you're at the ultimate goal of walking 50 minutes per session.

• **Cool down.** You should always finish by walking slowly for five minutes. Then stretch your calf and thigh muscles again to help minimize muscle soreness after walking.

Smart Strategies

To give yourself the best possible odds of succeeding at your walking program, you should also...

• **Track your progress.** To stay motivated, jot down the total time and distance of your walks. Or wear a fitness tracker, such as Fitbit, or use a phone app, like MapMyWalk, to help track your time, effort and distance.

• **Avoid boredom!** If you walk outside, vary your route. If you prefer a treadmill, listen to music or a podcast...or watch a 30-minute TV show.

Also helpful: Find a walking buddy—the social aspect can help keep you on target.

For an Extra Boost

Working with a physical therapist to start a walking program is smart, since supervised programs seem to be more effective by helping to ensure that you keep up with your walking program and hit the required pain thresholds. You're also likely to get help paying for your sessions with a physical therapist.

Recent development: Medicare Part B now covers comprehensive cardiac rehabilitation programs that include exercise, education and counseling for patients with PAD. The specific amount you'll owe may depend on several things, such as the Medigap insurance (if any) you have and the type of facility you choose. Check with your insurer.

An Alternative to Walking

If any amount of walking is too painful or too dangerous for you, don't give up. New research shows that you can get comparable results with arm exercises.

Important recent finding: In a study that was conducted at University of Minnesota School of Nursing in Minneapolis, researchers randomly divided 28 people with PAD (average age 65.6) into three different groups—no exercise...treadmill walking...or arm exercise. Participants assigned to arm exercises used an arm ergometer (a device with bicycle-like pedals that are operated by the arms). After three months of training for three hours a week, people in both exercise groups could walk farther without pain.

Other possibilities: It's likely that bike riding, dancing, swimming or pool walking, which haven't yet been tested in people with PAD, may also help relieve symptoms. If you enjoy those activities, talk to your doctor about giving them a try!

Don't Let the New Blood Pressure Guidelines Fool You

H. Gilbert Welch, MD, MPH, professor of medicine at The Dartmouth Institute for Health Policy and Clinical Practice, Lebanon, New Hampshire, and author of three books, including *Less Medicine, More Health: 7 Assumptions That Drive Too Much Health Care* and *Overdiagnosed: Making People Sick in the Pursuit of Health.* TDI.Dartmouth.edu

The definition of high blood pressure has reached a new low—130 is the new 140. According to guidelines set by the American Heart Association and the American College of Cardiology in late 2017, if your systolic (upper) number is 130 mm Hg or higher...and/or your diastolic (lower) number is 80 mm Hg or higher...you have high blood pressure, aka hypertension. The previous threshold was 140 mm Hg. (Diastolic, the lower number, is less important at predicting cardiovascular risk.)

Overnight, more than 30 million Americans "got" high blood pressure. Combined with those who met the earlier threshold, that's a total of about 103 million people. As an advocate for using less medicine whenever possible, I'm worried by these new guidelines. That's why I wrote an article in *The New York Times* titled, "Don't Let New Blood Pressure Guidelines Raise Yours." It's not that controlling very high blood pressure isn't important. It's critical. Treating very high blood pressure with medication is one of the most important preventive interventions doctors do.

But doctors also can do too much prescribing. Aggressive medical management to reach the new goals for people at the margin may have only modest benefits that don't outweigh the risks for side effects. In a blow to wide acceptance, the American Academy of Family Physicians (AAFP) declined to endorse the new guidelines because they don't meet that organization's standards for medical evidence. It's sticking with the previous guidelines.

When doctors disagree, it can be confusing for patients. *Here are some facts to help you and your physician make the right decision...*

Modest New Benefits

While the new guidelines emphasize lifestyle changes such as getting more exercise, losing weight if you need to and eating a healthful diet as the first line of defense—good advice for all of us—the likely practical effect will be to push many more people into drug treatment. So let's examine the benefits.

The new guidelines stem from a federally funded study called the Systolic Blood Pressure Intervention Trial (SPRINT). It covered people over age 50 at high risk for cardiovascular disease. Half were treated to bring their systolic blood pressure down to less than 140 and half to bring it down to less than 120.

Result: Compared with those treated to less than 140, those treated to less than 120 had 25% lower risk for heart attack, stroke, heart failure and death from cardiovascular causes. Sounds impressive, right? But in reality, over the course of the three-year study, about 6% of participants who aimed for 120 had cardiovascular "events" such as heart attacks—compared with 8% of those who aimed for 140. That's only a two-percentage-point difference.

The truth is, while reducing very high blood pressure—say, from 160 or 180 to 140—has enormous benefits, going from 140 to 130 doesn't. According to a review that included 74 trials and more than 300,000 patients that was published in *JAMA Internal Medicine*, bringing blood pressure levels below 140 did not help prevent a first heart attack or stroke, reduce the rate of cardiovascular disease or help prevent death overall.

Risks of Aggressive Treatment

In the SPRINT trial, getting to a blood pressure goal of less than 120 required an average of three different drugs per patient —compared with two drugs for a 140 goal. While that extra drug didn't substantially increase side effects in that trial, it's still true that 38% of patients in the 120-target group had adverse events, including abnormally low blood pressure, loss of consciousness and acute kidney injury. I'm concerned about adding even one extra prescription medication, especially for many elderly patients who already may take eight or even 10 medications a day.

Blood pressure drugs, like all drugs, have side effects. The type called beta-blockers can cause dizziness, weakness and fatigue, as can ACE inhibitors, angiotensin II receptor blockers and alpha blockers. Dizziness and lightheadedness can result in more falls, which is particularly dangerous for older people, making them more prone to fractures—including hip fractures, which can have devastating consequences for health and independence.

These concerns are among the reasons that the AAFP and the American College of Physicians came out with blood pressure treatment guidelines specifically for people age 60 and older in 2017.

Recommendations: Doctors should prescribe drugs for healthy patients only when systolic levels are 150 or higher. For patients at high cardiovascular risk, especially stroke patients, doctors are advised to start treatment at 140.

Over Diagnosis Risk

There's a bigger problem in extrapolating the results of the SPRINT trial to the real world. Blood pressure is an extremely volatile variable, and it can change within minutes in reaction to stress, activity or just the anxiety of sitting in a doctor's waiting room. (For how to get a good blood pressure reading, see next column.) To remove those stressors, the SPRINT researchers had patients measure their own blood pressure (using an automated cuff) after five minutes of quiet rest without staff in the room.

This may be an ideal way to measure blood pressure, but it's not what happens in the real world. You might have had a blood pressure reading of 130 in a situation such as the SPRINT trial, while it might be 140 or even higher when measured in your doctor's office. In practice, that may lead to many people being overmedicated.

What to Do Now

Have the new guidelines pushed you into the official "high blood pressure" range? I hope you now realize that it's not a medical emergency if they have. But it's an opportunity to talk to your doctor about what blood pressure goal is right for you, given your age and risk factors.

Even if you wind up needing medication, a lifestyle plan is enormously important. Limit alcoholic drinks to no more than one a day (two a day is OK for men). Revamp your diet to include plenty of fruits and vegetables and whole grains. Reduce your salt intake. Exercise regularly. If you smoke, quit. Lose weight if you need to. Find healthy ways to manage stress.

Ironically, the recent dramatic increase in the number of people with "high" blood pressure can distract patients and doctors from focusing on these important lifestyle changes. Doing those things is good for blood sugar, for better sleep and for overall well-being, regardless of blood pressure.

The Right Way to Measure Your Blood Pressure at Home

If you're concerned about your blood pressure, and especially if you've started to take medication to bring it down, consider measuring your blood pressure yourself at home. Many physicians recommend this do-it-yourself approach because it can help you become more aware of the things that move your blood pressure up or down.

Buy a monitor with an inflatable upper-arm cuff—more reliable than those with wrist cuffs or fingertip monitors. *Follow these tips when you measure your pressure...*

- **Relax.** Don't exercise or drink caffeinated drinks or alcohol for at least 30 minutes before measuring. Make sure your bladder is empty...sit quietly for five minutes before you take a measurement...sit still while you measure.
- **Watch your posture.** Sit with your back against a straight-back chair...feet flat on the floor, legs uncrossed. Support your arm on a flat surface with your upper arm at heart level. The middle of the blood pressure cuff should be placed just above where the elbow bends.

Place the cuff directly on your bare arm, not over clothing.

Take your pressure at the same time every day. Either morning or evening is fine. It doesn't matter whether you do it before or after taking medication—just be consistent.

Take two or three readings one minute apart. Print out or write down the results or store them in your device's built-in memory.

Ask your doctor's office if you can do a practice run there. That way you can be sure that you are using the monitor correctly at home.

Caution: Don't rely solely on your at-home readings. Compare them with the readings you get in your doctor's office as a backup.

The Real Secret to Lowering Your Blood Pressure

Janet Bond Brill, PhD, RDN, FAND, registered dietitian/nutritionist and nationally recognized expert in nutrition and cardiovascular disease prevention. She is a former director of nutrition for Fitness Together, one of the world's largest organizations of personal trainers, and has served as a nutrition consultant for several other large companies. She is author of *Blood Pressure Down: The 10-Step Plan to Lower Your Blood Pressure in Four Weeks—Without Prescription Drugs.* DrJanet.com

Forget everything that you have read about the latest "superfood" for lowering blood pressure. While it's true that certain foods do provide this remarkable benefit, many people mistakenly assume that there must be one nutritional magic bullet that will do the job on its own.

Is it possible to control high blood pressure (hypertension) with diet alone? Yes, many people can—but only when they take advantage of the additive benefits from multiple strategically chosen foods.

Example: Suppose you eat a lot of bananas because you know that this food is high in blood pressure–lowering potassium. That's great, but you'll shave only a point or two off your blood pressure.

To really leverage your diet, you need to also regularly consume other foods that help control blood pressure. When combined, the nutrients in these foods work synergistically to give the greatest blood pressure–lowering effects. Then the benefits accrue quickly—for some people, a five-point drop may occur within a week.

What you may not realize: By eating the right foods, losing weight if you're overweight and cutting sodium if you're salt-sensitive (see page 21), some people can achieve blood pressure drops that equal or exceed the effects of drug therapy—with none of the side effects. And if you must take medication, these foods may allow you to use a lower dose.*

Some of the best blood pressure–lowering foods are well-known—bananas, leafy green vegetables, etc. *Here are some lesser-known options to add to your hypertension-fighting diet…*

- **Beet juice/beet greens.** As a nutritionist, I usually advise clients to eat whole foods rather than drink juices because of the extra fiber. But beet juice is an exception. It's a concentrated source of nitrates, chemical compounds that quickly lower blood pressure.

When you drink beet juice or eat other high-nitrate foods (such as rhubarb, spinach, beet greens or chard), cells in the linings of blood vessels produce more nitric oxide, a molecule that dilates blood vessels and lowers blood pressure.

Scientific evidence: In a study that was published in *Hypertension* and looked at 64 adults with hypertension (ages 18 to 85), some of the patients drank a daily 8.4-ounce glass of beet juice, while others drank a juice with the active compounds removed (the placebo).

After one month, those given the real juice had average drops in systolic (top number) blood pressure of about eight points, while their diastolic pressure (bottom number) dropped five points. Blood pressure did not drop among those in the placebo group.

You can buy beet juice in health-food stores and juice shops. Or you can make your own by blending/processing cooked beets. To liven up the flavor, add a little lemon juice, ginger or a sweetener such as stevia.

**Caution*: If you take blood pressure-lowering medication, never change your dose or discontinue it without consulting your doctor.

Caution: If you have kidney disease, consult your nephrologist or a registered dietitian/nutritionist who specializes in kidney disease before regularly consuming beet juice—its high potassium level could worsen this condition.

• **Figs.** These delicious jewels are heart-healthy because they are super-high in potassium, with 232 mg in just two fresh figs. They also have a considerable amount of fiber and polyphenols, compounds that when consumed with additional blood pressure–lowering food can reduce systolic blood pressure by up to 12 points, in some cases.

Fresh figs are scrumptious, but dried figs are easier to find in grocery stores—and many people enjoy their intense sweetness.

What to try: Chop dried figs, and use them as a natural sweetener in oatmeal, pancakes, muffins or even soups.

• **Hibiscus tea.** If you enjoy chamomile and other herbal teas, you might like the delicate floral flavor of hibiscus tea, which is high in flavonoids, plant-based antioxidants with anti-inflammatory effects, and other heart-healthy compounds. One study, which compared hibiscus tea to *captopril* (Capoten), an ACE inhibitor blood pressure drug, found that the tea was just as effective as the medication.

• **Pistachios.** Even though most nuts are good sources of fiber, potassium and magnesium, pistachios are special because they are high in arginine, an amino acid that stimulates the production of nitric oxide (discussed earlier).

Important recent finding: A study at Pennsylvania State University found that people who ate 1.5 ounces of pistachios (about 70 nuts, unshelled) daily had drops in stress-related systolic blood pressure of nearly five points compared with those who ate nuts less than once a week.

Not fattening: Nuts are high in calories, but research has shown that people who eat them regularly actually tend to gain less weight than those who don't eat nuts—probably because the fiber and protein in nuts help dieters feel full longer. At roughly 260 calories per 1.5 ounces, you'll need to cut calories elsewhere to prevent weight gain but can likely do so easily because nuts give such a feeling of satiety.

• **Pomegranate juice.** Pomegranate juice contains many different flavonoids. The juice mimics the effects of ACE inhibitor drugs, such as *lisinopril* (Zestril, Prinivil, etc.), which dilate blood vessels and lower blood pressure.

A recent study found that people who drank a little less than two ounces of pomegranate juice daily for a year had average drops in systolic blood pressure of 12%.

The juice is tart, so some people buy sweetened versions.

My advice: Avoid the added sugar. Instead, add a little stevia or other natural sweetener. One pomegranate yields about half a cup of juice.

• **White beans.** Like many of the other foods described earlier, white beans are chock-full of potassium. One cup contains more than 1,000 mg of potassium. (A cup of black beans has about 800 mg.)

Potassium acts like a natural diuretic and removes sodium from the body. Many people are sensitive to sodium, which means that their blood pressure will rise if they consume too much (the standard recommendation is no more than 2,300 mg daily). Research has shown that one of the best ways to lower blood pressure is to increase your potassium–sodium ratio.

Is Salt Harmful for Everyone?

James J. DiNicolantonio, PharmD, a cardiovascular research scientist and doctor of pharmacy at Saint Luke's Mid America Heart Institute in Kansas City, Missouri. Dr. DiNicolantonio is also an associate editor of BMJ Open Heart, on the editorial advisory board of Progress in Cardiovascular Diseases and other journals and author of *The Salt Fix*. TheSaltFix.com

We've all been told that a high-salt diet is a leading cause of high blood pressure (hypertension), heart attack, stroke and heart failure. What doctors don't tell patients—what many doctors don't know themselves—is that salt doesn't have the same effect on everyone's blood pressure.

A surprising fact: Many people do better when they consume more than the USDA's recommended daily sodium limit of 2,300 mg (roughly the amount in one teaspoon of salt). *Other common misconceptions regarding sodium...*

MYTH #1: **Salt raises blood pressure in everyone.** It's true that doctors have a right to worry about the salt consumption for some patients. Salt sensitivity—generally defined as an increase of 5% or more in blood pressure when sodium is consumed—is most common in older adults, black people and people of Chinese descent.

Important: If you're sensitive to salt, exceeding the recommended daily limit of 2,300 mg of sodium can cause sharp rises in blood pressure.

But what's harmful for this subset of the population is not harmful for everyone. Research shows that salt sensitivity affects about half of people with high blood pressure and about 20% of people who have normal blood pressure.

MYTH #2: **Salt always increases heart disease.** If a high-salt diet increased blood pressure, it would obviously increase the risk for cardiovascular disease—but, as discussed earlier, this occurs only in some people. When researchers study whether eating highly salted foods increases the rates of high blood pressure and heart disease, the findings are mixed. Meanwhile, the correlation between high-salt diets and improved health is compelling.

Example: People consume staggering amounts of sodium in Japan, France and South Korea. The average South Korean, for example, consumes more than 4,000 mg of sodium a day. In France and other Mediterranean countries, very salty foods, such as prepared sardines, anchovies and many aged cheeses, are eaten with most meals. Yet these countries are among those with the lowest death rates from coronary heart disease in the world, and Japan and South Korea boast among the highest longevity.

Most people don't realize that a low-salt diet can sometimes raise blood pressure by stimulating the body's "rescue" system (the renin-angiotensin aldosterone system) that's designed to help the body retain salt and water. When this occurs, low salt intake can increase heart rate, blood clotting and the constriction of blood vessels. It's also been linked to insulin resistance and diabetes.

MYTH #3: **No one needs more salt.** The ubiquitous advice to reduce sodium intake might be justified if it helped some people and didn't hurt the rest. But this isn't always the case.

To remain in homeostasis, the physiological state that puts the least stress on the body, most people who are not salt sensitive need about 3,000 mg to 5,000 mg of sodium a day.

What's more, many of our food choices (sugar and caffeinated beverages, for example) deplete salt from the body. So do commonly prescribed medications such as some antidepressants, diuretics and diabetes drugs. In addition, the average nonathletic adult sweats out 600 mg of sodium a day.

MYTH #4: **Healthy diets are naturally low in salt.** The diets that experts recommend for disease prevention, such as the Mediterranean diet, do exclude many of the processed foods that happen to be high in salt (and other unhealthful ingredients)—but they're not low-salt diets overall. If anything, as mentioned above with such countries as Japan and South Korea, they contain more salt than Americans typically eat. Think seafood (clams, lobster, crab), olives, kimchi, etc.

Why do these countries have less cardiovascular disease than the US? While there is no definitive research that a high-salt diet is the reason, it's been my observation that people who indulge their salt cravings tend to eat more heart-healthy vegetables (particularly the bitter ones, such as bitter greens)...nuts...and seeds—most likely because these healthy foods taste better with salt.

What's more, there is often a lot of potassium in naturally salty foods—for example, spinach, Swiss chard and artichokes. When it comes to improving blood pressure and heart health, more potassium is probably more important than less sodium.

MYTH #5: **Everyone should check the sodium content on food labels.** Unless you eat a lot of pretzels, chips and other super-salty foods, you are unlikely to eat more salt than your body can handle—unless you're salt-sensitive (see below).

I do advise people to avoid processed foods—mainly because these foods tend to be high in sugar, which can increase the risk for high blood pressure, diabetes and obesity. Most processed foods also lack fiber, and a lack of fiber can cause sugar spikes. It's much better to indulge your salt cravings with foods that are naturally salty—for example, sea vegetables (kelp, seaweed and algae), seafood, cheese and olives.

Are You Salt-Sensitive?

There are no readily available tests to determine whether a person is salt-sensitive. So how do you know whether a low-salt diet would help you or hurt you?

Try this: With your doctor's OK, for two weeks, reduce your sodium intake to less than 2,300 mg of sodium per day. If your blood pressure drops by 5% or more, chances are you are salt-sensitive. If your blood pressure does drop, be alert for dizziness, fatigue, nausea, muscle spasms/cramps and blurred vision—signs that your blood pressure may be too low. In these cases, you may be better off listening to your body's salt cravings and eating the salt that it demands rather than adhering to a strict low-sodium diet.

Important: Discuss this with your doctor, and monitor your blood pressure closely.

Veggies Are a Healthy Recipe for Older Women's Hearts

Lauren Blekkenhorst, BHSc, research associate, School of Medical and Health Sciences, University of Western Australia, Perth.

Samantha Heller, MS, RD, senior clinical nutritionist, New York University Langone Medical Center, New York City.

Journal of the American Heart Association, online.

Eating lots of vegetables may help older women keep their blood vessels healthy, Australian researchers report.

The biggest benefit seems to come from cruciferous vegetables, including cabbage, brussels sprouts, cauliflower and broccoli. Eating these strong-smelling veggies was linked to less thickening of the carotid arteries, located in the neck.

Thickening of these major blood vessels is a sign of impending heart disease, the researchers said.

"These findings reinforce the importance of adequate vegetable intake to reduce your risk of atherosclerosis ['hardening of the arteries'], heart attacks and strokes," said lead researcher Lauren Blekkenhorst, BHSc. She's a research associate in the School of Medical and Health Sciences at the University of Western Australia.

The Study

For the study, Blekkenhorst's team had nearly 1,000 women 70 and older fill out questionnaires about how often they eat veggies.

Responses ranged from never to three or more times a day. Types of veggies included onions, garlic, leeks, shallots, beans, leafy green vegetables, cruciferous vegetables and yellow, orange or red vegetables.

The researchers used sonograms to measure the thickness of each woman's carotid arteries and the amount of plaque they contained.

The carotid artery walls of women who ate the most vegetables were about 0.05 millimeter thinner than those who ate the fewest.

That difference might be significant, Blekkenhorst said, because a 0.1 millimeter decrease in carotid wall thickness was linked to a 10% to 18% lower risk of stroke and heart attack.

On average, each additional half-ounce of vegetables eaten in a day was associated with nearly a 1% thinner carotid artery wall, she said.

The benefits found in the study were limited to vegetables like cabbage, brussels sprouts, cauliflower and broccoli, Blekkenhorst said. Other veggies did not show the same protective link.

She said the value of cruciferous veggies remained even after her team took into account a woman's lifestyle, heart disease risk, and other vegetable and dietary factors.

The report was published in *Journal of the American Heart Association*.

Implications

"Recommendations to include a couple of servings of cruciferous vegetables may optimize the health benefits of increasing vegetables in the diet," Blekkenhorst said.

She added, however, that this study doesn't prove a lack of vegetables caused carotid artery walls to thicken, only that there was an association between the two.

Benefits of Veggies

Veggies are good for you, Blekkenhorst said, because they're high in fiber, so you feel full without consuming many calories.

"They are also packed full of vitamins, minerals and phytochemicals, which have been shown to reduce inflammation and oxidative stress," Blekkenhorst said. Chronic inflammation plays a part in a number of age-related illnesses, including heart disease, she added.

Best of all, the benefits of vegetables exist whether you cook them or eat them raw, Blekkenhorst said. Though cooking reduces some nutrients, eating cooked vegetables aids digestion and absorption of these nutrients, she said.

Blekkenhorst said it's important to eat both raw and cooked vegetables throughout the day.

Any way you prepare them, you'll do your body good, according to a nutritionist not involved with the study.

"Whether raw, roasted, steamed, sauteed or boiled, vegetables offer an amazing array of health benefits," said Samantha Heller, MS, RD, a senior clinical nutritionist at New York University Medical Center.

Vegetables help you fight infection and reduce your risk for mental decline, some cancers, heart disease and diabetes, she said.

"Inflammation plays a big role in the development of atherosclerosis, so it makes sense that eating foods that help lower inflammation may lead to more supple arteries," Heller said.

Benefits in Men Unclear

Whether men also gain these benefits from vegetables isn't clear, the study authors said.

"We cannot be certain that the findings will be the same for older men, as the risk factors for vascular disease are different for men and women," Blekkenhorst said. "But it can't hurt for men to consume more cruciferous vegetables every day."

Heller said it seems reasonable to think that men would derive the same health benefits from eating a variety of vegetables.

To learn more about diet and heart health, visit the American Heart Association web site, Heart.org, and search "diet and lifestyle recommendations."

Stop Postsurgery Shivers to Help Your Heart

Tylenol calms postsurgery shivers. The teeth-rattling shivers that often occur after surgery are uncomfortable and can strain the cardiovascular system.

New finding: In a study involving 37 women undergoing surgery, just 22% of those who received intravenous *acetaminophen* (Tylenol) during surgery experienced shivering (believed to be related to the body cooling down), compared with 73.7% given a placebo. Oral acetaminophen taken before surgeries lasting less than two hours might also be effective in calming post-op shivers.

Takahiro Tadokoro, MD, anesthesiologist, University of the Ryukyus, Okinawa, Japan.

"Hot" Yoga Is No Better for Your Heart

Stacy Hunter, PhD, assistant professor, exercise & sports science, department of health and human performance, Texas State University, San Marcos, Texas.

Gregg Fonarow, MD, director, Ahmanson-UCLA Cardiomyopathy Center, codirector, UCLA Preventative Cardiology Program, and co-chief, UCLA Division of Cardiology, Los Angeles.

Experimental Physiology.

It's called "hot" yoga because it's practiced in sweltering temperatures, and some research has hinted that it might improve heart health more than traditional yoga.

But a new study suggests that adding heat to your Half Moon pose doesn't boost its cardiac benefits.

"We were surprised by the result that a non-heated practice seemed to have the same benefit on vascular health as the heated practice," admitted study author Stacy Hunter, PhD. She is an assistant professor of exercise and sports science in the department of health and human performance at Texas State University in San Marcos.

"Previous research has documented reductions in cardiovascular disease risk with sauna therapy alone," Dr. Hunter explained. "So we thought that the heated environment in Bikram [hot] yoga would cause a greater response and have more benefit."

About Bikram Yoga and Heart Effects

The researchers noted that Bikram yoga has a global following, and entails running through a sequence of 26 standard yoga poses in 105-degree heat.

At issue was whether Bikram yoga invigorated a process known as vasodilation, Dr. Hunter said. Vasodilation is associated with the production of nitric oxide, which helps to ward off inflammation. As such, vigorous vasodilation may ultimately slow or delay hardening of the arteries, which is a known risk factor for heart attack or stroke.

In an earlier study, Dr. Hunter's team found that middle-aged Bikram yoga participants experienced increased vasodilation.

But the question remained about whether this was sparked by the high-temperature environment of Bikram, or whether it might also happen among those performing yoga in normal temperatures.

The Study

To answer that question, the investigators focused on 52 sedentary but healthy adults aged 40 to 60.

Study participants were randomly assigned to one of three different groups. One group practiced Bikram in a hot environment; a second group practiced Bikram in a room that was 73 degrees; and a third "control" group wasn't assigned to either of the two Bikram classes.

For three months, the two Bikram groups engaged in three 90-minute yoga classes per week. In addition, the researchers measured each participant's vasodilation levels.

In the end, the investigators determined that both Bikram groups achieved similar improvements in their vasodilation levels, regardless of room temperature.

The study authors also noted that some older adults become less tolerant of heat as they age, so the finding could be of interest to seniors who are drawn to the potential heart health benefits of yoga but are leery of exposure to excessive heat.

The findings were published in the journal *Experimental Physiology.*

Expert Commentary

Gregg Fonarow, MD, codirector of the UCLA Preventative Cardiology Program in Los Angeles, cautioned there is no solid evidence to suggest that any form of yoga offers a leg up when it comes to heart health.

"There are multiple factors that can impact vascular dilation that do not translate to reduction in cardiovascular events. [And] these findings are not sufficient evidence to reach conclusions regarding potential benefits of yoga or Bikram yoga on heart or vascular health," Dr. Fonarow said.

"Individuals interested in improving heart and vascular health should follow evidence-based recommendations regarding physical activity, healthy diet, maintaining healthy body weight, blood pressure and cholesterol levels, and not smoking," he added.

There's more on yoga and heart health at the website of the American Heart Association, Heart.org. Search "yoga and heart health."

Heart Surgery Patients May Need Vitamin D

According to a recent study, when 75 open-heart surgery patients received 50,000 international units (IU) of vitamin D-3 just before and after surgery, their vitamin D levels rose to the normal range shortly after surgery. Six months later, they had fewer episodes of heart failure than patients who did not receive vitamin D.

If you have heart problems—especially before heart surgery: Ask your doctor about testing your vitamin D level.

Note: High-dose vitamin D should be given only under a doctor's supervision.

J. Brent Muhlestein, MD, cardiovascular researcher, Intermountain Medical Center Heart Institute, Salt Lake City.

Fewer Hospital Readmissions But More Deaths

Medicare penalties for hospitals that readmit patients with heart failure have had their intended effect of reducing the frequency of readmission...30-day readmission rates dropped from 20% before the penalties were instituted to 18.4% afterward. But this has not translated to better patient outcomes—it has had the reverse effect. The 30-day mortality rate for heart-failure patients rose from 7.2% to 8.6%. And one year after an inpatient stay, mortality rates rose from 31.3% before the penalty program to 36.3% afterward. Medicare officials say that they are monitoring the readmission penalty program.

Ankur Gupta, MD, research associate, Brigham and Women's Hospital, Boston, and leader of a study of 115,245 people, published in *JAMA*.

Thyroid Hormone and Heart Disease Link

Too much thyroid hormone now is linked to artery disease. Middle-aged and older adults with higher levels of free thyroxine (FT4) had twice the rate of calcified coronary arteries as those with normal levels—and an 87% higher risk for heart attack or stroke. Generally, elevated FT4 levels indicate hyperthyroidism. Symptoms include weight loss, anxiety, weakness, sleep difficulty and increased heart rate.

Arjola Bano, MD, MSc, DSc, a researcher in the departments of internal medicine and epidemiology at Erasmus Medical Center, Rotterdam, the Netherlands, and leader of a study of more than 9,400 people, published in *Circulation Research*.

Chapter 2

CANCER BREAKTHROUGHS

Stop Dreading Your Mammogram!

Not looking forward to your next mammogram? You're not alone. Many women experience anxiety in the days leading up to it.

In fact, the psychological distress surrounding mammograms (and the potential results) was a factor in the US Preventive Services Task Force's 2009 decision to change its recommendation to biennial (every other year), instead of annual, mammography screening for women of average risk, ages 50 to 74.

But mammograms do save lives. These X-rays help identify breast cancer in women with no signs or symptoms of the disease.

The Discomfort Factor

When researchers have studied mammogram pain or discomfort, their findings have varied wildly—based on numerous studies, anywhere from 1% to 77% of women report that the test was painful.

Meanwhile, an important study conducted at Beth Israel Deaconess Medical Center found that most women don't experience any pain or anxiety at all. Discomfort...perhaps. But pain is not a given—and quite subjective at that. Afterward, most women said the exam wasn't nearly as awful as they'd feared.

Simple Steps That Help

Besides understanding that mammograms are often not nearly as uncomfortable or painful as many women fear, there are some simple things you can do to reduce pre-mammogram anxiety and to make the experience itself less unpleasant. *For example...*

- **Limit caffeine intake.** Caffeine can make your breasts more tender. Try decreasing your intake starting a few days before the exam. Don't eliminate caffeine, though, or you'll risk having a caffeine-withdrawal headache.
- **Try Tylenol.** Most women can safely use *acetaminophen* (Tylenol), taken at a standard dose within four hours of the exam, to minimize discomfort.

Bonus: It will reduce any soreness you might experience afterward. Avoid aspirin and

Margarita Zuley, MD, FACR, chief of breast imaging and professor and vice chair of quality and strategic development for the University of Pittsburgh Medical Center department of radiology. A diagnostic radiologist specializing in breast imaging, she has been the principal investigator on multiple grants related to digital and 3-D mammography.

other nonsteroidal anti-inflammatory drugs (NSAIDs) such as *ibuprofen* (Motrin, Advil), which can increase the risk for bruising.

- **Exercise before the test.** A recent study conducted by researchers at Barretos Cancer Hospital in São Paulo State, Brazil, found that women who exercised for 20 minutes just prior to their mammograms reported less pain after screening compared with women who didn't exercise—perhaps because the physical activity promoted the release of endorphins, hormones that have a pain-relieving effect. Exercises included warm-ups and stretching...then a series of 10 upper-body moves, such as arm and shoulder circles or interlocking the fingers behind the back and raising the arms.

- **Know what to expect.** Women who feel armed with information about the procedure experience less pain and discomfort from mammograms—likely because they feel less anxiety.

What helps: For first-timers, ask your doctor to walk you through the procedure when he/she prescribes your mammogram. A few days prior to the test, do a dry run to the facility so you know exactly how to get there and, if you're driving, where to find parking.

If possible, bring a friend or family member with you to your appointment for support. The less you have to worry about the day of your mammogram, the more relaxed—and therefore the less pain—you will feel.

What Worsens Discomfort

Most women know that mammograms tend to be less uncomfortable during the first two weeks of the menstrual cycle when the breasts aren't as sensitive. Mammograms are also more accurate when performed on that schedule. This is likely because breast tissue is generally less dense at that time and more easily imaged.

What many women don't know: Certain health conditions can increase pain or discomfort during a mammogram. *What helps women affected by...*

- **Chronic pain.** When scheduling, alert the facility that you have chronic pain. There may be a technologist on staff who is trained in working with chronic pain patients. Continue taking any prescription medications as normal, and be sure to try the general tips above. Never be afraid to speak up if something hurts too much! The compression used for mammograms is based in part on the patient's tolerance.

- **Cold temperatures.** If you have trouble tolerating cold temperatures, ask the technologist for a robe or bring one from home. If your hands get cold, you can ask to wear surgical gloves.

- **Dense breasts.** Roughly 25% of postmenopausal women have dense breasts. This simply means that their breasts have denser, lumpier tissue. Dense breasts tend to be more sensitive to pain and are likely to benefit from a reduction in caffeine intake as described earlier.

- **A lumpectomy.** If you have had this procedure, which involves surgical removal of a suspected cancerous tumor and surrounding tissue, you should return to annual mammogram imaging after surgery.

Radiation and surgery can both cause changes in the breast tissue and skin that may make a mammogram less comfortable. The scar itself may be tender, and the skin may be more sensitive to the touch. Let your mammogram technologist know so that he/she can take any necessary precautions, such as making adjustments in position and compression.

- **Weight issues.** Obese women are nearly twice as likely to cite pain as a mammogram deterrent as nonobese women. The exact reasons are unknown, but being overweight has been associated with a lower pain threshold. Some obese patients also feel that having larger breasts or breast tissue that extends under the arms renders mammograms more painful. Be sure to try the general tips above.

Don't Let a Disability Stop You

Use of a wheelchair or scooter should not prevent you from getting screened for breast cancer.

What helps: When scheduling a mammogram, let the facility where you'll be tested know if you will need assistance undressing…standing…moving your arms…and/or transferring from your wheelchair or scooter. The technologist will work one-on-one with you to make the exam as comfortable as possible.

---

9 Ways to Prevent Breast Cancer—Before and After Menopause

Anne McTiernan, PhD, research professor at Fred Hutchinson Cancer Research Center in Seattle, Washington, and author of *Starved: A Nutrition Doctor's Journey from Empty to Full.* She was a member of the World Cancer Research Fund International/American Institute for Cancer Research panel that issued the report titled "Continuous Update Project Report: Diet, Nutrition, Physical Activity and Breast Cancer 2017."

What are the most effective things women can do to avoid getting breast cancer? A team of researchers at the World Cancer Research Fund asked that question. *Here's what they found…*

Background: Every year, 315,000 American women are newly diagnosed with breast cancer. Although new treatments have improved survival, breast cancer remains the second-leading cause of cancer deaths in American women. Many known risk factors are hard to change—such as getting your first period before age 12…not ever having children or having your first child after age 30...hitting menopause after age 55...a family history of breast cancer...being exposed to high levels of radiation. But many lifestyle factors do make a difference—some, a big difference.

Study: The World Cancer Research Fund International and the American Institute for Cancer Research gathered an international panel of experts to review 119 scientific studies involving 12 million women about the ways diet, weight and physical activity affect a woman's risk of developing breast cancer. They then determined which of those factors protected women the most from getting the disease—both before and after menopause. (Since men account for only 1% of breast cancer cases, the panel limited its recommendations to women.)

Convincing evidence found that…

- **Physical activity and breastfeeding decrease the risk for breast cancer.**
- **Drinking alcohol increases the risk.**
- **Eating certain kinds of vegetables and fruits reduces risk.**

Surprisingly, women who were overweight or obese between the ages of 18 and 30 were less likely to develop breast cancer, either before or after menopause, compared with women who were of normal weight between the ages of 18 and 30. The reasons aren't well understood. But while being overweight or obese throughout adulthood was still associated with less risk for premenopausal breast cancer, a pattern of adult weight gain—defined in different studies as after age 35 or age 50—was strongly associated with increased postmenopausal breast cancer risk.

Bottom line: These evidence-backed lifestyle habits can help prevent breast cancer…

Before Menopause

- **If you have children, breastfeed if you are able to.** The longer you nurse and the more children you nurse, the more you reduce breast cancer risk thanks to the resulting hormonal changes that reduce estrogen exposure throughout your life.
- **Watch out for weight gain in your 30s, 40s and 50s.** Being overweight before age 30 is protective against breast cancer. But take

steps to prevent the weight gain that tends to creep up after age 30.

After Menopause

• **Redouble efforts to manage your weight.** Once through menopause, obesity increases breast cancer risk by a whopping 40%, according to some studies. Women who get and eliminate breast cancer have a higher chance of their cancer returning and a higher chance of dying of the disease if they are obese.

• **Whittle your waistline.** It's not just how much you weigh, but where weight lodges on your body. Extra fat around your middle can lead to inflammation, increased levels of estrogen (produced by the fat) and higher insulin levels—all of which can set the stage for breast cells to mutate and turn cancerous. It's tough to avoid turning apple-shaped after menopause. Try to keep your waist measurement less than 32 inches by eating healthy foods and staying active.

At Every Age

These lifestyle factors can help prevent breast cancer throughout life—and it's never too late to start them…

• **Curb your drinking.** Even one drink a day increases breast cancer risk by 5% if you're premenopausal—and by 9% if you're postmenopausal. Each additional daily drink increases risk, on average, by the same percentages. So if you like to have a glass of wine with a meal, do not pour more than five ounces—that is one drink.

• **Step up your activity level.** Any type of exercise reduces breast cancer risk. Aim for about 30 minutes at least five days a week. While moderately intense activity such as brisk walking counts, exercising vigorously—running versus walking, kickboxing versus yoga—is particularly protective.

Higher-intensity workouts not only help you get rid of harmful belly fat but also boost the immune system so your body is better able to kill mutating cells before they form a tumor. (Exercise also can improve outcomes for people who have cancer, research finds.)

• **Get your calcium.** Diets rich in calcium protect against breast cancer both before and after menopause.

One reason: Calcium helps regulate cell growth, especially in breast tissue.

• **Load up on nonstarchy veggies.** There is evidence that eating nonstarchy vegetables—such as broccoli, leafy greens, summer squash, asparagus, tomatoes—is especially helpful in reducing the risk of estrogen-negative breast cancer, which tends to grow at a faster rate than hormone-positive cancers. Aim for at least one cup a day. (Starchy veggies such as potatoes don't count.)

• **Eat your carotenoids.** When choosing fruits and vegetables, go for color. Animal and test-tube studies have shown that carotenoids—fat-soluble pigments that give produce its coloring—have protective properties. Choose red, orange and yellow fruits and vegetables such as berries, beets, peppers and carrots.

How much can these healthy lifestyle habits help reduce breast cancer risk? By about one-third, the researchers estimate. That would be about 100,000 US women every year.

Don't Trust This Home Test

The first-ever home test for breast cancer genes is inadequate—akin to performing a mammogram on just one part of the breast. The test, from the company 23AndMe, checks for only three of the many hundreds of mutations in two BRCA genes that increase risk. Doctor-ordered tests are much more extensive. Most breast cancer is not hereditary, but if the disease does run in your family, discuss genetic testing with your doctor.

Anne McTiernan, MD, PhD, a cancer-prevention researcher at Fred Hutchinson Cancer Research Center and professor at University of Washington, both in Seattle.

Learn to Love Your Breasts

Love your breasts! Your life may depend on it. *New study*: Women who are unhappy with their breast size are less likely to perform self-exams and more likely to delay seeing a doctor when they notice changes.

Body Image: An International Journal of Research.

Newer Breast MRI May Be More Accurate and Easier

Sebastian Bickelhaupt, MD, head, Breast Imaging Research Group, German Cancer Research Center, Heidelberg, Germany.

Otis Brawley, MD, chief medical officer, American Cancer Society.

Radiology.

A new type of MRI (magnetic resonance imaging) that doesn't use a contrast agent appears better at detecting what's really cancer and what's likely just a harmless lesion, researchers report.

In a study in Germany, the new technique reduced false-positive findings by 70%. The scan was also able to detect 98% of breast cancers correctly, the researchers said.

"This more advanced imaging technique is very good at distinguishing things that might be invasive cancer and things that are likely not cancer," said Otis Brawley, MD, chief medical officer for the American Cancer Society. He wasn't involved in the study.

How the New Test Works

The new test is known as diffusion kurtosis imaging. To create it, the researchers altered another special type of MRI. Then they combined the new scanning technique with software that decides whether a suspicious breast lesion is benign (harmless) or malignant (cancerous).

The new MRI "basically maps the movement of water molecules in the tissue. If a malignant tumor grows in the tissue, it disrupts the healthy tissue structure, which changes the movement of water molecules in this area," explained the study's lead researcher, Sebastian Bickelhaupt, MD. He's the head of the Breast Imaging Research Group at the German Cancer Research Center in Heidelberg.

Benefits of New MRI Versus Current MRI

Currently, MRI scans are used as part of screening for women with a particularly high risk of breast cancer.

This may include women with a breast cancer gene or genes, women with a family history of a breast cancer gene who haven't been tested themselves, those who've had radiation to the chest to treat lymphoma, and women with certain syndromes that raise the risk of breast cancer significantly, according to the American Cancer Society.

The problem is that MRIs currently find a lot of areas in the breasts that are deemed suspicious.

"I advise patients to ready themselves emotionally. MRI delivers a lot of false positives and there's a high probability that you will need several biopsies," Dr. Brawley explained.

Along with reducing the need for unnecessary biopsies due to false positive findings, the benefits of the new MRI type include no contrast agent, the researchers. A contrast agent is a substance introduced intravenously that makes it easier to see certain areas on an imaging test.

The new test also has a shorter imaging time. Dr. Bickelhaupt said the test only takes about 10 minutes. And unlike mammography or CT scans, there is no exposure to radiation.

These two factors—no need for an IV contrast agent and shorter test—potentially could reduce MRI costs.

Study Details

The study included 222 women from two sites in Germany. Ninety-five of the women were only included in the training portion of the study. The second group included 127 women. Their average age was 59. All had undergone X-ray mammography that indicated potential cancer.

All the women underwent the new MRI test, then had a biopsy to see if the suspicious area was cancer. The researchers then compared the findings from the new test to the biopsy results. They also assessed the results of conventional MRI images.

The investigators found that the new test was significantly better than standard MRI at detecting breast cancers.

The study was published in the journal *Radiology*.

Implications

"Although the numbers are pretty small in this study, this technique is an exciting thing. My gut is that if larger studies continue like this, this technique will be available in hospitals in the next decade or so," Dr. Brawley said.

Dr. Bickelhaupt and Dr. Brawley said this technique isn't designed to replace current standards, such as mammograms or ultrasounds.

Instead, Dr. Bickelhaupt said this test would expand the options available to women based on their clinical needs.

"Implementing such imaging approaches into the clinical routine might expand the diagnostic toolbox of the radiologist in the future," he said.

Learn more about new imaging tests to detect breast cancer from the American Cancer Society. Visit Cancer.org and search "experimental breast imaging."

Death Is a Good Incentive for Fighting Cancer

A loved one's cancer experience impacts prevention decisions.

Recent study: Half the women at high risk for breast cancer who had experienced the death of a loved one from any type of cancer were likely to choose aggressive measures—such as mastectomy—to prevent their own cancer. By comparison, just 3% of women with a loved one who survived cancer chose aggressive measures.

If you have risk factors for breast cancer: Make sure your doctor fully explains all preventive treatments before you choose which is best for you.

Tasleem Padamsee, PhD, assistant professor of health services management and policy, The Ohio State University, Columbus.

Extra Body Fat May Raise Breast Cancer Risk, No Matter Your Weight

Neil Iyengar, MD, medical oncologist, Memorial Sloan Kettering Cancer Center, New York City.

Mia Gaudet, PhD, strategic director, breast and gynecologic cancer research, American Cancer Society, Atlanta.

Graham Colditz, MD, DrPH, associate director, prevention and control, Siteman Cancer Center at Barnes-Jewish Hospital and Washington University School of Medicine, St. Louis.

American Association for Cancer Research conference, Austin, Texas.

Older women who carry some extra body fat may face a heightened risk of breast cancer—even if their weight is normal, a new study finds.

"This suggests women should not just concentrate on weight," said Mia Gaudet, PhD, strategic director of breast and gynecologic cancer research for the American Cancer Society.

"Instead, they should focus on doing things that can help reduce body fat levels—like a healthy diet and regular exercise," said Dr. Gaudet, who was not involved in the study.

Background

Past research has found that overweight and obese women generally have a higher risk of developing breast cancer after menopause.

But doctors have long relied on body mass index (BMI) to tell whether people are normal weight or not.

The problem is, BMI does not distinguish between fat, muscle and bone. So, it's an imprecise gauge of body composition—and disease risks, recent studies have shown.

"It's now 'fairly well established' that BMI is not the best indicator of a person's risk of conditions like type 2 diabetes and heart disease," said lead researcher Neil Iyengar, MD. "And now it seems that may also be true for breast cancer."

New Study

The findings are based on 3,460 women ages 50 to 79 who were part of a large study called the Women's Health Initiative. The women all had a normal BMI at the outset, and all had their body fat measured with dual energy X-ray absorptiometry, or DXA.

DXA is a whole-body scan that gives a snapshot of a person's body composition.

Over 16 years, 182 women developed breast cancer; most had tumors that were estrogen receptor-positive, which means estrogen helps fuel their growth.

On average, the study found, women with higher body fat levels had a greater risk of developing ER-positive breast cancer—women whose fat levels were in the top 25% were twice as likely to develop the cancer, compared to women in the bottom 25%.

The findings do not prove definitively that body fat caused the cancers, according to Dr. Iyengar. But his team accounted for many other factors—including the women's family history of breast cancer, use of hormone therapy, and their exercise and drinking habits.

And still, extra body fat was a risk factor.

The findings were presented at an American Association for Cancer Research conference in Austin, Texas.

Possible Explanation

Why would body fat matter? Fat is "active tissue," Dr. Iyengar explained, and when it accumulates in excess, it outgrows its blood supply and fat cells start to die. When that happens, he said, there is inflammation, and substances called growth factors are churned out.

"Those growth factors can potentially support cancers," Dr. Iyengar said.

"On top of that, fat is a source of continued estrogen production in postmenopausal women," said Graham Colditz, MD, DrPH, of the Siteman Cancer Center at Barnes-Jewish Hospital, in St. Louis.

Dr. Colditz, who was not involved in the study, said the findings make sense.

Expert Advice

But practically speaking, he added, it will still be much easier for women to monitor their weight on the bathroom scale, versus having their body fat levels tracked.

Dr. Colditz echoed Dr. Gaudet's advice: Even if women have a normal BMI, they should still strive for a healthy diet and regular exercise—including, he said, resistance exercises to maintain and build muscle.

In fact, Dr. Iyengar said, study participants with higher body fat levels did generally exercise less often than other women did.

The study looked only at postmenopausal women, so the findings do not necessarily apply to breast cancer in younger women, Dr. Iyengar said.

In general, he noted, premenopausal breast cancer differs from cases that arise later in life—and it's not clear whether weight

Hair Products and Breast Cancer Risk

The use of brown or black hair dyes by black women was tied to a 51% greater risk for breast cancer. White women who used dark dyes had 31% higher risk. The study found an association between using hair products and the risk of being diagnosed with breast cancer, but it does not prove cause and effect.

Adana Llanos, PhD, MPH, assistant professor of epidemiology with Rutgers School of Public Health, New Brunswick, New Jersey, and leader of a study of more than 4,000 women, published in *Carcinogenesis*.

or body composition have any bearing on that risk.

For more information on the link between body weight and cancer, visit the American Cancer Society website, Cancer.org, and search "body weight and cancer risk."

Heavier Women May Need More Frequent Mammograms

Women with a BMI (body mass index) of 25 or more (about 150 pounds for a five-foot, five-inch woman) are more likely to be diagnosed with a breast tumor larger than 2 cm, compared with women who have a lower BMI. The findings were especially pronounced among heavier women diagnosed with cancer that was detected between regular screenings. These women also had a worse prognosis than those who were thinner.

Fredrik Strand, MD, radiologist, Karolinska University Hospital, Stockholm, Sweden.

High Fruit Consumption, Low Breast Cancer Risk

Women who ate at least three servings a day of apples, bananas and grapes as teenagers were 25% less likely to have developed breast cancer in middle age than women who said that they ate only a half serving of those fruits daily. There also was some benefit—but less of it—linked to eating oranges and/or kale. Fruit juice of any type did not seem linked to lower breast cancer risk.

Study of the questionnaires of more than 44,000 women by researchers at Harvard T.H. Chan School of Public Health, Boston, published in *The BMJ*.

Birth Control–Cancer Link

Women who are using or have recently used birth control pills, implants, injections or intrauterine devices that release hormones are at increased risk for breast cancer. In a study of 1.8 million women, ages 15 to 49, breast cancer risk was increased by 20% among women who used hormonal birth control. Still, risk is low in these ages, so absolute risk was small—an extra 13 cases for every 100,000 women using hormonal contraceptives for one year. Women should balance breast cancer risk with the health risks of nonhormonal contraceptive methods, such as IUDs.

Anne McTiernan, MD, PhD, is a cancer prevention researcher at Fred Hutchinson Cancer Research Center, Seattle, and author of ***Starved: A Nutrition Doctor's Journey from Empty to Full.***

Rare Cancer Linked to Breast Implants

Mark W. Clemens II, MD, FACS, associate professor in the department of plastic surgery at MD Anderson Cancer Center, University of Texas in Houston. He has published numerous journal articles about BIA-ALCL. MDAnderson.org

The Food and Drug Administration has identified a link between a specific type of breast implant and a rare form of cancer that's being called breast implant-associated anaplastic large-cell lymphoma (BIA-ALCL).

Nearly all the women who have experienced this cancer of the immune system have had "textured" breast implants, which have a rough surface. Textured implants are sometimes recommended by plastic surgeons because they are less likely than smooth implants to later move out of position. (Their textured surface is not visible through the skin.)

What to do: Women who have breast implants—either textured or smooth—should see their doctors if they have swelling and/or asymmetry in the area. This could be a buildup of fluid, which could be a symptom of BIA-ALCL.

Fortunately, the survival rate of this cancer is very high when it is diagnosed and treated promptly. Treatment typically involves a test to determine whether this cancer is indeed the cause of the fluid collection, followed by surgical removal of the implant if it is. In around 85% of cases, the cancer can be cured with surgery without even subjecting the patient to chemotherapy.

It is not necessary to have textured implants removed simply to avoid the possibility of developing BIA-ALCL in the future. This cancer is very rare even among women who have textured implants—as of July 2017, there have been only 464 known cases worldwide among the millions of women who have had textured implants—and very treatable when it does occur.

Risk of Breast Cancer's Return Can Linger for Decades

Daniel Hayes, MD, professor, breast cancer research, University of Michigan Comprehensive Cancer Center, Ann Arbor.

Harold Burstein, MD, medical oncologist, Dana-Farber Cancer Institute and Brigham and Women's Hospital, Boston.

Neil Iyengar, MD, medical oncologist, Memorial Sloan Kettering Cancer Center, New York City.

New England Journal of Medicine.

Women treated for early-stage breast cancer still face a substantial risk of recurrence up to 20 years later, a large, new study shows.

Cancer experts say the findings should help inform women's treatment decisions.

Fewer Women Need Chemo

Fewer women need chemotherapy for early-stage breast cancer. For women with stage 1 or stage 2 breast cancer, rates have dropped from 35% to 21% in recent years. More oncologists now order genetic profiling of these early-stage tumors, which helps predict which tumors will not recur after treatment (surgery, radiation and sometimes hormones). Women with these tumors often are able to skip chemo, sparing them grueling side effects.

Allison W. Kurian, MD, associate professor of medicine at Stanford University School of Medicine in Stanford, California, and lead author of a study published in *Journal of the National Cancer Institute.*

Recurrence Risk Higher Than Expected

Specifically, the researchers followed women with estrogen-receptor-positive breast cancer, which means the hormone helps fuel the cancer's growth. Standard treatment includes hormonal therapy—with drugs that block estrogen's effects—to help prevent a return of the cancer.

All of the women in the study, nearly 63,000, were scheduled to receive the typical five years of hormonal therapy.

Researchers found that while the women remained cancer-free for those five years, the risk for recurrence over the next 15 years was still significant.

It was greatest for women whose initial cancer had spread to multiple lymph nodes near the breast by the time it was diagnosed. Their odds of eventually having a distant recurrence—meaning the cancer spread to such tissue as the bones, liver or lungs—were as high as 41%.

Doctors have long known that women with estrogen-sensitive breast cancer often have recurrences many years later, said Harold Burstein, MD, a cancer expert affiliated with the American Society of Clinical Oncology. He was not involved in the research.

"But the risks in this study are probably higher than many of us would've thought," said Dr. Burstein, who's an oncologist at the Dana-Farber Cancer Institute in Boston.

He stressed, though, that the women in the study started their treatment more than 20 years ago, and many advances have been made since.

"We're doing a better job of treating this disease now," Dr. Burstein said. "These numbers are probably worse than what women today would face."

Senior researcher Daniel Hayes, MD, agreed.

"These data are scary," said Dr. Hayes, a professor at the University of Michigan's Comprehensive Cancer Center. "But women with ER-positive cancer are doing better now than 25 years ago."

Still, he said, the findings give doctors and women more information for making treatment decisions.

That's because women can opt for more than five years of hormonal therapy. Studies have shown that longer treatment further cuts the risk for recurrence.

However, that can also mean additional years of side effects—like hot flashes, sexual dysfunction and joint pain, Dr. Hayes said. If women have a clearer picture of their future odds of recurrence, he said, that could help them decide whether the treatment is worth the downsides.

Study Details

For the study, Hayes's team combined the results of 88 trials that included almost 63,000 women, all with estrogen-sensitive breast cancer. After their initial treatment with surgery, and sometimes chemotherapy, all were prescribed five years of hormonal therapy. Most received the drug *tamoxifen*, sometimes with newer hormonal drugs called aromatase inhibitors.

Overall, the study found, the odds of a distant recurrence varied greatly, depending on how far the original cancer had spread to nearby lymph nodes.

Women with no affected lymph nodes faced a 13% to 19% chance of a distant recurrence in the 15 years after their hormonal therapy ended. For those with one to three affected nodes, the odds of a distant recurrence were 20% to 26%. Women with four to nine nodes affected, the chances of such recurrence were 34% to 41%.

The findings were published in the *New England Journal of Medicine.*

Study Implications

The study, Dr. Hayes said, was not designed to tell anyone what to do. "I could show these same data to two different women and get two different treatment decisions," he said.

But, he added, "there's no question" that women in these situations should discuss longer-term hormonal therapy with their doctor.

Neil Iyengar, MD, who specializes in treating breast cancer at Memorial Sloan Kettering Cancer Center in New York City, described the research as "a very useful study for patients and doctors."

Dr. Iyengar said he sees many women with earlier-stage cancers struggle with the issue of whether the side effects of hormonal therapy are worth it. The new findings, he said, might offer some women more motivation to continue—at least for the first five years, if not beyond.

But Dr. Burstein pointed out that additional hormonal therapy does not erase the possibility of a recurrence.

It won't turn that 13% risk into zero risk," he said. "But it can reduce it."

The American Cancer Society has more information on treating breast cancer with hormone therapy at Cancer.org. Search "hormone therapy for breast cancer."

Surprising Cancer Risk

Women who eat lots of high-calorie, low-nutrient foods, such as chips, fast food and candy, are 10% more likely, on average, to develop obesity-related breast, colon, ovarian, kidney or endometrial cancer.

The big surprise: The increased cancer risk was identified even among those of normal weight, according to the 15-year study that tracked 92,000 women.

Cynthia Thomson, PhD, RDN, professor, health promotion sciences, University of Arizona's Zuckerman College of Public Health, Tucson.

Acupuncture May Ease Pain Tied to Breast Cancer Care

Lauren S. Cassell, MD, chief of breast surgery, Lenox Hill Hospital, New York City.

Dawn Hershman, MD, leader, Breast Cancer Program, NewYork-Presbyterian/Columbia University Medical Center, New York City.

Cynara Coomer, MD, chief of breast surgery, director of the Florina Rusi-Marke Comprehensive Breast Center, Staten Island University Hospital, New York City.

San Antonio Breast Cancer Symposium, news release.

Some common breast cancer medications can trigger joint pain, but new research suggests acupuncture may ease that side effect.

The finding could be a win-win for breast cancer patients, said one oncologist who reviewed the study.

"Acupuncture has been around for thousands of years and has no real downside," said Lauren Cassell, MD, chief of breast surgery at Lenox Hill Hospital in New York City.

"If something so simple as acupuncture can improve upon these symptoms and the patients' quality of life, we will have more women becoming compliant in taking their medication, and one would expect improved outcomes," Dr. Cassell added.

The Study

The new study was led by Dawn Hershman, MD, who heads the Breast Cancer Program at NewYork-Presbyterian/Columbia University Medical Center in New York City.

Dr. Hershman's team tracked outcomes for 226 postmenopausal women with early-stage breast cancer who were taking drugs called aromatase inhibitors.

These drugs—which include Arimidex, Femara and Aromasin, among others—are often used to treat women with estrogen-sensitive breast tumors, Dr. Hershman said.

But she added that "many patients suffer from side effects that cause them to miss treatments or stop treatment altogether. We need to identify strategies to control these side effects, the most common of which is debilitating joint pain and stiffness."

Dr. Hershman's team wondered if the ancient practice of acupuncture might help. Of the patients in the study, 110 received true acupuncture, 59 were given fake acupuncture (needles placed at ineffective spots on the body), and another 57 were placed on a waiting list.

The patients in the true and fake acupuncture groups underwent twice-weekly sessions for six weeks, followed by one session a week for six more weeks.

After six weeks, patients in the true acupuncture group reported much lower pain scores than those in either the fake acupuncture or waiting list groups, Dr. Hershman's team reported.

The study was presented at the annual San Antonio Breast Cancer Symposium, in Texas.

Implications

The finding may mean that women with pain related to aromatase inhibitor use might stick to their meds longer if acupuncture eases their joint pain, "but we need to conduct further studies to determine if this is indeed the case," said Dr. Hershman.

In the meantime, the findings suggest that "health-care practitioners should discuss the possibility of acupuncture with patients experiencing aromatase inhibitor-related joint pain and stiffness, because it has the potential to improve their quality of life," Dr. Hershman said.

Expert Commentary

Cynara Coomer, MD, directs the Florina Rusi-Marke Comprehensive Breast Center, at Staten Island University Hospital in New York City. Reading over the findings, she agreed that "the integration of Western and Eastern medicine is an important path to explore" in breast cancer care.

And with an opioid-addiction crisis sweeping the United States, "it is important for physicians to find other means of pain control for our patients," she added.

"This is yet another study that reveals the benefits of acupuncture in treating pain," Dr. Coomer said.

Breastcancer.org has more information on aromatase inhibitors. Search "aromatase inhibitors" at Breastcancer.org.

New Breast Cancer Care

A device that treats early-stage breast cancer tumors by targeting them with precisely focused beams of radiation, minimizing damage to surrounding tissue, has received FDA clearance. The GammaPod is expected to shorten the standard three-to-six-week radiation treatment and may eliminate the need for surgery. To find a hospital using GammaPod, go to Xcision.com and click on "patients."

William F. Regine, MD, Isadore and Fannie Schneider Foxman Endowed Professor and Chair of Radiation Oncology, University of Maryland School of Medicine, Baltimore, and GammaPod coinventor.

Breakthrough Cancer Therapy

Caron A. Jacobson, MD, medical oncologist and assistant professor of medicine at Dana-Farber Cancer Institute and Harvard Medical School, both in Boston. She is the medical director of the Immune Effector Cell Therapy Program at Dana-Farber, which houses its CAR T-cell program. Dr. Jacobson, who specializes in lymphoma treatment and is affiliated with Brigham and Women's Hospital in Boston, is the principal investigator of CAR T-cell trials in lymphoma there and at Dana-Farber.

When it comes to the development of cancer treatments, the decades-long arc of progress is slow and incremental. Then something truly significant happens to change the course of the disease. What's happening now appears to be one of those moments.

Latest development: A type of blood-cancer treatment that has already shown remarkable success in clinical trials is beginning to receive FDA approvals. Two of these treatments, for example, have recently been approved (see page 37).

With the new treatment, known as CAR T-cell therapy, blood is drawn from a patient to isolate his/her T-cells, the powerhouses of the body's immune system. The T-cells are genetically altered and reprogrammed to recognize and kill tumor cells and then infused back into the patient.

The treatment has been called a "living drug" because it's hoped that the enhanced T-cells will continue to multiply and remain active in the body, possibly providing lifelong protection against the cancer.

A Game Changer

Researchers at universities and pharmaceutical companies have now developed CAR T-cell therapy for leukemia, multiple myeloma and lymphoma—blood cancers that account for about 10% of all cancer cases diagnosed in the US each year.

The hope is that similar treatments eventually will be used for tumors affecting the breast, lung, prostate and other parts of the body.

Important: The treatment of "solid" tumors with this type of gene therapy still presents formidable obstacles that will have to be overcome.

CAR T-cell therapies have mainly been studied in patients with lymphoma or other blood cancers that didn't respond well to standard treatments or that later recurred.

Example: Lymphoma patients are typically given several types and/or protocols of standard chemotherapy without a sure result. These patients are thought to be good candidates for CAR T-cell therapy—and the early results are promising. Studies show that up to

80% of such patients respond to CAR T- cell therapy, and about 30% to 40% of patients were still in remission after six months. In earlier studies, some patients have remained in remission for more than five years.

Important caveat: So far, hundreds of patients have been treated with CAR T-cell therapy. We're seeing remarkable response rates, with many patients achieving a "complete" response—meaning that no cancer is detectable in the body with current methods. But the treatments are too new—and patients haven't been followed for a long enough time—to say for sure that the treatments promise a cure.

How It Works

Except for cases for which FDA-approved CAR T-cell therapy now is available (see below), adult patients who are eligible for this treatment receive it by participating in a clinical trial. They report to a laboratory or clinic, where they undergo a four-to-six-hour process to collect blood cells, which are then sent to a company that reengineers the patient's T-cells, giving them the ability to recognize a protein (for example, CD19) on the surface of blood-cancer cells. The engineering process takes two to four weeks.

The patients are given several days of routine chemotherapy. After that, the engineered T-cells are given back to the patient via infusion. This treatment, which takes about 15 minutes, usually is administered just once, though some studies allow a second infusion if there is a partial response or relapse. The cell infusion and period of observation thereafter are typically done on an inpatient basis.

The reengineered cells circulate throughout the body and quickly begin to multiply and attack the tumor cells. Even though it's hoped that the reengineered cells will stay active in the body indefinitely, it's too early to know if this will happen. The cells might last for six months, 12 months...or forever.

Not Risk-Free

With the treatment beginning to get FDA approval, it is expected to be very expensive—possibly costing hundreds of thousands of dollars. At this point, it's unclear the extent to which insurance will cover the cost.

For now, the CAR T-cell treatments are somewhat risky. The genetically altered T-cells, when activated by cancer cells, can trigger a condition known as cytokine release syndrome. Many patients experience intense flulike symptoms, including a high fever, aches and fatigue. About 10% to 15% will get sick enough that they require ICU-level care, but these side effects can be treated with steroids and other drugs. Mild-to-severe confusion may develop in up to 30% of patients. While this too is reversible, there have been cases of fatal brain swelling.

The cardiac stress and respiratory distress due to the "inflammatory cascade" that is triggered by the treatment also can be life-threatening. The risks will undoubtedly decline as doctors gain more experience with the therapy.

How to access this therapy...

Latest development: Based on the results of trials of CAR T-cells in children and young adults with acute lymphoblastic leukemia, in August 2017, the FDA approved a CD19-targeted CAR T-cell therapy called *tisagenlecleucel* (Kymriah). In October 2017, a second CAR T-cell therapy, *axicabtagene* (Yescarta), was approved for patients with large B-cell lymphomas who have not responded to other treatments.

For patients with lymphoma, leukemia or multiple myeloma for whom an FDA-approved CAR T-cell therapy is not available, a clinical trial may be an option. If your doctor believes that you're a candidate for CAR T-cell therapy, discuss whether it makes sense for you to participate in an ongoing study. Your oncologist can advise you about clinical trials in your area. If accepted into the trial, the CAR T-cell therapy is covered but supportive care is billed to insurance.

Got Cancer? Protect Your Heart from Harmful Therapies

Anju Nohria, MD, director of the Cardio-Oncology Program at Dana-Farber/Brigham and Women's Cancer Center in Boston. Dr. Nohria is also a cardiovascular medicine specialist at Brigham and Women's Hospital, an assistant professor of medicine at Harvard Medical School and the author of more than 60 peer-reviewed articles. BrighamAndWomens.org

First, the good news: Thanks to advancements in prevention, detection and treatment, the overall number of cancer deaths has been significantly reduced.

Now, some bad news: For some patients, this success comes at a high cost—many cancer treatments are considered cardiotoxic, meaning they can damage the heart.

In fact, 99% of 303 oncologists included in a 2017 study published in the *International Journal of Cardiology* said that they prescribe cardiotoxic therapies.

While these are among the most effective treatments for cancer, they can cause dangerous heart conditions such as high blood pressure (hypertension), heart failure, arrhythmia and more...or make preexisting conditions worse—either during treatment or years later.

Protecting Your Heart

The risk for heart damage from these treatments depends on such factors as the type of treatment and dose...the location of the cancer...and the patient's age, preexisting cardiac risk and overall health status.

When developing a treatment plan for cancer, an oncologist should carefully weigh the risks and rewards of treatments that are considered to be cardiotoxic and discuss this in detail with his/her patient.

Cancer therapies that have been shown to have negative effects on the heart—and how to protect yourself...

- **Anthracyclines,** such as *doxorubicin* (Adriamycin) and *epirubicin* (Ellence). This class of chemotherapeutic drugs, commonly used to treat lymphoma, ovarian cancer and breast cancer, kills cancer cells by damaging their DNA. However, in the process of attacking the cancer, these drugs can weaken the heart, increasing the risk for heart failure. About 9% of patients taking an anthracycline medication will experience a weakening of the heart muscle known as cardiomyopathy. Cardiomyopathy tends to occur within the first year after treatment but may not manifest for 10 to 20 years.

To protect your heart: Your oncologist should check for cardiomyopathy with a baseline echocardiogram (ultrasound of the heart) prior to anthracycline chemotherapy, and again within one year of completing treatment. If cardiomyopathy is caught early, heart medication, such as a beta-blocker combined with an ACE inhibitor, can be started. New research suggests that this drug combination may have a protective effect on a patient's heart during cancer treatment. Ask your doctor if this strategy is right for you.

- **Radiation.** Radiation to the chest—especially the left side, where the heart is—can damage the blood vessels that bring blood to the heart, the heart valves and the heart muscle, contributing to coronary artery disease, heart failure and arrhythmia. Thanks to advancements in targeted radiation (radiating only the tumor, not the entire chest), the risk of having a heart issue after radiation is lower than ever. Still, many patients who have had radiation will experience cardiac issues sometime in the 40 years following treatment. For this reason, the effect is more concerning for younger cancer patients than older patients.

To protect your heart: If you have had radiation treatment to the chest, see your cardiologist or internist annually for a thorough physical and make sure that any cardiovascular risk factors you might have—such as hypertension, diabetes and/or excess weight—are addressed.

My advice: Ten years after radiation treatment, have an echocardiogram and stress test, repeating these tests every five to 10 years, or sooner if you're experiencing any of the cardiac symptoms mentioned on page 39.

• ***Trastuzumab* (Herceptin).** This cancer medication, used to treat more aggressive breast cancers (HER2-positive, specifically), causes weakening of the heart muscle, typically during treatment. Thirteen percent of patients taking trastuzumab plus an anthracycline drug experience heart issues. Most at risk are those who have a prior history of cardiac risk factors such as hypertension and diabetes and those who are over age 65.

To protect your heart: You'll need an echocardiogram before and after treatment, and possibly during treatment as well, to check for warning signs. Fortunately, cardiomyopathy caused by this drug tends to be reversible—if your oncologist notices any problems, he can halt treatment, begin medication such as a beta-blocker and ACE inhibitor to help heal the heart, then restart trastuzumab. (For more information on how breast cancer therapies can affect your heart health, see page 4 in "Heart Health for Women," chapter 1.)

Important: Recent research suggests that taking a combination of trastuzumab and an anthracycline along with a blood pressure drug called *candesartan* (Atacand) successfully treats early breast cancer while protecting the patient's heart. And a new study indicates that women with early, localized breast cancer can now take trastuzumab for just nine weeks instead of the customary year with the same anticancer effect but much less cardiotoxicity.

• **Tyrosine kinase inhibitors,** such as *bevacizumab* (Avastin) and *sunitinib* (Sutent). These newer cancer medications, used to treat kidney, esophageal, stomach and colon cancers, block a receptor required for new blood vessel formation, starving tumors of blood needed for growth. That's bad news for tumors and for the heart, which needs a steady blood supply to thrive. Because of this, 20% to 60% of patients taking a tyrosine kinase inhibitor will experience hypertension during treatment and, in some cases, cardiomyopathy and heart failure.

To protect your heart: Your oncologist will monitor your blood pressure throughout treatment with this drug, adding blood pressure medication if necessary. No echocardiogram is needed. Once treatment is complete, your blood pressure usually returns to normal.

Note: Patients who have a preexisting heart condition or cardiac issues while receiving these therapies should get treated at a cardio-oncology program or see a cardio-oncology specialist. To find one near you, check with your oncologist.

Watch Out For...

Anyone receiving cardiotoxic cancer therapy who has symptoms such as shortness of breath, chest pain, difficulty breathing when walking or lying down or changes in heart rhythm should alert his/her doctor.

Note: Many cardiotoxic effects cannot be felt by the patient, so vigilant monitoring of cardiac function during (and sometimes after) treatment is also vital.

What You May Not Know About Ovarian Cancer

Douglas Levine, MD, director, division of gynecologic oncology, Perlmutter Cancer Center, NYU Langone Health, New York City.
NYU Langone Health, news release.

In a report that will likely surprise many women, researchers say most cases of ovarian cancer originate in the fallopian tubes, not the ovaries.

"Based on a better understanding of its origins, our study suggests new strategies for the prevention and early detection of ovarian cancer," said senior study author Douglas Levine, MD. He is director of the division of gynecologic oncology at the Perlmutter Cancer Center, which is part of NYU Langone Health in New York City.

About Ovarian Cancer

Ovarian cancer is difficult to diagnose in its earliest—and most treatable—stages. Fewer than 50% of women diagnosed with the disease survive more than five years after diagnosis, according to the American Cancer Society.

The Study

For the study, Dr. Levine and his colleagues performed genetic analyses of ovarian cancer cells from 96 patients.

Eggs from the ovaries travel through the fallopian tubes on their way to the uterus. The researchers discovered that ovarian cancer cells have more in common with cells covering the tips of fallopian tubes (tubal cells) than with those on the surface of ovaries.

"We found no differences in the 20,000 genes that we can identify. This leads us to believe that these ovarian cancers all originate in the fallopian tubes," Dr. Levine said.

The report was published in the journal *Nature Communications.*

Implications

The good news is that if markers for these tubal cells can be found, then blood tests, advanced Pap smears, or direct tests on tubal tissue might spot ovarian cancer earlier, the study authors said.

It might also turn out to be feasible to remove a woman's fallopian tubes, but not her ovaries, to reduce the risk of ovarian cancer in those at high risk for the disease, the study authors suggested.

For more information on ovarian cancer, visit the website of the American Cancer Society, Cancer.org/cancer/ovarian-cancer.

Dad Can Pass on Ovarian Cancer Genes, Too

Kevin Eng, PhD, assistant professor of oncology, Roswell Park Comprehensive Cancer Center, Buffalo, New York.

PLoS Genetics, news release.

A gene mutation that's passed down from a father is associated with earlier onset of ovarian cancer in daughters and prostate cancer in the father and his sons, a new study suggests.

Previous research had shown that sisters of women with ovarian cancer have a higher risk for the disease than their mother, but the reasons for this were unclear.

"Our study may explain why we find families with multiple affected daughters: Because a dad's chromosomes determine the sex of his children, all of his daughters have to carry the same X chromosome genes," said study author Kevin Eng, PhD. He's an assistant professor of oncology at Roswell Park Comprehensive Cancer Center, in Buffalo, New York.

Dr. Eng's team decided to look at whether genes on the X chromosome passed down from the father might influence a daughter's risk of ovarian cancer.

Study Details

The researchers examined data about pairs of granddaughters and grandmothers. They also sequenced portions of the X chromosome from 186 women affected by ovarian cancer.

The investigators discovered that women with ovarian cancer linked to genes inherited from their father's mother developed the cancer much earlier than those with ovarian cancer linked to genes from their mother. In addition, the same genes from the father's mother are also associated with higher rates of prostate cancer in fathers and sons.

Further investigation led the researchers to a previously unknown mutation on the X chromosome that may be associated with cases of ovarian cancer that develop more than six years earlier than average.

The study was published in the journal *PLoS Genetics.*

Implications

The findings suggest that a gene on the X chromosome may increase a woman's risk of ovarian cancer, independent of other known risk genes, such as the BRCA genes. But the researchers did not prove that this gene causes ovarian cancer risk to rise.

Further research is needed to confirm the identity and function of this gene, the study authors added.

"What we have to do next is make sure we have the right gene by sequencing more families," said Dr. Eng.

"This finding has sparked a lot of discussion within our group about how to find these X-linked families," Dr. Eng said. "It's an all-or-none kind of pattern: A family with three daughters who all have ovarian cancer is more likely to be driven by inherited X mutations than by BRCA mutations."

The American Cancer Society has more information on ovarian cancer at Cancer.org. Search "ovarian cancer."

Some Blood Pressure Meds Tied to Pancreatic Cancer Risk in Women

Zhensheng Wang, MPH, PhD, postdoctoral associate, Duncan Comprehensive Cancer Center, Baylor College of Medicine, Houston.

Victoria Manax Rutson, MD, chief medical officer, Pancreatic Cancer Action Network, Manhattan Beach, California.

American Association for Cancer Research meeting, Chicago.

Certain drugs prescribed to treat high blood pressure may boost a woman's risk for developing pancreatic cancer after menopause, new research suggests.

In a large study of postmenopausal women, those who had ever taken a short-acting calcium channel blocker (CCB) saw their pancreatic cancer risk shoot up by 66%.

And women who had used a short-acting CCB for three years or more faced more than double the risk for pancreatic cancer, compared with those who had taken other types of blood pressure drugs.

This class of drugs includes short-acting *nifedipine* (brand names Procardia, Adalat CC), *nicardipine* (Cardene IV) and *diltiazem* (Cardizem).

The short-acting CCBs were the only blood pressure drugs linked to higher pancreatic cancer risk, according to study lead author Zhensheng Wang, MPH, PhD.

Risk for Pancreatic Cancer

However, people taking this class of drugs shouldn't panic, because their absolute risk of developing pancreatic cancer still remains very low. According to the US National Cancer Institute, just 1.6% of Americans will develop the cancer during their lifetime. That means that—even after accounting for a bump up in risk from taking a CCB—an individual's odds for the disease remains minimal.

Still, the new finding was unexpected, said Dr. Wang, a postdoctoral associate at Baylor College of Medicine in Houston.

Prior investigations had hinted that CCBs might even protect against pancreatic cancer by boosting levels of a protein (sRAGE) known to keep inflammation in check, said Dr. Wang.

Reduced inflammation is typically associated with a lower risk for a range of cancers.

So what might explain the current results?

Possible Explanations for Increased Risk

Dr. Wang noted that short-acting CCBs are "the least effective" blood pressure drug available. That could mean many of the women in the study had not achieved good blood pressure control to begin with, which could have boosted their risk for diabetes. And diabetes is a known risk factor for pancreatic cancer.

Dr. Wang also said blood samples taken from more than half the pancreatic cancer patients revealed that those who had ever taken a short-acting CCB also had notably lower levels of the sRAGE protein, compared with women who had taken other types of blood pressure drugs. That would mean less inflammation control and, therefore, potentially higher cancer risk.

Finally, he hypothesized that women who are prescribed short-acting CCBs might differ in some way from patients prescribed other types of blood pressure control.

CCBs tamp down blood pressure by preventing calcium from entering cells in the heart and blood vessel walls, thereby decreasing cardiac stress and workload.

In 1996, the US Food and Drug Administration took steps to discourage doctors from prescribing short-acting nifedipine. It warned that some researchers had linked the drug to an increased risk for heart attack and stroke.

New Study Detals

The current study followed more than 145,000 participants in the Women's Health Initiative study. They were between 50 and 79 years old at the start of the study, and medication use—but not dosage—was monitored between 1993 and 1998.

By 2014, more than 800 had developed pancreatic cancer, with risk up only among those who had been prescribed a short-acting CCB, Dr. Wang's team found.

For those who'd used the drugs three years or more, risk of pancreatic cancer was 107% higher than for those who took other blood pressure drugs.

Longer-acting CCB drugs were not associated with any risk elevation. Neither were beta blockers, diuretic drugs or ACE inhibitors.

Dr. Wang and his colleagues presented their findings at a meeting of the American Association for Cancer Research in Chicago. He said the findings need to be reconfirmed.

Expert Advice

One cancer specialist agreed that more investigation is warranted.

"There is no doubt more research needs to be done on this," said Victoria Manax Rutson, MD, chief medical officer for the Pancreatic Cancer Action Network in Manhattan Beach, California.

But for now, Dr. Rutson advised patients to "consult with their doctors before removing or adding any medications."

"Removing hypertension medications can be extremely dangerous, especially if someone has a history of high blood pressure," she warned.

Dr. Rutson also said if pancreatic cancer runs in your family, you might want to consult a doctor.

"If you have a familial history of pancreatic cancer, it is important to visit with a gastroenterologist, especially if you begin to exhibit any symptoms that are new or out of the ordinary," Dr. Rutson added.

Pancreatic cancer is the fourth leading cause of cancer deaths in the United States. Dr. Wang said it typically strikes older adults with chronic medical conditions, such as high blood pressure.

There's more on blood pressure medication at the American Heart Association web site, Heart.org. Search "blood pressure medications."

Nuts Fight Stomach Cancer

A study involving 566,000 older adults found that regularly eating nuts and peanut butter was associated with a 27% lower risk for gastric noncardia adenocarcinoma (cancer of the lower stomach), compared with people who reported consuming these foods infrequently.

Possible reason: The beneficial polyphenols, fiber, vitamins and minerals in nuts and peanuts (which are technically legumes).

Christian C. Abnet, PhD, MPH, senior investigator, division of cancer epidemiology and genetics, National Cancer Institute, Bethesda, Maryland.

Unusual Signs of Brain Cancer...and New Hope

Keith Black, MD, chair and professor of the department of neurosurgery at Cedars-Sinai Medical Center and director of the Maxine Dunitz Neurosurgical Institute and the Johnnie L. Cochran, Jr. Brain Tumor Center. Dr. Black has operated on more than 6,000 patients with brain tumors. He is author of *Brain Surgeon: A Doctor's Inspiring Encounters with Mortality and Miracles.*

Senator John McCain made headlines after being diagnosed with a glioblastoma, the deadliest of all brain tumors. That grim description makes it sound like it's over for those who are afflicted.

But survival rates vary widely. Some of these tumors respond better than others to treatment, so it's important to recognize easy-to-miss symptoms of this disease. Early diagnosis means treatment can start sooner. And while it can't be cured, there are advances that may improve the odds of living longer.

What Is a Glioblastoma?

This cancer is a primary brain tumor—it originates in the brain in contrast to cancers such as lung cancer, skin cancer or breast cancer that start somewhere else and may spread to the brain.

About half of primary brain tumors are benign (not cancerous)—and these have a high cure rate. The rest are malignant and tend to be aggressive and life-threatening. A glioblastoma is both the most common and the most aggressive kind of malignant primary brain tumor. It is a tumor that grows from cells that make up the gluelike supportive tissue of the brain, and tumor cells migrate throughout the brain, so it's hard for a surgeon to remove it entirely. Average survival after diagnosis is only 18 to 24 months, with 25% of patients alive after two years and 10% alive after five years.

Glioblastomas strike both men and women, often in their 40s, 50s or 60s. Few causes are known—exposure to high levels of radiation to treat a childhood cancer is one, and cell-phone use is a suspected cause (see page 44). There is rarely an identifiable genetic predisposition. The frustrating reality is that most cases, like Senator McCain's, are seemingly spontaneous—no one knows what brings them on.

Signs and Symptoms

With a glioblastoma, as the malignant cells spread, they increase pressure in the cranium, which leads to headaches in about half of patients. Blurry vision and/or seeing double can also occur. So can mood changes such as sudden-onset depression or anger. Muscle weakness or numbness in the arms and/or legs, which can lead to trouble walking, is another possible symptom. *More symptoms...*

- **Seizures.** Brain tumors can interfere with communication between nerve cells, causing abnormal electrical activity that manifests as seizures. Nearly one-third of brain tumor patients will experience at least one seizure. A seizure can range in intensity from a subtle twitching on one side of the body to a loss of consciousness. It may be preceded by an aura, an abnormal change in sensation such as tingling, sensing flickering lights or smelling an unpleasant odor.
- **Trouble reading.** While memory loss and confusion can be glioblastoma symptoms, some are more specific. Other commonly affected areas of the brain are the frontal, temporal or parietal lobes, which are responsible for language comprehension, math or spatial orientation. If a tumor grows in the left frontal or temporal lobes, a person may have difficulty speaking or understanding others or comprehending sentences containing cross-references or comparisons. With tumors in the parietal lobe, math may become unusually challenging and so may interpreting material shown in formats such as columns or charts—the parietal lobe also governs recognition of left-right or up-down positioning.

Just having one of these symptoms, or even more than one, does not mean that you have brain cancer, of course. One clue is how quickly symptoms come on. With a glioblastoma, several serious symptoms often arise in a matter of weeks or at most a few months.

New Treatments

The first option after discovery of a glioblastoma is often surgery, followed by radiation and chemotherapy. A glioblastoma can't be cured, but it can be managed to extend life. *Some promising newer treatment options now being studied in humans...*

- **Immunotherapy.** A cutting-edge class of drugs known as checkpoint inhibitors ignite the immune system by blocking certain signals released by tumors. That allows tumors to be "seen" and attacked by the immune system. Several clinical trials are now under way to test immunotherapies for glioblastomas.

- **Drugs that cross the blood-brain barrier.** There is a dense lining of cells that surrounds and protects the brain. Most drugs can't cross it, including many chemotherapy drugs. But the budding field of nanomedicine—including the use of drugs as tiny as molecules—is leading to investigational agents that breach the barrier, enter tumor cells and block key proteins.

- **Brain tumor vaccine.** Vaccines containing a patient's own immune cells—specifically, dendritic cells (cells that identify foreign invaders in the body)—may be able to activate a patient's immune system to attack the tumor. In a small 2017 study of 16 glioblastoma patients who received such a vaccine plus chemotherapy, published in *Clinical Cancer Research*, four were still alive after five years. More trials are under way.

On the horizon...

- **Blood test before symptoms arise.** Changes in tumor protein activity indicative of a future brain tumor may one day be detectable via a blood test.

- **Could Zika help?** Scientists are exploring whether the Zika virus, which can cross the blood-brain barrier, might in a deactivated form destroy brain tumor cells.

More from Dr. Black

The Cell-Phone/Brain Cancer Connection

Wireless devices including cell phones emit radiation, which we know can penetrate into the brain and, over time, may cause normal cells to become cancerous. Some studies have found a link between cell-phone use and brain cancer, including glioblastomas. But others have failed to do so. It makes sense to err on the side of caution...

- **When speaking on a cell phone,** minimize radiation exposure by using wired earphones (not a wireless version) or use the speakerphone function.

- **Limit use to areas with good reception,** which enables your phone to function at reduced power and therefore with reduced radiation.

Gum Disease Linked to Cancer

Postmenopausal women with a history of periodontal disease have a 14% higher risk for any cancer—and a risk for esophageal cancer three times higher than that in women without gum disease. Periodontal disease also is associated with a higher risk for lung, breast and gallbladder cancers and melanoma. The study did not prove cause and effect, but it is known that periodontal disease can cause general inflammation, which increases risk for cancer.

Jean Wactawski-Wende, PhD, dean of the School of Public Health and Health Professions, department of epidemiology and environmental health, University at Buffalo, New York.

Melanoma Danger

Nearly 20% of people who had once had melanoma, the deadliest form of skin cancer, reported getting sunburned in the last year, and only 62% said they "often or always" wore sunscreen.

Protect Your Face from Skin Cancer

Do you love the outdoors during winter? Don't forget sunscreen, especially on your eyelids and the area surrounding your eye sockets. These spots are prone to skin cancer, yet people often miss them when applying sunscreen.

Tip: Sunscreens labeled "for sensitive skin" are less likely to sting if they get in your eyes.

Study by researchers at University of Liverpool, UK, published in *PLOS ONE*.

The danger: Melanoma survivors have a nearly ninefold risk for a recurrence.

Rachel Isaksson Vogel, PhD, assistant professor, department of obstetrics, gynecology and women's health, University of Minnesota Masonic Cancer Center, Minneapolis.

Melanoma Alert: Don't Wait

Waiting to remove melanoma can be deadly. Patients with stage 1 melanoma were 5% more likely to die over an eight-year period if they were operated on 30 to 59 days after their biopsies than those treated sooner. Risk for death rose to 41% for those who waited longer than 120 days. See your dermatologist if you notice any moles that are asymmetrical, bigger than a pencil eraser or changing in size, shape or color.

Brian Gastman, MD, plastic surgeon and director of melanoma surgery, Cleveland Clinic, Ohio, and leader of an analysis of 153,218 American adults, published in *Journal of the American Academy of Dermatology.*

Protection from UV rays

Are dark- or light-colored clothes better for protecting against UV rays?

Color is less important than fabric weave. To protect your skin from ultraviolet (UV) rays, go for tightly woven fabrics such as denim or twill. Sheer fabrics allow more UV rays to reach your skin. Synthetic fabrics are more protective than natural fabrics such as cotton, flax or linen, unless these fabrics have been treated with a chemical sunblock. You can find sun-protective clothing at many outdoor clothing retailers.

Some manufacturers add an ultraviolet protection factor (UPF) label to their clothing, a rating based on the fabric's weight, construction and fiber content. A UPF rating of 50 provides excellent protection.

Barney J. Kenet, MD, dermatologist specializing in skin cancer and cofounder of the American Melanoma Foundation, New York City.

For Cancer Fatigue, Try Exercise

If you suffer from cancer-related fatigue, consider skipping antifatigue medications. A recent meta-analysis of 113 studies including 11,000 men and women found that exercise alone (such as walking or yoga) reduced cancer fatigue significantly, especially when started before or during treatment. Psychological counseling, such as cognitive behavioral therapy, was also effective.

Karen M. Mustian, PhD, MPH, University of Rochester Medical Center, New York.

Cancer Survivors Can Develop PTSD, Too

Caryn Mei Hsien Chan, PhD, National University of Malaysia, Bangi.

Cancer, news release.

People usually imagine post-traumatic stress disorder (PTSD) as happening to war veterans or assault victims.

But new research shows the trauma of a cancer diagnosis often leaves survivors with the condition.

Many may not want to admit how they feel, the study's lead author said.

"Many cancer patients believe they need to adopt a 'warrior mentality,' and remain positive and optimistic from diagnosis through treatment to stand a better chance of beating their cancer," explained Caryn Mei Hsien Chan, PhD, of the National University of Malaysia.

"To these patients, seeking help for the emotional issues they face is akin to admitting weakness," she said.

The Study

In their study, Dr. Chan and her colleagues tracked outcomes for 469 adults with different types of cancer. The research showed that nearly 22% had symptoms of PTSD six months after their cancer diagnosis. And about 6% still had the condition four years after diagnosis.

And while overall rates of PTSD did seem to decrease over time, a third of patients who had the condition six months after their cancer diagnosis had either persistent or worsening PTSD four years later, the study found.

The study was published in the journal *Cancer.*

Possible Explanation

Dr. Chan noted that many patients live in fear that their cancer will return, and may believe that any lump or bump, pain or ache, fatigue or fever indicates a return of the disease.

Implications

PTSD can have a real impact on cancer care, she added. Some survivors may skip visits with doctors to avoid triggering memories of their cancer experience, leading to delays in seeking help for new symptoms or even refusal of treatment for unrelated conditions.

Counseling and support are key. For example, the study found that breast cancer patients were 3.7 times less likely to have PTSD six months after diagnosis than patients with other types of cancers. This may be because the breast cancer patients received support and counseling in the first year after cancer diagnosis.

"We need psychological evaluation and support services for patients with cancer at an initial stage and at continued follow-ups because psychological well-being and mental health—and by extension, quality of life—are just as important as physical health," said Dr. Chan. "There needs to be greater awareness that there is nothing wrong with getting help to manage the emotional upheaval—particularly depression, anxiety and PTSD—post-cancer," she added.

For more information about PTSD, visit the website of the National Institute on Mental Health, NIMH.nih.gov. Search "PTSD."

Drink Your Joe for Cancer Survival

People with colorectal cancer who drank at least four cups a day of regular or decaf coffee after their diagnosis had 52% lower risk for death from colorectal cancer, compared with people who drank no coffee. Previous studies have shown that drinking coffee may prevent colon cancer in the first place.

Yang Hu, a doctor of science candidate, department of nutrition and epidemiology, Harvard T.H. Chan School of Public Health, Boston, and leader of a study published in *Gastroenterology.*

Get an Extra Edge Against Cancer

Mark A. Stengler, NMD, a naturopathic physician and founder of The Stengler Center for Integrative Medicine in Encinitas, California. He is coauthor of *Prescription for Natural Cures* and *Prescription for Drug Alternatives* (Bottom Line Books). MarkStengler.com

More than one-third of American adults reach for vitamins, herbs or other natural medicines when they have colds or other routine (and hopefully mild) health problems. Similar remedies can help when you have cancer.

To learn more about the best and safest ways to use natural therapies—also known as complementary and alternative medicine (CAM)—to fight cancer and its complications, we spoke with Mark A. Stengler, NMD, a naturopathic physician who treats cancer patients.

How CAM Can Work

Research has shown that many so-called "alternative" treatments can enhance the effects of conventional cancer care such as surgery, radiation or chemotherapy...reduce treatment side effects...and possibly improve survival.

This type of integrative care doesn't replace conventional cancer treatments. Rather, with the guidance of a doctor, complementary therapies are added to a patient's treatment plan.

Important: To ensure that the therapies described below would be appropriate for you, consult the Society for Integrative Oncology (IntegrativeOnc.org) to find an integrative oncologist near you...or check with The American Association of Naturopathic Physicians (Naturopathic.org) to locate a naturopathic doctor who also treats cancer patients.

Also: Be sure to ask the doctor you choose to be in touch with your oncologist. *Here's how CAM can help with problems that plague most cancer patients...*

- **Get relief from "chemo brain."** It's estimated that three-quarters of cancer patients will experience some degree of mental cloudiness. Known as "chemo brain," it can include mood swings, memory loss and mental fatigue. It eventually improves, but some patients will feel like they're in a mental fog years after their treatments have ended.

What helps: The omega-3 fatty acids in fish oil supplements—a typical daily dose is 1,000 mg total of eicosapentaenoic acid (EPA) and docosahexaenoic acid (DHA) combined—help regulate acetylcholine, a neurotransmitter that increases nerve growth factor and improves memory as well as energy levels.

The omega-3s also increase the effectiveness of 5-fluorouracil and other chemotherapy drugs, according to a study published in *Clinical Nutrition Research*. In research published in *Cancer*, lung cancer patients who took fish oil along with chemotherapy had a greater one-year survival rate than those who didn't take the supplements.

Note: Fish oil may cause stomach upset in some patients, along with bleeding in those who are taking anticoagulant medications such as *warfarin* (Coumadin), *apixaban* (Eliquis) and *rivaroxaban* (Xarelto).

- **Boost energy levels.** Ginseng is one of the more effective supplements for cancer patients. A number of studies have shown that it reduces treatment-related side effects, including weakness and fatigue. A double-blind study in *Journal of the National Cancer Institute* found that patients who took ginseng had less fatigue than those given placebos.

My advice: The American form of ginseng (Panax quinquefolius) is more effective than the Asian form.

Typical dose: 1,300 mg to 2,000 mg daily. It rarely causes side effects, although it may lower blood sugar in those with diabetes.

Also helpful: Glutathione, a "super antioxidant" that can be combined with chemotherapy to reduce toxin-related fatigue and other side effects. It's usually given in an IV solution. Side effects are unlikely, but it may interfere with some chemotherapy drugs. Be sure to consult an integrative oncologist to see whether you will/won't benefit from glutathione.

- **Improve immune response.** Turkey tail is one of the best-studied medicinal mushrooms. Available in capsule form, the supplement has chemical compounds (beta-glucans) that stimulate many aspects of the immune response, including antibody activity—important for inducing the death of cancer cells.

Impressive research: A study published in *Cancer Immunology and Immunotherapy* found that postsurgical remissions in colorectal cancer patients were twice as common in those who were given turkey tail.

Typical dose: 3,000 mg daily. Side effects are unlikely.

Healing Garden

A gardening program helps cancer survivors adopt healthier lifestyles. In a study, Master Gardeners mentored cancer survivors to set up vegetable gardens. Compared with non-gardening people, participants ate more vegetables, gained fewer inches and had improved self-worth. Search online for "cooperative extension" plus your zip code to see if there are gardening classes for cancer survivors nearby.

Wendy Demark-Wahnefried, PhD, RD, professor of nutrition sciences at University of Alabama at Birmingham.

A Nutritional Boost

Conventional oncologists receive little training in nutrition, but it's a critical issue for cancer patients. One study found that 91% of cancer patients had nutritional impairments, and 9% were seriously malnourished. Research shows that malnutrition contributes directly or indirectly to a significant number of cancer deaths due to poor appetite and the disease process of advanced cancer.

Loss of appetite is a major cause of malnutrition and muscle loss (cachexia). I advise patients who are losing weight to address these problems by getting more calories.

With every meal, include high-fat foods such as olive oil, coconut oil, avocado, nuts and seeds. A 10-year study, published in *Archives of Internal Medicine*, looked at more than 380,000 adults and found that a Mediterranean-style diet, which is high in olive oil and other healthy fats, reduced cancer deaths in men by 17% and 12% in women.

Also helpful: Protein shakes. They can provide the extra protein that's critical for cancer patients. Up to 80% of those with advanced cancer experience muscle loss. Protein shakes can help reverse it.

Best option: Ready-made whey protein or pea protein shakes—both are nutritious, have 5 g of sugar or less per serving and are readily available in health-food stores.

My advice: Get 1 g to 1.2 g of protein per kilogram (2.2 pounds) of body weight daily. This means that someone who weighs 150 pounds will need about 68 g to 82 g of protein daily. You can get that much from two or three servings of a typical whey protein beverage, which comes ready-mixed or in powdered form.

Caution: If you have moderate or severe kidney disease, check with your doctor for advice on your protein intake.

The Right Team to Treat Your Cancer

Richard A. Ehlers II, MD, associate professor, department of breast surgical oncology and associate vice president in the Division of Houston Area Locations at The University of Texas MD Anderson Cancer Center. He is also adjunct assistant professor in the department of surgery at The University of Texas Medical Branch at Galveston.

If you or a loved one is being treated for cancer, you may not be aware of so-called "tumor boards." But if you're getting care at a major academic or cancer-specific medical center, these regular face-to-face gatherings of cancer specialists—oncologists, radiologists, surgeons, pathologists, psychologists and others—play a key role in assessing individual cases. This may involve reviewing the pathology report...tracking disease progression...and discussing the treatment options for different types of cancer.

What gets reviewed: If your case comes before a tumor board, the doctors likely will address a variety of issues. Is surgery an option or will radiation and/or chemotherapy be more appropriate? If surgery can be done, should it or chemotherapy be used first, followed by other treatments? Is this patient battling mental health issues...or getting the runaround from insurance to get coverage for certain drugs?

How Tumor Boards Help

Cancer care is rarely a straightforward process. From the time you are diagnosed until your treatments end, your care will depend on the opinions of a surprising number of specialists—and good communication among those experts can strongly affect how well you do.

Important recent finding: Among nearly 5,000 patients with colorectal and lung cancers, those whose doctors participated in weekly tumor boards lived longer, according to a study presented at a symposium of the American Society of Clinical Oncology.

To ensure that the medical center where you're being treated relies on a tumor board's guidance, you should seek out a cancer center designated by the National Cancer Institute or accredited by the Commission on Cancer.

Large cancer centers usually have separate tumor boards for different types of cancer. At smaller programs, a single board will review all or most cancer cases.

Tumor boards provide important oversight because what seems like a perfect treatment plan can fall short in real-world circumstances. For example, chemotherapy might be the recommended treatment for a specific cancer, but a tumor-board oncologist might argue that a particular patient isn't healthy enough to withstand the treatment. A psychologist or social worker at a meeting might point out that the patient will need transportation to and from the chemotherapy clinic.

Who Gets Reviewed?

At MD Anderson Cancer Center and other large cancer centers, virtually all cases are discussed at a tumor board, although doctors give most of their attention to rare/complicated cases. There's no separate charge to patients for the review.

My advice: If you're not sure that your case has been discussed at your treatment center's tumor board, ask your doctor whether it has been (or will be). Your doctor should not be offended by this question—especially if he/she will be presenting the case. If your case hasn't been reviewed, ask why not. You have the right to request a tumor board review, but it might not be available at a smaller medical center.

Most tumor boards meet weekly or twice a month and are comprised of a dozen or more specialists, including surgeons, medical oncologists, radiation oncologists and pathologists. Depending on the cancer, other doctors—gynecologists, urologists, etc.—may participate. Meetings often include a nutritionist, nurses, mental health experts and a social worker.

The Benefits

Your case might go before a tumor board prior to treatment...after a preliminary treatment plan has been initiated...or during treatment when there is an important change in clinical circumstances.

Important finding: When the records of more than 200 pancreatic cancer patients collected from various institutions without tumor boards were later evaluated by a panel at Johns Hopkins University School of Medicine that included medical and radiation oncologists, surgical oncologists, pathologists and other experts, treatment changes were recommended in nearly 25% of these cases.

Research also shows that patients tend to have better outcomes in terms of treatment responsiveness, recovery times and survival, among other factors, when their cases are discussed at a tumor board.

Also: Patients whose cases are reviewed are more likely to be guided to a clinical trial—one that their primary oncologist might not be aware of. Many cancer patients are eligible for these trials, which provide excellent care...yet only about 3% of patients ever participate. The more patients there are enrolled, the more quickly important clinical questions can be answered.

The National Cancer Institute website lists thousands of clinical trials that are looking for participants—to compare drug treatments, study new surgical techniques or radiation treatments, etc. Most tumor boards have a "checklist," which includes the question of whether there is a trial for which the patient might be eligible.

The Personal Touch

The services provided by tumor boards go beyond the nuts and bolts of treatment. For example, many cancer patients lose weight during chemotherapy or radiation treatments. If poor nutrition is threatening your recovery—or even your ability to continue treatments—a nutritionist might recommend nutritional counseling, or even help you find a free meal service in your area.

Many cancer patients suffer from mental health issues—depression, bipolar disorder, etc. The best cancer plan won't help if you're unable (or unwilling) to continue treatments. A tumor board will attempt to address—or correct—all the issues that can affect how well or poorly you respond to treatments.

Patients don't typically attend tumor boards. Many different cases are reviewed at any one meeting. The presence of a patient would affect the confidentiality of others' personal health information.

"One-Stop" Blood Test for Cancer Shows Early Promise

Anne Marie Lennon, MD, PhD, director, multidisciplinary pancreatic cyst program, Johns Hopkins Kimmel Cancer Center, Baltimore.

Len Lichtenfeld, MD, deputy chief medical officer, American Cancer Society, Atlanta.

Science.

In an early step toward "one-stop" screening for cancer, researchers report they've developed a blood test that can detect eight types of the disease.

The blood test is dubbed CancerSEEK. It was able to catch cancer cases anywhere from 33% to 98% of the time, depending on the type. The accuracy range was better—69% to 98%—when it came to five cancers that currently have no widely used screening test, the scientists reported in a new study.

Those cancers included ovarian, pancreatic, stomach, liver and esophageal cancers.

The researchers said the findings are an "exciting" initial step.

The hope is to eventually have a single blood test that can screen people for a range of common cancers.

Background

In recent years, researchers have been studying "liquid biopsies"—tests that look for cancer markers in the blood or other body fluids. Those markers can include, for instance, mutated genes or abnormal proteins shed from tumors.

But it can be like looking for "less than a needle" in a haystack, said Len Lichtenfeld, MD, deputy chief medical officer for the American Cancer Society.

So far, liquid biopsies have mostly been tested in patients with advanced cancer. Early stage cancers shed fewer markers.

"You have to detect smaller and smaller molecules that are swimming in a sea of background noise," Dr. Lichtenfeld said.

CancerSEEK is different because it combines tests that look for 16 genes and 10 proteins linked to cancer, explained Anne Marie Lennon, MD, PhD, one of the researchers.

"That's a big move forward," she said.

The researchers also tested blood samples from 812 healthy people, to see how often the test gave "false-positive" results. That happened less than 1% of the time.

That's promising, Dr. Lennon said, because for any test to be useful for screening, its false-positive rate has to be low.

As for cost, the researchers estimate the blood test could run less than $500.

The findings were published in *Science*.

Implications

Ultimately, Dr. Lichtenfeld said, the big question will be: Does this kind of testing save people's lives?

"Just because we're able to detect a protein, that doesn't mean we'll save everyone's life," he noted.

Still, he said he's "hopeful" that this or similar tests will eventually offer a way to catch particularly deadly cancers, such as ovarian and pancreatic tumors, earlier.

For more information on liquid biopsies, go to the National Cancer Institute website, Cancer.gov, and search "liquid biopsy."

Chapter 3

LUNG HEALTH AND ALLERGIES

Lung Disease Can Strike Anyone

You notice that you're feeling tired all the time, short of breath and can't get rid of a nagging mucus-filled cough. These all could be symptoms of chronic obstructive pulmonary disease (COPD). But you've never smoked a cigarette in your life and that's a smoker's disease, right? Yes...but not always.

What few people realize: About 25% of people who show signs of lung disease and airway obstruction don't smoke and never have...and about 10% of people formally diagnosed with COPD have never smoked.

Since most never-smokers are unaware that they could be at risk, they tend to blame early COPD symptoms on ailments such as allergies, asthma or lingering colds. Even doctors may fail to consider COPD in never-smokers. As a result, many patients with early—and mild—COPD aren't taking the necessary steps to protect their lungs. That's a problem because undiagnosed COPD not only can affect one's quality of life, it also can lead to flare-ups, hospitalizations and even early death. *What you need to know...*

A Major Threat

COPD is the third-leading cause of death in the US, and it affects 15 million adults—more if you count those with impaired lung function that has gone undetected.

COPD is a broad term that's used to describe a number of lung diseases, including emphysema (damage to the alveoli, small air sacs in the lungs)...chronic bronchitis (inflammation of the large bronchial tubes)...and some cases of severe asthma that do not completely reverse between flare-ups or exacerbations. COPD is a progressive disease—it develops slowly (often over decades), and the symptoms always worsen over time.

Risks for Nonsmokers

Giving up cigarettes is the best way for smokers to guard against COPD. For nonsmokers, many common COPD risk factors are tricky (or impossible) to avoid. *For example...*

David M. Mannino, MD, the Kurt W. Deuschle endowed chair in preventive medicine and environmental health at the University of Kentucky, Lexington, where he directs the Pulmonary Epidemiology Research Laboratory and the Southeast Center for Agricultural Health and Injury Prevention. He is chief scientific officer of the COPD Foundation. COPDFoundation.org

• **Asthma.** Roughly 40% of COPD patients have a history of chronic obstructive asthma, and many of them have never smoked.

• **Pneumonia or other severe respiratory infections.** People who have these illnesses in childhood experience lung damage that increases their risk for COPD.

• **Genetics.** Among nonsmokers with COPD, 1% to 3% have alpha-1 antitrypsin (AAT) deficiency, a genetic defect that can lead to damaged alveoli and emphysema. Anyone who has a first-degree relative with COPD is at increased risk for this genetic defect.

• **Environmental factors.** These can include smoke (for firefighters)...dust (agricultural workers and miners)...chemical fumes (manicurists and janitors)...and air pollution (everyone). Scented products, such as candles or air fresheners, can irritate the lungs, too. Anything that chronically irritates your lungs, such as secondhand smoke, can increase risk for COPD.

Smoking Is Worse Than You Think!

Smoking causes even more diseases than previously thought. In addition to the well-known risks for lung cancer and other lung diseases, heart attacks and stroke, smoking now is linked to increased risks for infection, kidney disease, intestinal disease caused by poor blood flow, and some heart and lung diseases not previously thought to be caused by tobacco use. The additional diseases are believed to add 60,000 deaths from tobacco per year in the US.

Analysis of health data on almost one million people by researchers at the American Cancer Society, published in *The New England Journal of Medicine.*

Should You Get Tested?

If you have any of the symptoms described earlier, you should ask your doctor to test you for COPD. Past-smokers and those who work in high-risk industries—coal miners, for example—might want to get tested even if they don't have symptoms. Anyone with asthma should be tested for pulmonary function at least once every five years.

Red flag: It takes you longer than expected to recover from colds, the flu or other respiratory illnesses. Someone who's healthy will generally start feeling better—with less coughing and shortness of breath—within a week or two. In my practice, I've noticed that those with early COPD take several weeks or even months before they're fully recovered. Other symptoms include a nagging cough, wheezing and tightness in the chest.

The most common lung test is called spirometry. With this test, you blow into a tube that's connected to a machine that measures both your lung capacity and how quickly you're able to exhale air. The test takes only a few minutes, and it can detect early COPD even when you don't have symptoms.

If spirometry shows your lung function to be normal, you won't need other tests unless your doctor feels there's a strong chance that you have COPD based on your symptoms. In that case, he/she might recommend other lung-function or imaging tests (such as a chest X-ray or CT scan).

Exception: If your lung function is impaired but you don't have any obvious COPD risk factors, your doctor will want to know if there's a genetic cause. A blood test for AAT deficiency is done routinely for those who test positive for impaired lung function, as well as for those who develop COPD symptoms at an early age or have a family history of the disease.

What Can You Do?

Most patients with COPD will need to use treatments such as bronchodilators and inhaled steroids—and perhaps use supplemental oxygen when the disease advances.

Patients with AAT deficiency can take a synthetic form of the missing protein, given weekly in IV infusions. Some studies have shown that the treatments help protect the lungs...others have been less conclusive.

To keep your lungs healthier...

• **Try to breathe clean air.** If you have a smoky fireplace, clean the chimney, or don't use the fireplace at all. Wear a dust mask or respirator (see below) if you're tilling a field or working in a woodshop. Do your best never to breathe secondhand smoke.

Helpful: Check the Air Quality Index (AQI) in your area by going to the EPA website AirNow.gov. People with COPD or other lung diseases may be advised to stay indoors on days when the AQI is elevated.

If you're moving: Go to Lung.org, click on "Our Initiatives," then "Healthy Air," then "State of the Air" and plug in possible zip codes to see where the air is cleanest—and where it's not.

• **Avoid toxic fumes.** This includes fumes from oven cleaners, drain cleaners, paint, etc. If it makes you cough or burns your nose, you shouldn't be breathing it.

If you must use such products, wear a respirator. A respirator labeled N95 will protect you from particulate matter (such as dust or sawdust), while respirators that contain chemical cartridges will protect you against fumes from cleaning supplies and similar products.

If you have COPD, also eat a healthy diet, with lots of fruits and vegetables, and exercise if you can. Doing so can reduce symptoms and add to your quality of life.

Statins and COPD

People with COPD live longer with statin drugs.

Recent study: Patients with chronic obstructive pulmonary disease (COPD) who used statins were 45% less likely to die from lung-related issues than other COPD patients and had a 21% lower risk of dying from any cause.

Possible reason: Statins, used to reduce cholesterol levels, have anti-inflammatory properties that may benefit certain people with COPD.

Larry Lynd, PhD, professor of pharmaceutical sciences at University of British Columbia, Vancouver, Canada.

E-Cigarettes Can Help You Quit

It still is best to quit all nicotine-containing products, including e-cigarettes, using FDA-approved smoking-cessation aids (such as nicotine gums and patches) to wean yourself off nicotine addiction. But e-cigarettes are less harmful than cigarettes, according to the American Cancer Society's review of evidence—and research suggests that e-cigarettes may help some smokers quit all nicotine products.

Jeffrey Drope, PhD, vice president of economic and health policy research at the American Cancer Society, Atlanta.

Don't Clean with This

Regular use of bleach is linked to lung disease. Nurses who used disinfectants such as bleach...glutaraldehyde, a strong disinfectant for medical instruments...hydrogen peroxide...or cleaning alcohol at least weekly were 22% more likely to develop chronic obstructive pulmonary disease (COPD) over an eight-year period than ones who did not use disinfectants. The preliminary, unpublished study showed association but not cause and effect.

Study of 55,185 working nurses by researchers at the French National Institute of Health and Medical Research, presented at a recent meeting of the European Respiratory Society International Congress.

10 Common Mistakes People Make When Using an Inhaler

Richard Firshein, DO, director and founder of The Firshein Center for Integrative Medicine in New York City and author of *Reversing Asthma*.

Imagine that you were prescribed one pill a day, and on some days you swallowed only one quarter...on other days, only one half. It doesn't sound good, right?

If you use a "metered-dose" inhaler, the most commonly used medication dispenser for a wide variety of lung conditions, odds are that you're getting less than half a full dose with each puff. Research suggests that up to 80% of patients incorrectly use this type of inhaler, which delivers a premeasured aerosol dose of medication. If you inhale a partial dose often, you may assume that the medication isn't working...or you may wind up with some serious side effects, such as a racing heart, a chronic sore throat or stomachaches. Or you could develop a condition called *tachyphylaxis*—when more of the medication gets in your bloodstream and less in your lungs, you develop a resistance to the medication.

Here are 10 mistakes you may be making with your metered-dose inhaler...

Preparation Mistakes

• **Not shaking the inhaler well enough before each spray.** Because the canister contains both your medication and a propellant, without thorough mixing, you cannot be sure that the proportions will be the same from puff to puff.

Better: Just before taking your dose, shake the inhaler vigorously for about 10 seconds.

• **Positioning the mouthpiece incorrectly.** Tilt your inhaler five degrees too high, and you'll send most of the medicine to the roof of your mouth rather than into your lungs. Five degrees too low, it'll hit your tongue. Either way, you'll swallow more of it than you inhale.

Better: Think about how you're holding the inhaler before beginning. Is it perpendicular to your windpipe? If not, adjust the position. The nozzle should be pointing directly to the back of your throat.

• **Tilting the chin.** Just as the inhaler's angle matters, so does the angle of your head. Even a slight shift up or down can change that angle, which will cause a considerable amount of medication to miss the target.

Better: If you're sitting, stand up—it's much easier to align your head and neck properly that way. Then make sure you're facing straight ahead with the bottom of your chin parallel to the floor.

Coordination Mistakes

• **Releasing the medicine at the wrong time.** Aerosol lung medications are supposed to enter your lungs while you breathe in. If you dispense your medication too early, you won't have inhaled deeply enough to adequately pull the medicine into your lungs. Too late, and the dose may be sprayed into your mouth after you've completed most of your inhalation.

Better: Start your breath (through your mouth, not your nose!) before depressing the canister. About a second after you begin breathing in, squeeze the canister while inhaling deeply.

• **Jerking when dispensing a dose.** You've taken care to angle both the mouthpiece and your chin correctly, but a sudden movement when you dispense the medicine—such as when you press down on a canister-type dispenser—can move everything out of alignment exactly when the medication is spraying.

Better: Each time you use your inhaler, pay attention to how much force it takes to activate the spray—it may be less force than you've been using. Do your best not to move your hand or head while squeezing the inhaler between your forefinger and thumb.

• **Taking a breath too quickly.** If you pay attention exclusively to the "deep" part of the breath, you may inhale so fast that the medicine reaches only partway into your lungs.

Better: Picture your lungs expanding as you draw in the medication for about five seconds. Once your lungs are filled, hold your breath for 10 seconds, then breathe out slowly through pursed lips—not through your nose—as if you are whistling.

Post-Dose Mistakes

• **Leaping into a panicky second puff.** When you're struggling to breathe and the first dose from a quick-acting inhaler doesn't help, you probably want to put it right back up to your mouth and try again. But if you've misdirected the medication the first time—which could explain why you didn't feel relief—moving fast on the next round probably won't help, either. And if you've accidentally swallowed your medication, it could leave you feeling shaky. Trembling hands make it even less likely that you'll use the inhaler correctly, and things can snowball from there.

Better: For your second puff, pay close attention to your form. Shake the inhaler again. Stand up, look straight ahead and hold the device perpendicular to your windpipe. Begin to breathe in, and after one second, squeeze the canister. Keep breathing in slowly, as deeply as you can, then hold your breath for 10 seconds before exhaling.

• **Forgetting to rinse your mouth.** Even if you use your inhaler perfectly, odds are that some medication still will land in your mouth and on your tongue. Swallowing it can lead to sore throats and other side effects.

Better: After completing your exhalation, fill your mouth with water, swish it around and gargle briefly, then spit it out. Do not swallow.

• **Not cleaning the inhaler.** Although you can't see it, with each use your inhaler leaves a trace of propellant and medication in the mouthpiece. In time, that can build up and partially block the spray.

Better: At least once a week, remove the canister and rinse the plastic mouthpiece and cap under warm running water. If you see any residue, use soap as well. Do not rinse any other parts. Allow it to air-dry completely before replacing the canister and cap.

Biggest Mistake of All

• **Ignoring the signs that you're doing it wrong.** If you regularly taste bitterness after a puff of an inhaled medication or if you use the inhaler and don't see improvement, don't just continue on. Continued misuse can lead to long-term side effects such as feeling jittery or developing stomachaches from swallowing more than you inhale. It also encourages the development of oral thrush, a yeast infection that can be stimulated by certain asthma medications. Thrush produces spotty white blotches on your mouth and can leave you with a chronic sore throat and difficulty swallowing. Even if you're using your inhaler correctly, you still may develop thrush—but the likelihood increases dramatically when medication winds up on the surface of your mouth, tongue and throat.

Better: When you notice any of the signs mentioned above, go back to the drawing board and review the advice in this article. If you still are concerned that you are not using your inhaler correctly, ask your doctor about using a spacer attachment. It's a tube that connects to the mouthpiece so that you can dispense a complete, single dose into it. Once all the medication is in the spacer tube, you breathe it in when you're ready—so there's no need to worry about clicking at exactly the right moment.

Oxygen for Asthma? No!

Sessions at oxygen bars—where you pay to inhale highly concentrated oxygen through tubes placed in your nose—have been touted as relieving stress, alleviating hangovers and providing relief from asthma. However, there have been no long-term studies backing up these claims. For a person with asthma, a visit could trigger an attack due to the scent, or "flavoring," that some bars add to the oxygen (such as lavender to "relax").

When experiencing asthma symptoms, use an inhaled bronchodilator or anti-inflammatory agent (such as an inhaled corticosteroid) to open your airways. Oxygen does not relax the bronchial tubes or prevent inflammation in this way.

George M. Boyer, MD, FACP, FCCP, chairman, department of medicine, Mercy Medical Center, Baltimore.

The Safest Vacation Spots for People with Asthma

Melanie Carver, vice president of digital strategy and community services, Asthma and Allergy Foundation of America, Landover, Maryland.

Spending your long-anticipated time off laid low with asthma symptoms isn't anyone's idea of a fun vacation.

So the first thing to keep in mind when you're poring over glossy brochures of dream locales is to know and recognize your asthma triggers. For example, if hot, humid air makes you breathless and wheezy, a week on the Gulf coast is a riskier getaway for you. Or if cold, windy air brings on symptoms, then you'd be better off skipping the sites in locales with those kinds of climate.

But besides your specific triggers, anyone with asthma should avoid exposure to bad air quality and pollution. In fact, when air quality is very poor, people with asthma are advised to stay indoors with their windows closed—most likely not exactly the vacation itinerary you had in mind.

If your asthma is triggered by pollen, it's a good idea to check out the pollen count where you're traveling on AccuWeather.com and Pollen.com. If you have to drive in an area that has a high count for the particular pollen that triggers your symptoms and/or bad air quality, keep your car windows rolled up and the air-conditioning on.

To find places that you might particularly want to avoid, check the list of Asthma Capitals on the Asthma and Allergy Foundation of America (AAFA) website (AAFA.org/page/asthma-capitals.aspx). The list ranks the 100 largest cities in the US according to how challenging they are for people with asthma. AAFA looks at 13 factors, including air quality, pollen counts and smoking laws. A recent Asthma Capitals report names Memphis, Richmond (Virginia), Philadelphia, Detroit and Oklahoma City as the five worst US cities for asthma sufferers.

Be prepared: Before heading off on your vacation, be sure to follow your treatment plan so your asthma is under control before you go. If you take medications, bring enough to last at least the length of your trip—and, ideally, a bit longer in the event that your return home is delayed. Also, keep emergency medications (such as rescue inhalers) on you at all times. If you depend on an inhaler, bring an extra in case one runs out…or you leave it behind in a hotel room or restaurant. If you're flying or traveling by train, pack some sanitizing wipes to wipe down tray tables and armrests to remove pet dander.

Note: Even if there is no pet on board, pet dander is always present on planes and trains because the dander travels on people's clothing. AAFA has more tips for traveling safely with asthma.

Wishing you happy, healthy trails—and easy breathing!

Natural Treatments for a Difficult Allergy Season

Holly Lucille, ND, RN, a nationally recognized naturopathic doctor, author and educator practicing in Los Angeles. DrHollyLucille.com

If your nose is stuffed up and your eyes are watering, you're not alone. What's an allergy sufferer to do—especially when the usual remedies for allergies (whether conventional medications or natural remedies) don't seem to be helping? We asked Holly Lucille, ND, RN, who practices naturopathic medicine in Los Angeles, how she helps her allergy patients when pollen, mold and other allergies are at their worst. *Here's her advice…*

Conventional vs. Natural Remedies

One of the problems with taking conventional medications such as Claritin, Zyrtec or Allegra is that they offer only temporary relief for allergy symptoms and can produce

Vitamin D for Asthma

In a meta-analysis of 955 asthma patients, vitamin D (400 IU to 4,000 IU daily) taken with an asthma medication, such as an inhaled bronchodilator, reduced the need for steroids by 30% and the need for emergency or hospital care by 50%, compared with the use of asthma medication alone.

Why: Vitamin D boosts immune response to respiratory viruses and reduces airway inflammation.

Adrian Martineau, PhD, professor of respiratory infection and immunity, Queen Mary University of London, UK.

uncomfortable side effects, such as fatigue, headache and dry mouth, among others. In addition, when an allergy season lasts many weeks or even months, like this one, you may be on these medications for longer than you want or longer than feels good.

Here's where the benefit of natural remedies comes into play. Natural treatments generally are much easier on the body—which means that you can take them for longer periods of time.

There are many natural treatments available in supplement form that work to control allergies. They often work in different ways. *For symptom relief, try the following combination...*

A detoxifier...

• **Milk thistle** *(Silybum marianum),* a flavonoid that helps the liver process toxins more efficiently, thereby helping to clear out potential allergens.

A remedy for symptom relief...

Try one of the four remedies below. If it doesn't help your allergy symptoms within two weeks, try the next one on the list.

• **Quercetin,** a flavonoid antioxidant, reduces the inflammation caused by allergens.

• **Stinging Nettle** *(Urtica dioica),* a plant that has been found to reduce the amount of histamine created in response to an allergen.

• **Butterbur** *(Petasites hybridus),* an herb that prevents the release of chemicals that cause inflammation in the nasal passages.

Caution: Butterbur is related to ragweed, so if you have a ragweed allergy, taking butterbur can make your symptoms worse. Also, some butterbur preparations contain pyrrolizidine alkaloids (PAs), which can damage the liver. Use only butterbur products that are certified and labeled "PA-free."

An immune booster...

• **A probiotic.** These are "good bacteria" in supplement form that boost health and the immune system. They are especially helpful for people fighting allergies because they improve immune function and reduce inflammation associated with allergies. There are specific types of probiotic species that help specific ailments. When it comes to boosting the immune system, one combination to consider is *Lactobacillus acidophilus* and *Bifidobacterium.* Taking a probiotic can help the immune system year-round, not just during allergy season.

All of these remedies, which are available online and in health-food stores, are safe for adults. Follow label instructions. Pregnant women should not use these supplements—and should speak to a physician before taking probiotics.

Combining Natural and Conventional Remedies

What about taking both conventional medications and natural remedies? While the goal is to avoid drugs, it's OK to add a drug to your natural therapies when symptoms are very severe. It's best to do this for the shortest possible time—for example, only a few days. Conversely, for allergy sufferers who rely on drugs, adding one or two natural treatments may eventually enable them to lower the dosage or even wean themselves off of the drugs altogether.

Getting to the Root of the Problem

In addition to helping patients find the remedies that work best for them, holistic doctors believe in getting to the root cause of a patient's allergy problem. Often, a diet high in sugar, processed foods or mucus-producing foods such as dairy can make a patient more susceptible to allergies. Stress and lack of sleep can depress the immune system—and contribute to allergies. If your allergies are particularly stubborn this year, consult a holistic doctor who can help you get to the root of your problem.

What Causes Watery Eyes

Robert Latkany, MD, ophthalmologist and founder, The Dry Eye Clinic, New York City.

Allergies—particularly seasonal allergies—are a common source of watery eyes, but the problem typically resolves once the allergen is removed. However, an often-overlooked source of watery—and frequently bloodshot—eyes is ocular rosacea, an eye inflammation that's a cousin to the skin condition that causes irritated skin. Treating ocular rosacea (with warm compresses, prescription eyedrops or oral antibiotics) and avoiding triggers such as alcohol and spicy foods should help.

Other common causes of watery eyes: Droopy eyelids, which allow excess tears to pool and then spill down the cheeks, rather than drain down the back of the nose to the throat. Cosmetic surgery on upper or lower lids or a blocked tear duct (caused by scar tissue, debris or narrowed ducts due to age) also can prevent tears from draining properly.

Ironically, dry eye syndrome, in which the tear glands produce inadequate moisture, can cause excessive wateriness—scratchy, burning dry eyes trigger the tear glands to make tears in order to soothe the irritation. Ointments for dry eye may alleviate wateriness.

Bottom line: See an ophthalmologist to identify the cause and determine the best course of treatment.

Bad Hot Flashes, Sleep Apnea Often Go Together

JoAnn Pinkerton, MD, executive director, North American Menopause Society.

North American Menopause Society, news release.

As if severe hot flashes alone weren't enough of a problem for menopausal women, a new study finds these symptoms may also be tied to a greater risk for sleep apnea and related heart issues.

The Study

The study included nearly 1,700 middle-aged women, about 25% of whom were at intermediate or high risk for obstructive sleep apnea—for instance, they generally were older, had higher levels of body fat and had high blood pressure.

Compared with women who had mild or no hot flashes, those who reported severe hot flashes were nearly twice as likely to have obstructive sleep apnea, the researchers found.

The study was published in the journal *Menopause*.

About Sleep Apnea

In sleep apnea, pauses in breathing or shallow breathing prevent a person from getting a good night's sleep.

Sleep apnea has been linked to a significantly increased risk for heart disease, high blood pressure, stroke, depression and early death, said the study authors.

According to JoAnn Pinkerton, MD, executive director of the North American Menopause Society, "Sleep disruption is a common complaint at menopause. It is important to recognize the high number of undiagnosed sleep disorders, including obstructive sleep apnea."

Although the study found an association between severe hot flashes and the chronic sleep disorder, it did not prove a cause-and-effect relationship.

Advice

"Early morning headaches or excessive daytime sleepiness should raise concern for obstructive sleep apnea, and signal a possible need for sleep apnea testing," Dr. Pinkerton suggested.

The National Heart, Lung, and Blood Institute has more information on sleep apnea at NHLBI.nih.gov.

Why You May Need a Sleep Study

Michael J. Breus, PhD, a sleep specialist with a private practice in Los Angeles. Dr. Breus is also author of *The Power of When: Discover Your Chronotype—and the Best Time to Eat Lunch, Ask for a Raise, Have Sex, Write a Novel, Take Your Meds, and More.* TheSleepDoctor.com

There's no sugarcoating it—sleeping in a lab feels strange. You've got electrodes attached to your scalp, face and legs…you're in an unfamiliar bed…and a night-vision camera is recording your every move.

So why would you leave the comfort of your own bed to do such a thing? If your sleep is being disrupted but you're not sure why, a sleep study can be the best way to finally get the answers you need.

Here's what to expect during a sleep study—and how to ensure that you get the most accurate results…*

Inside a Sleep Lab

People who have problems during sleep often end up in the office of a sleep specialist (usually an otolaryngologist, a pulmonologist, a cardiologist or a neurologist) who is board-certified in sleep medicine and trained to evaluate patients for sleep disorders. When it comes to diagnosing most sleep problems, the gold standard is a sleep study (also known as a polysomnogram).

During a sleep study, your brain waves, heart rate, breathing, blood oxygen levels and leg and eye movements are measured. This important data helps your doctor not only diagnose your condition but also determine the best treatment.

What a sleep study can identify…

• **Sleep apnea.** Your doctor may suspect obstructive sleep apnea (OSA)—which affects one-quarter of all American adults between the ages of 30 and 70—if you have morning headaches, awaken with a dry mouth and/or suffer from excessive daytime drowsiness. If your bed partner complains that you snore, that also can be a red flag.

With OSA, your upper airway closes during sleep, temporarily halting your breathing. This can happen for 10 seconds or longer dozens or even hundreds of times a night.

The sleep study calculates the number of times breathing either stops or becomes abnormally slow. For example, OSA would be assessed as mild if you stop breathing five to 14 times per hour…moderate (15 to 30 times per hour)…or severe (more than 30 times per hour).

• **Periodic limb movement disorder (PLMD).** This condition is suspected if you have uncontrollable leg movements when you are trying to sleep. It is closely related to restless legs syndrome (RLS), which causes an overwhelming urge to move your legs during periods of inactivity (during the day or night). PLMD causes similar symptoms—along with telltale muscle twitches—that occur only at night.

Because RLS occurs when you're awake, it usually can be diagnosed based on symptoms alone. A sleep study identifies PLMD and its severity, which helps determine the best treatment approaches.

*A sleep study should be performed at a center that is accredited by the American Academy of Sleep Medicine. To find such a center, go to SleepCenters.org.

Many people get relief from PLMD by massaging their legs, walking and stretching. If those approaches aren't effective, *pramipexole* (Mirapex) is a prescription medication that is effective for both RLS and PLMD.

• **Narcolepsy.** You or your doctor may suspect this condition if you suffer from excessive daytime sleepiness, nap attacks and/or hallucinations as you fall asleep or awaken.

Testing takes a total of about 20 hours and typically consists of an overnight polysomnogram, immediately followed by a multiple sleep latency test, which consists of a series of five 20-minute naps scheduled at specific intervals throughout the following day. Your doctor will evaluate how quickly you fall asleep, what stages of sleep you enter and for how long. Narcolepsy is typically treated with medications, including stimulants such as *modafinil* (Provigil)...or antidepressants such as *fluoxetine* (Prozac)...and/or scheduled napping.

Important: You may assume that a sleep study would be the best way to diagnose insomnia, but the test is not used for this purpose—people who suffer from insomnia tend to sleep even less in a sleep study environment than in their own beds, making an accurate diagnosis more difficult. Instead, your sleep specialist will make the diagnosis after taking a thorough inventory of your physical and mental health, discussing your sleep routine and reviewing your sleep diaries.

How to Get Accurate Results

To get the most accurate results from your sleep study...

• **Don't use hair products.** These products can prevent electrodes from properly sticking to your scalp and body.

• **Bring your favorite pillow,** as well as a pair of comfortable pajamas (preferably button-down so the technician can access your chest to place electrodes), a good book or anything else that gives you comfort.

• **Ask about sleep medications.** If you feel anxious and want to take a medication to make you feel sleepy, discuss this beforehand with your doctor and tell the lab technician who is administering the test if you have taken anything for sleep.

You can typically use an over-the-counter product, such as Tylenol PM. You should avoid a benzodiazepine such as *alprazolam* (Xanax)—this type of drug can worsen sleep apnea.

• **Use caution with alcohol.** Some labs advise against drinking alcohol before your test. However, if you normally have a drink in the evening, ask your doctor about continuing that practice so the study will accurately assess what is happening in your brain and body. Most labs won't allow alcohol, so enjoy it at home and have someone drive you to and from your appointment.

Rather Stay at Home?

Even though they are not as reliable as a sleep study in a lab, home sleep tests (HSTs) are becoming an increasingly popular option to identify OSA.

How it works: Your doctor sends you home with a small kit that contains the equipment you need. Before bed, you secure a belt and a small data recorder around your chest. The recorder attaches to an airflow sensor that's worn under your nose to monitor your breathing during sleep. A pulse oximeter placed on your finger records oxygen saturation levels to

False Penicillin Allergy?

About 95% of patients who believe they're allergic to penicillin are not.

Recent finding: When researchers reviewed the medical records of 8,400 surgical patients, those who had surgery without penicillin were 50% more vulnerable to surgical-site infection—even if a different antibiotic was prescribed.

Why: Alternative antibiotics aren't as effective as those related to penicillin. If you've been told that you're allergic to penicillin, get an allergy evaluation prior to surgery.

Kimberly G. Blumenthal, MD, assistant professor of medicine, division of rheumatology, Harvard Medical School, Boston.

identify times when you stop breathing during sleep. After one to three nights of recording, your doctor uploads and reviews the data.

About 10 companies manufacture HSTs, including ApneaLink Air and NovaSom. A home sleep test costs about $150 to $500 versus $1,300 and up for a sleep study conducted in a lab. Like standard sleep studies, an HST is usually covered by insurance as long as you have OSA symptoms.

What about apps? Some smartphone apps claim to wirelessly test for sleep apnea at home by detecting and analyzing snoring or by emitting sound waves from the phone's speakers to track breathing patterns.

Beware: These products are not sensitive enough to provide accurate results. You could get a false reassurance by using one of these apps, which would delay an accurate diagnosis.

Common Seasonal-Allergy Mistakes

Clifford Bassett, MD, founder and medical director, Allergy and Asthma Care of New York, quoted at LiveScience.com.

Common seasonal-allergy mistakes and what to do instead...

Mistake: Opening windows, which lets pollen in.

Better: Run the air conditioner, and use high-efficiency filters to trap pollen.

Mistake: Not taking regular antipollen steps.

Better: Wash hair at the end of every day, keep pets clean, avoid hanging laundry outdoors.

Mistake: Neglecting your eyes, through which pollen often enters the body.

Better: Wear sunglasses and a brimmed hat when outdoors, and use eye rinses regularly.

Mistake: Waiting too long to start on allergy medicines.

Better: Take them at the start of pollen season instead of waiting for symptoms to get worse.

Mistake: Overusing nasal sprays.

Better: Use them for no more than five days in a row to avoid irritating sinuses and the lining of the nose.

Food Allergies Affect Adults, Too

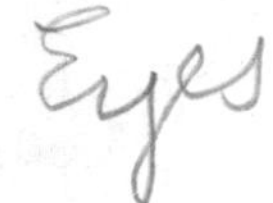

Ruchi Gupta, MD, MPH, associate professor of pediatrics and medicine at Northwestern University Feinberg School of Medicine, Chicago, and clinical attending physician at Ann & Robert H. Lurie Children's Hospital of Chicago. Dr. Gupta is author of *The Food Allergy Experience*.

Shrimp may have always been your favorite indulgence. But one night, after a luscious dinner at a seafood restaurant, you break out in itchy hives or, even worse, find yourself struggling to breathe. What's the problem?

It could be a food allergy...completely out of the blue. Because food allergies are so commonly associated with children, many adults are shocked to learn that a food that they have enjoyed for decades can suddenly trigger alarming—or even life-threatening—symptoms.

Surprising statistic: In a recent national survey that included more than 40,000 American adults, an astounding 45% of those with a food allergy developed the condition after age 18.

Even though the research showed that more adults are developing new food allergies, science hasn't yet pinpointed why. Researchers theorize that the uptick could be due to a number of different factors, including changes in our environment...increased hygienic practices...increased exposure to antibiotics or antibacterials...changes to our microbiome (microorganisms, such as bacteria and fungi, in an environment)...and/or overall changes in dietary habits.

Culprit Foods

What food allergies are most common in adulthood? Shellfish tops the list, with just under 4% of study participants reporting that they developed this allergy after age 18. In addition to shellfish, seven other foods (milk, peanuts, tree nuts, fish, eggs, wheat and soy) are responsible for 90% of food allergies in adults and children.

But this list is by no means complete. You can develop a food allergy to many other foods.

Symptoms to Watch Out For

How do you know that a food allergy is making you feel lousy—or even putting your life at risk by making it difficult to breathe?

Unlike a food intolerance or sensitivity, which tends to cause milder symptoms, such as abdominal discomfort (stomach pain and bloating, for example), that can occur even a day later, a food allergy triggers symptoms that are acute, more immediate and tough to ignore.

Within a few hours or even minutes of eating the questionable food, you might experience itching, swelling, rash or hives... wheezing, difficulty breathing and/or a feeling that your throat is closing...vomiting (combined with hives or rash)...and even a precipitous drop in blood pressure that can lead to fainting.

Important: If someone is experiencing any of these symptoms due to a known or possible food allergy, it's imperative for the person to be given epinephrine as soon as possible to reverse an allergic reaction. Call 911 to get medical help. Whether epinephrine is self-administered or given by another person, the treated individual should receive medical care immediately following its use.

Guesswork Isn't Enough

Why are food allergies in adulthood so frequently missed?

The symptoms, of course, aren't easily overlooked. But what often happens is that the sufferer simply stops eating the problematic food. If shrimp makes you break out in hives, you can just stop eating it, right? (This tactic is why the incidence of food allergies in adults is likely underdiagnosed.) Or you simply may not recognize what is behind some annoying symptom, such as a chronic cough.

But food avoidance—without knowing for sure why the reaction occurred—isn't always the answer. Getting a proper diagnosis is crucial, because completely dodging a food isn't always realistic (hidden ingredients, anyone?) and you need to know how to manage the problem in any circumstance.

Identifying a Food Allergy

The first step to unearthing a food allergy is to keep a food diary that documents the food(s) you're eating that cause symptoms. This will give you an accurate history to discuss with your physician—ideally an allergist,* who has special training in diagnosing and treating allergies. You also can record the information with an app on your phone.

To make an actual diagnosis, your physician may draw from an array of clinical tests. However, it is important that this testing be based on a supportive clinical history after ingestion of an allergen. *The different types of testing that are useful in confirming a clinical food allergy are...*

- **Skin prick tests** involve placing a drop of allergen onto the surface of the skin, then pricking it through to introduce the allergen into the top layer of the skin on the forearm or back. If specific immunoglobulin E (IgE) antibody toward the allergen is present and attached to the allergy cells, then redness and an itchy bump should develop within about 15 minutes. Some doctors prefer this type of testing over blood tests (see below) because they consider skin prick tests to be more accurate.
- **Blood tests** that measure the presence of IgE antibodies to questionable food(s) in the blood.
- **Oral food challenge,** considered the gold standard to identify food allergies. Increasing amounts of the problematic food

*To find an allergist near you, consult the American Academy of Allergy, Asthma & Immunology at Allergist.AAAAI.org or the American College of Allergy, Asthma & Immunology at ACAAI.org/locate-an-allergist.

are consumed in the doctor's office, where you're observed for a reaction in a controlled environment.

Note: You do not need the oral food challenge if you get a positive test result from a skin prick or blood test and you've had a past reaction to the offending food. Because the blood test and skin prick test have a high false-positive rate, you need both the positive test result and a past food reaction to be considered to have that allergy.

If you're diagnosed with a food allergy, your allergist will advise you on the foods to avoid and give you coping strategies in case of an allergic reaction. For example, you'll get a prescription for an epinephrine auto-injector, along with specific instructions on how and when to use it. If you have a known food allergy, you also may want to wear a medical ID bracelet, available online.

On the horizon: Several exciting treatment advances soon may offer other options. These include oral or skin patch–based immunotherapies that slowly release an allergen into the body in small quantities, desensitizing the immune system to its effects...and vaccines to prevent a food allergy from taking hold among those considered at risk.

Why Some Fruits Make Your Mouth Itch

Beth Corn, MD, associate professor of medicine at Icahn School of Medicine at Mount Sinai, New York City. She also is a spokesperson for the American College of Allergy, Asthma and Immunology and past president of the New York Allergy and Asthma Society. ACAAI.org

Some people who suffer from pollen allergies also suffer from an underreported condition called "oral allergy syndrome"—their mouths, lips, tongues and/or throats feel tingly or itchy and sometimes swollen after they eat certain fruits or vegetables. Symptoms can be so severe that they feel like their throats are closing. On very rare occasions, oral allergy syndrome can cause a potentially fatal allergic reaction.

The first thing to know is that these people typically are not allergic to the fruits and vegetables they react to. They have this reaction because of their pollen allergies—the proteins in the fruits or vegetables are so similar to the proteins in pollens that their immune systems mount an allergic response to them.

Apples, pears, peaches, nectarines, plums, cherries, apricots, carrots, celery, cantaloupe and honeydew are among the most common triggers, but this can vary by person and depends in part on which pollen someone is allergic to. People who are allergic to ragweed pollen might experience oral allergy syndrome when they consume bananas, cucumbers, melons, sunflower seeds and/or zucchini. People allergic to grass pollen are more likely to cite celery, melons, oranges, peaches and/or tomatoes. And people allergic to birch pollen can experience this with apples, almonds, cherries, hazelnuts, peaches, pears and/or plums.

What to do: Stop eating the food, and take an antihistamine such as Benadryl immediately.

Important: If your symptoms include difficulty breathing or dizziness, call 911.

If you wish to continue consuming a fruit or vegetable that causes you mild symptoms, talk to your health-care provider. He/she may suggest cooking it first. The heat will break down the proteins that are confusing your immune system.

Example: Eat a baked apple rather than a raw apple.

Lactose Intolerance vs. Milk Allergy

National Institute of Diabetes and Digestive and Kidney Diseases.
Johns Hopkins Medicine.
FARE (Food Allergy Research & Education).
KidsHealth.org
Oregon Dairy and Nutrition Council.

Are you thinking of breaking up with milk and ice cream because you're convinced you're allergic to dairy...or are lactose intolerant? Before you steer your shopping cart away from the dairy aisle forever, let's get the terms straight. Lactose intolerance is not the same as milk allergy, and what works for one won't necessarily work for the other. *Here's what you need to know...*

What Is Lactose Intolerance?

Lactose is a sugar that's present in cow's milk. People with lactose intolerance have low levels of lactase, an enzyme that helps digest lactose. If your body doesn't make enough lactase, your morning bowl of cereal with milk, that pizza you have at lunch or the bowl of ice cream for dessert can leave you bloated, gassy and experiencing constipation or diarrhea...or both.

Who has lactose intolerance? Mostly adults —and, indeed, most adults. Worldwide, about 65% of adults lose all or some of their ability to digest lactose in adulthood. In these people, the ability to produce lactase declines gradually throughout childhood and adolescence, so symptoms usually don't occur until adulthood.

There's a strong genetic component: 90% of adults of East Asian descent are lactose intolerant, and the condition is prevalent in African-Americans, other Asian Americans, Hispanics, Native Americans and people of Arab, Jewish, Greek and Italian descent.

The exception: Only 5% of people of Northern European descent are lactose intolerant.

How do you know you have it? Most people with lactose intolerance easily pinpoint some or all of the above symptoms between 30 minutes and two hours after consuming dairy. If you want to be a little more scientific about it, keep a food diary to track your symptoms—record what you eat and when and then how you feel over the next couple of hours. Still not sure? Your doctor can give you a breath test for a definitive diagnosis of lactose intolerance.

What's the health risk? You might think that people with lactose intolerance would be more prone to osteoporosis because they avoid calcium- and vitamin D–rich foods. The good news is that research hasn't found this link to osteoporosis to be true. Still, if you can't digest most dairy foods, you need to consume alternative sources of these nutrients, such as soy milk fortified with calcium and vitamin D.

What can you do about lactose intolerance? Not everyone with lactose intolerance has to eliminate dairy...it depends on your symptoms. You can try an elimination diet—cut out all dairy for two to four weeks, then gradually reintroduce small amounts to see how much and what types you can handle. You might also try consuming low-lactose milk and other dairy products that have had lactose reduced...adding a lactase supplement to your diet to help you digest lactose-containing dairy foods...eating dairy products in combination with other foods... or enjoying naturally lower-lactose dairy, such as hard cheeses and yogurt.

Bonus: Eating fermented dairy foods with active live cultures, including yogurt and kefir, has an added benefit—the lactose-digesting bacteria may last for weeks in the gut, helping you digest other dairy foods like milk or ice cream.

What Is a Milk Allergy?

A true milk allergy means your immune system reacts to specific proteins in milk, especially casein, as though they are harmful invaders. The defense an allergic person's body mounts against the misidentified "enemy" triggers symptoms ranging from the mild, such as diarrhea, stomach cramps or hives, to more severe—indeed, potentially fatal—such as swelling in the throat and difficulty breathing.

Who has a milk allergy? Allergy to cow's milk is most often seen in babies and children and is often outgrown. Infants may have an allergic reaction to a milk-based formula, and even strictly breastfed babies can have an allergic reaction to cow's milk proteins that enter breast milk through the mother's diet.

How do you know you have it? Via allergy testing, such as a skin or blood test. If you suspect your baby has a milk allergy, take the child to a pediatric allergist for testing.

Can adults have a milk allergy? Yes—in fact in one study, more than half of adult patients who had problems digesting dairy foods in spite of being on a low-lactose diet tested positive for a milk allergy. If you have trouble digesting dairy foods, and a breath test shows that you don't have lactose intolerance, ask your doctor to test you for a milk allergy.

What can you do? In the case of a true allergy, you (or your child, more likely) will have to avoid all dairy products and foods containing them until the allergy is outgrown—or permanently if it is not outgrown.

This Herb Nixes Allergies and Coughs

Jamison Starbuck, ND, a naturopathic physician in family practice and writer and producer of Dr. Starbuck's Health Tips for Kids, a weekly program on Montana Public Radio, MTPR.org, both in Missoula. She is a contributing editor to *The Alternative Advisor: The Complete Guide to Natural Therapies and Alternative Treatments.* DrJamisonStarbuck.com

Stinging nettle, with its odd-sounding name, grows throughout the US and is thought by some to be nothing more than a weed. This deep green, leafy plant can indeed grow to six feet tall or more. And if you're hiking in a damp forest or taking a stroll past a weed-filled, untended lot, you'll likely happen upon nettle. But don't be deceived—stinging nettle is a nutritious spring food and is widely considered to be one of the most useful of botanical medicines. As a food, stinging nettle is often eaten like spinach. It contains calcium, potassium, iron and plant protein. The irritating needles are destroyed by steaming. Some people harvest stinging nettle on their own or buy it at a local farmer's market.

As a medicine, I frequently recommend stinging nettle to treat...

- **Seasonal allergies.** When allergy season begins (or up to a month before, if possible), patients who suffer from annoying seasonal allergy symptoms can start using nettle in tea or tincture form. The typical dose is 16 ounces daily of nettle tea or one-quarter teaspoon of tincture in two ounces of water, twice a day—taken at least 15 minutes before or after eating. The herb helps strengthen the body's immune system to reduce common allergy symptoms such as runny nose, watery eyes, sneezing and fatigue.

For prompt allergy relief: Freeze-dried nettle in capsule form is an effective and convenient way to help fight symptoms. A typical dose is two capsules three or four times a day when you have allergy symptoms. Many of my patients find that they need more nettle at the beginning of allergy season and that they are able to reduce the dose after a few weeks. Once allergy season is over, you can stop taking this herbal medicine.

- **Cough.** Nettle also acts as an expectorant, a medicine that helps push mucus out of your throat and lungs. For patients who have a simple cough or cough due to bronchitis, for example, I often recommend nettle tea or tincture. A typical dose is four ounces of tea, four times a day...or one-quarter teaspoon of tincture in two ounces of water, four times a day.

Scientists aren't entirely sure how stinging nettle works, but because it has multiple medicinal uses, it continues to be studied in North America and Europe. Because the plant is considered generally safe to use as medicine, you can purchase it over-the-counter and follow the manufacturer's instructions. But if you want to try nettle, it's wise to visit a health-care practitioner who is knowledgeable about botanical medicines. This includes naturopathic physicians. To find one near you, consult The American Association of Naturopathic Physicians, Naturopathic.org.

Caution: If you are allergic to any type of weed, don't use stinging nettle. If you have diabetes, high blood pressure, kidney disease or take a blood thinner, lithium or a sedative, talk to your doctor before taking nettle. This herb can interact with certain medications—especially those listed here and used for the conditions above. Pregnant women should not use nettle.

Natural Cough Remedies That Work Better Than OTC Drugs

Gustavo Ferrer, MD, a pulmonologist in private practice in Weston, Florida. He is the author of *Cough Cures: The Complete Guide to the Best Natural Remedies and Over-the-Counter Drugs for Acute and Chronic Coughs*. Dr. Ferrer grew up in Cuba, a culture that effectively utilizes herbal teas and folk remedies for coughs and colds.

It's enough to make you dizzy—hundreds of boxes and bottles lining the drugstore shelves, all promising to eradicate your cough...and perhaps also chest congestion, postnasal drip, sneezing and other related symptoms. Americans spend billions a year on over-the-counter (OTC) respiratory medications—including cough suppressants, decongestants and antihistamines. Coughs are also one of the top reasons why we see a doctor.

Here's a surprise...most of the time, it's all unnecessary. Why? Most acute coughs brought on by a cold or the flu go away on their own within a few days and don't require a doctor's care. Sometimes, though, a cough can linger as long as two or three weeks, so you want to take something for relief.

Here's the real bombshell: Most OTC cough remedies just don't work! Back in 2006, the American College of Chest Physicians concluded that there's no strong evidence of effectiveness for the vast majority of drugstore cough medications. In 2014, a Cochrane review of 29 clinical trials involving nearly 5,000 people reached the same conclusion. But they are heavily advertised, so people still buy them.

But don't despair. There is real help out there. Some OTC remedies really do relieve coughs—though not in the way you'd expect. Even better are natural cough remedies, using readily found ingredients, which are both effective and safe.

These OTC Products May Help

Nine times out of 10, acute cough symptoms are triggered by post-nasal drip—that annoying mucus trickling down the back of your throat. *These OTCs decrease secretions to ease postnasal drip...*

- **Antihistamines.** *Loratadine* (Claritin), *fexofenadine* (Allegra), *cetirizine* (Zyrtec) and *diphenhydramine* (Benadryl) block histamine, a naturally occurring chemical that provokes mucus production. They dry up mucus and decrease nasal secretions—even if you don't have an allergy.

Caution: They can cause water retention as a side effect. Avoid if you have glaucoma or prostate enlargement or are taking diuretics. Also, because these old-fashioned antihistamines can make you drowsy, you can become dependent on them to fall asleep.

My advice: Take half the recommended dose, for no more than a week.

- **Saline nasal spray.** Salt plus water—it doesn't get much more natural than that! The simple act of spraying this combination into nasal passages usually alleviates the stuffiness that can trigger constant hacking. Try versions that contain only these two active ingredients, such as Ocean Nasal Spray, Ayr Saline Nasal Mist or Little Remedies Saline Spray/Drops.

Caution: Avoid sprays containing *oxymetazoline* (Afrin), *phenylephrine* (Sudafed) or *xylometazoline* (Triaminic), which lead to "rebound congestion" when they wear off.

Natural Remedies for the Win

These natural cough relief remedies are your best bet for cough relief. They calm throat irritations, dry up mucus and boost the immune system—safely. *My top picks…*

• **Warm lemon and manukah honey "tea."** Everyone knows about the lemon/honey combo, which calms a cough while cutting mucus. But you can make it even more effective with manukah honey, a special kind from New Zealand that has strong antimicrobial properties, so it protects against the underlying cold virus. Regular raw honey also has antimicrobial properties. Blend a tablespoonful of honey with the juice from half a lemon in a cup of just-boiled water. For optimal benefit, drink it just before bedtime, when coughs typically rev up…and again in the morning.

• **Dark chocolate.** Most people have no idea that one of their favorite treats is also a natural cough suppressant—thanks to *theobromine*, a chemical component in chocolate. The darker the chocolate, the more theobromine, so aim for versions containing more than 65% cocoa. Eat a small square—about one-half to one ounce—two or three times a day.

Caution: Chocolate has caffeine, so don't eat it in the evening.

• **Beet and/or pineapple juice.** Both beet and pineapple juices have long been standbys for coughs due to bronchitis. Both help open bronchial passages and make it easier for your body to bring up excess mucus. Whichever you choose, a half cup (four ounces) is enough. It's fine to drink it two or three times a day. (*Note*: If you've been told to limit nitrates, avoid beet juice.)

• **Elderberry syrup.** Elderberry syrup, readily available in health-food stores, is a traditional remedy for colds, coughs and the flu. It acts as an expectorant and also has anti- viral and antiflu properties. Take as directed on the package, up to three times a day. Dilute in water if that makes it easier to take.

Important: If your cough lasts beyond three weeks—or includes symptoms such as coughing up blood, significant shortness of breath, chest pain or persistent fever—see a doctor.

Avoid these OTC cough products…

• **Cough suppressants.** A common ingredient is dextromethorphan (DXM), first introduced 60 years ago. It's found in popular brands including NyQuil, Coricidin HBP Cough & Cold, Delsym and Dimetapp DM. Not only is there no evidence that it works, it can provoke a narcotic-like "high" when taken in large amounts, leading to potential for abuse.

• **Cough expectorants.** Guaifenesin, the active ingredient in Mucinex, Robitussin, Tussin and Guaifenesin LA, doesn't have the narcotic-like downside of DXM, but there's no evidence that it works, either.

• **Combination products.** Most OTC remedies combine ingredients in the same product to treat a variety of symptoms.

Example: DXM, guaifenesin, an antihistamine, plus acetaminophen. This kitchen-sink approach is a bad idea—you're treating symptoms you don't have with drugs you don't need. The biggest pitfall? You might be taking acetaminophen for a headache or fever and don't realize that it's also in your combo cough remedy…so you may exceed the safe daily limit, which increases the risk for liver damage.

4 Surprising Facts About Mucus

Neil L. Kao, MD, a board-certified specialist in internal medicine, allergies and immunology and an attending physician at Greenville Health System and Spartanburg Regional Medical Center, both in South Carolina.

Mucus. It's hard to even say the word without curling a lip in disgust. But this much-maligned secretion is really a superhero in disguise—a stoic defender of the unprotected parts of your body. Sound like too much horn-blowing for such a yucky substance? Not so.

Few people understand the important role that mucus plays in keeping us healthy…and how to keep one's supply of this gooey substance functioning optimally. *What you need to know...*

What Mucus Does

Mucus is a watery, slick secretion that forms a physical and chemical barrier on many of the body's internal surfaces. Mucus protects the entire respiratory tract—that is, your nose, sinuses, mouth, throat, trachea, bronchial tubes and lungs—against foreign invaders such as bacteria and viruses. Mucus lubricates the surface and prevents excessive dryness.

The entire gastrointestinal tract, from mouth to colon to anus, as well as the genital tract in both males and females, produces mucus to perform these same functions. The principle of producing secretions like mucus is also present elsewhere in the body. For example, your eyes constantly produce a protective film of secretions that function just like mucus. We call them tears.

Your Protector

When your body senses danger, mucus is part of a defense system that kicks into gear. All mucus contains disease-fighting enzymes, chemicals and sometimes white blood cells called neutrophils. They work together to trap, inactivate or kill the foreign substances.

One purpose of mucus is to prevent these substances from entering the body. Having lots of mucus helps to wash away any offensive microorganisms and particles, such as bacteria and pollen. We blow our noses to eliminate mucus from our bodies. The remaining mucus is swallowed, digested and reabsorbed by the intestines. Stomach acid or enzymes from the pancreas should inactivate and destroy any disease-causing substances.

What you may not know: Any perceived attack—not only viruses, bacteria or allergens (such as pollen or pet dander) but also chemicals—can increase mucus production.

When this occurs, your mucus-making machinery can get busy when you least expect it. For example, the chemical compound capsaicin, which is found in chili peppers, will temporarily ramp up mucus production in the nose (making the nose "run") in an effort to clear the irritant from the body.

And what about dairy products? Studies have not shown that dairy increases mucus production. When the question was investigated, researchers found only that milk causes phlegm (a sticky form of mucus) to thicken. However, in my practice, I've observed that mucus does increase in some patients—perhaps due to the individual's reaction to the proteins in milk.

My advice: If you feel that dairy increases your mucus production, you may be more comfortable if you cut back or eliminate your dairy intake.

A Color Change

Healthy mucus is usually clear and thin. Sometimes, however, nasal mucus may change from clear to a deep yellow-green. This color change is due to the heavy presence of neutrophils. They are naturally light green in color, even though they're considered "white" blood cells.

Anytime there is a greater concentration of neutrophils, secretions may appear green. This can happen, for instance, during a respiratory infection when extra neutrophils are dispatched to fight the infection...or if your mucus dries out due to dehydration.

What you may not know: Contrary to popular belief, greenish-yellow mucus does not always mean that you have a bacterial infection. You may have a viral infection. Yet many people make that faulty assumption and demand antibiotics from their doctors. Antibiotics, as most people know, do nothing to eliminate a viral infection.

A nasal or throat swab or sputum test can be performed to tell whether your infection is caused by bacteria (which may necessitate antibiotic treatment) or a virus (which you'll have to live with until it passes).

Danger Signs

In rare instances, mucus can signal a serious health problem.

What you may not know: If your nasal mucus turns brownish-black, it may be caused by a fungal infection (aspergillosis) of the lining of the nose. Aspergillus is a common mold found on dead leaves, rotting vegetation and in some heating and air-conditioning systems. When aspergillus particles are inhaled, an infection can develop in people with weakened immunity or lung disease. The infection also causes shortness of breath, fever and fatigue. Aspergillosis requires prompt treatment with steroids and antifungal medication or it can become fatal.

When your eye is the target of disease or irritation, mucus can alert you to a potential danger. With conjunctivitis (pink eye), the eye usually produces a watery discharge or white or light yellow mucus.

While most cases of pink eye are benign, some may progress and cause permanent damage to your vision. To prevent such damage, see a doctor promptly if you have green or yellow mucus coming from your eye or if you wake up with eyes sealed shut from dry, crusty mucus.

When the Body Ages

As we get older, we lose our ability to control how much mucus we produce, leaving mucus-containing organs more prone to disease-causing organisms.

For example, decreased mucus production results in an increased risk for ear, nose, sinus, throat and lung infections, including pneumonia, because the body is less able to efficiently kill and clear away bacteria and viruses. To help maintain the full function of mucus-producing cells, it's important to treat allergies and not smoke or snort products.

What you may not know: Mucus protects the sensors in the nose that are responsible for smell and taste. If the body does not make enough mucus to keep the inside of the nose moist, sensors in the nasal passages don't function well and food tastes bland. One way to help retain these senses is with regular nasal washes (see below).

Note: If the inside of your nose feels dry, it can also be a sign that you are dehydrated and need to drink more fluids.

A One-Two Punch

Nasal irrigation may sound like a messy proposition, but it's a healthy habit for most people. Irrigation can remoisten dry nasal passages if there's not enough mucus...or it can help remove excess mucus when you have a bad cold or congested sinuses.

How nasal irrigation can help: If you have a runny nose with thick mucus, it's a good idea to perform a nasal wash at least once a day. It helps remove excess mucus and whatever elements may be causing this excess, such as viruses, bacteria, allergens (such as pollen and molds) and irritant particles such as the chemicals in smoke. Also, don't worry about leaving yourself "dried out"—the body simply produces more mucus.

A worthwhile daily habit: Even for those who are not battling an overabundance of mucus, a daily nasal wash can assist breathing and promote healthy nasal passages.*

You can use a bottled nasal irrigation product or saline solution. Such products include Ayr, Ocean, Simply Saline and drugstore brands. But this approach can become expensive with daily washes.

Many people prefer to use a teapot-shaped device called a neti pot. They're available at drugstores and online for around $15. Follow label instructions.

To avoid infection, the FDA advises against using tap water, which may contain low levels of organisms such as bacteria and protozoa. Instead, the agency recommends using bottled distilled or sterile water...boiled and cooled tap water (boiled for three to five minutes, cooled to lukewarm and used within 24 hours)...or water passed through a filter designed to trap potentially infectious organisms.

*If your immune system is compromised for any reason or if you've had recent nasal or sinus surgery or have a structural abnormality such as a deviated septum, consult your doctor before practicing nasal irrigation.

Important: Make sure to wash your neti pot with hot water and soap after each use, rinse thoroughly and dry with a paper towel or let it air-dry to keep it free of mold, bacteria or other contaminants.

Marijuana for Sleep Apnea

A marijuana-based drug could be the first medication for sleep apnea. *Dronabinol* (Marinol), an antinausea drug, reduces breathing interruptions in apnea patients, a study reports.

University of Illinois at Chicago and Northwestern University.

Keep Smelling Smoke...

Ronald Devere, MD, FAAN, director, Taste and Smell Disorder Clinic, Austin, Texas.

D*ysosmia* is the condition of smelling something (generally unpleasant, such as smoke or garbage) that simply isn't there. Such episodes typically last 10 minutes to an hour.

It's commonly caused by medications (such as diuretics, cardiovascular drugs or neurology medications such as the Parkinson's drug *levodopa*), pregnancy, a zinc deficiency, diabetes or even severe colds or recurrent sinus infections. Dysosmia also has been linked to migraines—in these cases, the smell disappears when the headache resolves.

For most people, dysosmia is not a serious issue and will generally go away after several months. If it doesn't, consult an ear, nose and throat specialist, who may suggest a nasal endoscopy to rule out abnormalities such as a polyp in your nasal passageways (often the result of chronic inflammation due to asthma or allergies). Corticosteroid medications can shrink polyps, but if that doesn't work, they can be removed surgically. In rare cases, an MRI may be required to determine if the cause is a brain tumor, stroke or head trauma (following an injury such as a concussion)—in some cases, all of these conditions can trigger abnormal electrical discharges in the brain that result in dysosmia.

Many people find relief by "cleaning out" the nasal passageways with saline drops or the regular use of a neti pot (a teapot-like device used to irrigate your nasal passages with a saline solution). Medications such as *gabapentin* (Neurontin), generally prescribed for seizure disorders, may be prescribed to block abnormal electrical discharges in patients whose quality of life is affected by these smells.

Chapter 4

STROKE PREVENTION AND RECOVERY

Women Who Are Most at Risk of Stroke

Stroke affects more women than men in the United States. And a new study pinpoints stroke risk factors unique to females.

"Many people don't realize that women suffer stroke more frequently than men, and mortality is much higher among women," said Kathryn M. Rexrode, MD, the study's corresponding author.

Background

"As women age, they are much more likely to have a stroke as a first manifestation of cardiovascular disease rather than heart attack," said Dr. Rexrode, who is with Brigham and Women's Hospital in Boston.

The study attempts to better understand susceptibility, she said.

"Why do more women have strokes than men? What factors are contributing and disproportionately increasing women's risk?" said Dr. Rexrode.

Stroke affects 55,000 more women than men each year in the United States. It's the leading cause of disability and the third leading cause of death in women, the researchers said in background notes.

Study Findings

Dr. Rexrode's team analyzed the scientific literature and identified several factors that increase stroke risk in women. *These include...*

- **Menstruation before age 10.**
- **Menopause before age 45.**
- **Low levels of the hormone dehydroepiandrosterone (DHEA).**
- **Use of birth control pills.**

A history of pregnancy complications can also indicate higher stroke risk. These problems include gestational diabetes and high blood pressure during or immediately after pregnancy, the researchers said.

The paper was published in the journal *Stroke*.

Expert Advice

Some of these risk factors are common, and the researchers stressed that few women who have one or more will suffer a stroke. How-

Kathryn M. Rexrode, MD, assistant professor of preventive medicine, Harvard Medical School and Brigham and Women's Hospital, Boston.

Brigham and Women's Hospital, news release.

ever, they said it's important for health care providers to be aware of any heightened risk.

"These women should be monitored carefully and they should be aware that they are at higher risk, and motivated to adhere to the healthiest lifestyle behaviors to decrease the risk of hypertension (high blood pressure) and subsequent stroke," Dr. Rexrode said.

The National Stroke Association's website, Stroke.org, has more information on women and stroke. Search "women."

Are Stroke Symptoms Different for Women?

Suzanne Steinbaum, DO, attending cardiologist and director of Women's Heart Health, Lenox Hill Hospital, New York City, writes the menopause blog "At the Heart of It All" for Bottom Line. She is the author of *Dr. Suzanne Steinbaum's HeartBook*. SRSheart.com

Are you confused about which stroke symptoms are specific to women? Should you look for the same symptoms that men experience or different ones?

The answer is you should look for both—but start with the "classic" stroke symptoms that both men and women experience. Knowing these common symptoms is an essential starting point. *These include...*

- **Sudden severe headache.**
- **Numbness or weakness on one side of the body.**
- **Paralysis on one side of the face or one arm or leg.**
- **Loss of balance or coordination.**
- **Dizziness or confusion.**
- **Trouble speaking.**
- **Difficulty understanding what others are saying.**
- **Blurred or double vision in one or both eyes.**

The American Heart Association developed the acronym "F-A-S-T" to help boil down key symptoms and what to do...**F**acial drooping, **A**rm weakness, **S**peech difficulty and **T**ime—call 911 immediately!

But recent research has found that women can also show different signs of stroke. It's particularly important to pay attention as you get older, as stroke risk starts to rise in the years just before menopause.

Women are more likely than men to...

- **Feel disoriented, confused or agitated.**
- **Experience sudden shortness of breath with no apparent cause.**
- **Feel nauseated or even vomit.** How to tell that it's a sign of a stroke? If it's GI-related, it will likely be accompanied by diarrhea and/or fever. But if it is accompanied by more classic symptoms such as being unsteady when walking or dizziness, suspect stroke.
- **Fainting**—even hallucinating.
- **Hiccups**—this could be a sign of a disruption of the breathing center in the brain. Pay attention to accompanying symptoms such as dizziness, numbness or weakness. These will be clues that the hiccups may be stroke-related.

Knowing the stroke symptoms that are specific to women may help you identify the need for emergency help sooner. And, when it comes to stroke, every second counts.

Are You Stroke-Ready?

Michael Frankel, MD, professor of neurology at Emory University School of Medicine, Atlanta. His team played a major role in the DAWN trial, published in *The New England Journal of Medicine* in January 2018. This study provided critically important data showing the benefit of thrombectomy within 24 hours of stroke onset.

Of course, no one wants to have a stroke. But about 800,000 times a year someone in the US has one. Most often, it's an acute ischemic stroke—blood flow to the brain is interrupted, starting a cascade of damage that can lead to death or disability.

The good news: Today's stroke is not your grandfather's stroke. Your chances of surviving and thriving have increased dramatically, thanks to recent advances. To have the best chance of recovering from a stroke, you need to act quickly—and smartly. *Here are four mistakes that can make the difference between life and death…*

MISTAKE #1: **Not recognizing stroke symptoms.** A stroke often causes multiple symptoms, but some people have only one. However, to spot one or more stroke symptoms, you need to recognize them.

Most people can name at least one of the many stroke symptoms. Classic symptoms include a droopy face on one side…numbness or weakness of the face, arm or leg (especially on just one side)…and trouble walking or balancing. *But there are other symptoms that are also important to watch for…*

- **Trouble seeing in one or both eyes.**
- **Sudden confusion.**
- **A severe headache with no known cause.**
- **Sudden, unexplained dizziness.**

Helpful: If you think someone near you may be having a stroke, think FAST. The letters stand for…

F: Face. Ask the person to smile to see if one side of the face droops.

A: Arms. Ask the person to raise both arms to see if one drifts downward or can't be moved at all.

S: Speech. Ask the person to repeat a simple phrase and listen for slurring or other difficulties.

T: Time. If you see any of these signs, call 911 right away—and make note of the time. Medical personnel will want to know when the symptoms started.

MISTAKE #2: **Ignoring a stroke symptom that lasts only a few minutes.** You may have had (or witnessed) a transient ischemic attack, a so-called TIA or "ministroke." That can be a warning that a bigger stroke is coming. You should still call 911.

Important: If you witnessed a person who had possible stroke symptoms, be sure that the hospital team has your cell phone number so you can be reached to confirm what you observed in the patient.

MISTAKE #3: **Getting a ride to the hospital.** In a medical emergency, you may be tempted to wait to see what happens or have someone drive you to a hospital or doctor's office. With a possible stroke, this is a very bad idea. Instead, call 911 and tell the operator you are seeing or having possible stroke symptoms. Don't worry about being wrong.

Emergency medical workers will assess you and look for other conditions (such as low blood sugar, low blood pressure or a seizure) that could mimic a stroke. They can start treating such conditions right away. If the emergency crew suspects a stroke, they will call ahead to the nearest appropriate hospital so the medical team can prepare.

MISTAKE #4: **Going to any hospital.** With a stroke, it does matter what hospital you go to—and that's another reason to call 911.

Under an accreditation system maintained by The Joint Commission, hospitals can get certifications ranging from "acute stroke ready" for those with basic supports in place…to "primary stroke centers" for those offering more advanced care…to "comprehensive stroke centers" for those offering the most advanced state-of-the-art care.

A new approach: According to new guidelines from the American Heart Association/American Stroke Association (AHA/ASA), if the patient is having severe stroke symptoms, emergency personnel can travel an additional distance (up to 15 minutes) to reach a comprehensive stroke center. In some regions, the distance may need to be longer. And in some states, medics are required to take patients to the hospital of their choice, while other states leave this decision to emergency personnel. Medics are trained to make the best hospital choice for the patient's needs.

Getting the Right Treatment

If you are taken to the hospital as a possible stroke patient, ideally you will arrive with a loved one who can describe the onset of your symptoms and share your medical history.

Important: Keep a cell phone number for a family member in your wallet—this is critical so that someone who knows you well can give medical information if you are alone and cannot speak for yourself.

If the hospital team determines that you may be having symptoms of an acute stroke, you will receive brain imaging—most often in a CT machine, ideally within 20 minutes of arriving at the hospital.

If your scan rules out bleeding in or around your brain (a hemorrhagic stroke) and you meet other criteria—including onset of your stroke no more than three to four-and-a-half hours earlier—you will get immediate intravenous treatment with a clot-busting medication called a tissue plasminogen activator, or tPA, to break up the clot in your brain, limiting damage and potential disability.

Beyond tPA

There's now an alternative to tPA called *mechanical thrombectomy*. This procedure physically removes the blood clot. It is sometimes done after or instead of clot-busting drug treatment. In some cases, you will need to be transferred to another hospital, by ambulance or helicopter, to get it.

Under guidelines from 2015, the procedure had to start within six hours of your initial stroke symptoms. This was a problem for people far from well-equipped and well-staffed hospitals or who woke up with symptoms (a so-called "wake-up stroke") or had stroke symptoms of uncertain duration.

Now: The treatment window has been expanded. Studies show that some patients with blockage in a major artery leading to the brain can benefit from thrombectomy 16 to 24 hours after the stroke began.

Again, doctors will try to determine whether you are in that time window by asking when your symptoms started (or when you were last seen symptom-free). Patients also are screened with advanced brain-imaging tests to find those who still have large areas of brain tissue healthy enough to benefit from restored blood flow.

The Stroke Treatment You May Need to Ask for

Sameer Ansari, MD, PhD, associate professor of radiology, neurology and neurological surgery at Northwestern University Feinberg School of Medicine, Chicago. NM.org

A surgical procedure called thrombectomy dramatically improves the odds that many stroke victims will survive and return to independent lives.

Problem: Many hospitals don't offer it. Compelling evidence for its effectiveness is so new that many aren't geared up for it yet. But there are ways to make sure you get it if you need it.

Background: Every year, about 800,000 people in the US have a stroke and 130,000 die. The vast majority (87%) of strokes are ischemic—caused by a clot that blocks blood flow to the brain. The go-to treatment offered by virtually every hospital is the clot-dissolving drug tissue plasminogen activator (tPA), given as soon as possible intravenously.

But if the clot is large—a kind often resistant to tPA treatment—a neurosurgeon can do a thrombectomy, a procedure that physically removes the clot. A surgeon uses a device called a stent-retriever to remove the clot from a blood vessel in the brain. This procedure is not brand new, but only in the past few years have studies made it obvious that it often is the best treatment option when a large clot blocks blood flow to the brain. Compared with standard stroke care, this reduces the death rate from 26% to 14%—and patients who survive score 26% higher on a post-stroke independence scale, on average. Recent improvements to the surgical tools used in thrombectomies likely are increasing survival rates as well. New research finds that the procedure can be effective as long as 24 hours after a stroke—not just six hours, as previously believed—although the sooner, the better.

What to do: Before you or a loved one has a stroke, get familiar with the "thrombectomy-capable stroke center" nearest to you. This hospital will have undergone a rigorous certification process for stroke care, including this procedure. You can do this by calling area hospitals or searching the database at StrokeCenter.org/trials/centers.

If you or a loved one experiences potential stroke symptoms, call 911. The EMS team should transport the patient to the nearest stroke center if one is close enough, but you can always ask to be sure. Wherever you wind up, ask if the patient is a candidate for a thrombectomy. If the answer is yes but the hospital can't perform it, ask how quickly the patient can be transferred to such a hospital—by helicopter, if necessary.

This Is Your Brain on Cigarettes

Smoking increases the risk for brain hemorrhages. New study results show that female smokers are at a much greater risk for bleeding in the lining of the brain than nonsmokers. Women who smoked 21 to 30 cigarettes a day were 8.35 times more likely to have a subarachnoid hemorrhage than nonsmokers. While the risk increased for men, it was not as great—men who smoked the same number of cigarettes a day were 2.76 times more likely to have a brain hemorrhage than nonsmokers.

Analysis of data on 65,521 adults, average age of 45, who had taken part in a Finnish national survey beginning in 1972 and who were followed up for an average of 21 years, led by researchers at University of Helsinki, Finland, and published in *Stroke*.

Anemia Increases Death Risk in Stroke Patients

Anemia—a low level of red blood cells—was associated with up to a two times higher risk for death for up to one year following either a hemorrhagic (bleeding in the brain) or an ischemic (blood clot in the brain) stroke. The study emphasizes the need for increased awareness of this condition in stroke patients.

Meta-analysis of nearly 30,000 stroke patients led by researchers at University of Aberdeen, Scotland, UK, published in *JAMA*.

Blood Thinner Update

Steven Swiryn, MD, clinical professor of cardiology, Feinberg School of Medicine, Northwestern University, Chicago.

Adults with atrial fibrillation (irregular heartbeat) often use blood thinners to prevent stroke.

New study: AFib patients with a pacemaker or defibrillator implant who have very brief and infrequent episodes are at low risk for stroke and may not need blood thinners unless episodes become longer or more frequent. Blood thinners increase risk for bleeding.

Caution: Do not discontinue this drug without discussing with your doctor.

Full-Fat Dairy Is Good for Your Heart

Consuming full-fat dairy is associated with lower cardiovascular risk than previously thought. Eating full-fat cheese, milk or yogurt does not raise the risk for heart attack or stroke. These dairy products neither help nor harm cardiovascular health.

In-depth analysis by researchers from England, Denmark and the Netherlands, published in *European Journal of Epidemiology*.

Eat Fat, Live Long

High-fat foods help you live longer, while high-carb intake is linked to increased risk for death.

Recent finding: People who had the highest carbohydrate consumption were 28% more likely to die than those who ate the least amount of carbs.

But the opposite was true for high-fat foods: Those with the highest total fat intake, averaging about 35% of calories from fat, were 23% less likely to die than those with the lowest intake. Higher-fat diets also were associated with lower stroke risk. Increased intake of all types of fat—saturated, polyunsaturated and monounsaturated—was associated with a lower risk for death.

Study of 135,335 people, ages 35 to 70, in 18 countries, led by researchers at McMaster University, Ontario, Canada, published in *The Lancet.*

Recover Faster from a Stroke

Steven R. Zeiler, MD, PhD, head of stroke research at Johns Hopkins Bayview Medical Center in Baltimore.

You already know that the most important thing you can do if you are having a stroke (or suspect that you are) is to get to an emergency room as fast as possible. Every second that you save may stop precious brain tissue from dying.

But what you and your care team do in the days immediately after a stroke also is critical—especially for recovering from motor deficit and regaining control of your muscles.

Two important new findings...

First finding: In animal studies in a lab, waiting just one week to start rehab led to significantly worse outcomes.

Second finding: A certain medication can prevent that stroke recovery window from closing so quickly.

The overall window for stroke recovery in people continues well past the first week, of course. Many people who have had strokes can continue to improve for months, even years. So never give up! *But here's what to do immediately after the emergency phase...*

- **Start rehab quickly.** Take advantage of that early recovery period—the sooner you begin, the greater your recovery. If your doctors don't start your rehab in the hospital a day or two after the stroke, ask about it and push for it—even if there are medical issues that make it difficult.

- **Ask about the drug *fluoxetine.*** Other recent research has shown that this antidepressant, aka Prozac, started within one day after a stroke, not only improves recovery but also extends the length of the recovery window. An earlier randomized clinical trial showed that patients with moderate-to-severe motor deficit after ischemic stroke (the most common kind, caused by a blood clot) who took fluoxetine every day for three months, starting five to 10 days after a stroke, had significantly greater improvement than patients who received a placebo. Other drugs in the same class also seem to improve stroke recovery, but the most data exist for fluoxetine—and the new research adds to the urgency of that prescription. While more and more physicians are prescribing fluoxetine, it is not yet a standard of care—so ask.

- **Engage your brain right away.** What you do matters, too—so don't rely solely on rehab services. Do your best to stimulate your brain by playing games on a tablet or working on a puzzle. When people visit you in the hospital, rather than just watching TV together or exchanging pleasantries, have a real conversation about current events or a book you recently have read. In animal studies, mice kept in enriched and stimulating environments after stroke had greater recovery than those kept in simple cages. You want as much of your brain back as possible...so use it as soon as possible!

Women Fare Worse Than Men After a Stroke

Lynda Lisabeth, PhD, professor, epidemiology, University of Michigan School of Public Health, Ann Arbor, Michigan.

Marc Fisher, MD, editor-in-chief, *Stroke,* and professor, neurology, Harvard Medical School, Boston.

Stroke.

Women tend to have a tougher time recovering from a stroke than men do, though the reasons aren't completely clear, researchers say.

Study Findings

On average, female stroke survivors reported more limitations in their day-to-day activities than male survivors did, according to a review of 22 studies. Female survivors also were more likely to develop depression after their stroke and rate their health-related quality of life as low.

Possible Explanations

As for why, the researchers point to some possible explanations. Women tend to be older and in poorer health when they suffer a stroke, compared with men. Also, strokes in women are typically more severe.

But those differences only partly explained the findings, said senior researcher Lynda Lisabeth, PhD.

"There are other things going on here that we just don't understand yet," said Dr. Lisabeth, a professor at the University of Michigan School of Public Health, in Ann Arbor.

One possibility, she said, is that "social factors" are at work. Compared with men, women who have a stroke are more likely to live alone and be otherwise socially isolated.

When they have a stroke, there may be no one around to recognize it and call 911, Dr. Lisabeth said. After the stroke, they may lack help at home, or someone to get them to doctor appointments and rehabilitation therapy sessions.

Chocolate vs. Stroke

Good news for chocolate lovers! In a new study of 55,000 people, those who ate two to six one-ounce servings of chocolate per week had a 20% lower risk for atrial fibrillation (AFib), an irregular heartbeat that raises risk for stroke, heart attack and dementia, than those who indulged only once a month.

Why: Flavonoids in cocoa may improve blood vessel function.

Important: It's the cocoa—not milk and sugar—that's good for you, so the higher the cocoa content, the better.

Elizabeth Mostofsky, MPH, instructor in epidemiology, Harvard T.H. Chan School of Public Health, Boston.

Beyond that, elderly women may be worse off financially than elderly men, the researchers suggested. From studies so far, though, it's not clear whether that plays a role in women's poorer stroke recovery.

Dr. Lisabeth said more research is needed to better understand what's going on.

If social isolation, for example, is part of the problem, there could be ways to change that, she said. For instance, technology could be used to connect stroke survivors with health professionals or other women going through the same thing.

Depression After Stroke

Marc Fisher, MD, is a neurologist and editor of the journal *Stroke,* which published the findings.

Dr. Fisher said the results bring to light some important issues—including the fact that women may be particularly vulnerable to depression after a stroke. Across the studies, women were up to three times more likely to suffer depression than men were.

That's a fact that might get lost in everything else that's happening during post-stroke care—where the main focus is to prevent a second stroke, Dr. Fisher said.

He suggested that stroke survivors with depression symptoms bring it up to their family and their doctor.

Dr. Lisabeth agreed, noting that depression could hinder patients' recovery from the stroke itself.

Prevention, Signs and Fast Treatment of Stroke

Ideally, strokes would be prevented in the first place, she said.

That makes it important for women (and men) to get any risk factors for stroke under the best control possible. Those include high blood pressure, diabetes and the irregular heartbeat known as atrial fibrillation.

A healthy diet, regular exercise and not smoking are critical, too, according to the American Stroke Association.

Dr. Fisher said, "You also need to be aware of the signs of stroke and have a plan in place for what to do."

He pointed to the stroke association's "FAST" acronym as a way for people to remember the stroke warning signs. The first three letters refer to facial drooping, arm weakness and speech difficulty; if a person has any of those symptoms, the advice is to call 911 and say, "I think it's a stroke."

Quick treatment—represented by the last letter—is vital, Dr. Lisabeth explained, because it may minimize brain damage from the stroke and, therefore, the long-term effects.

If a blood clot has caused the stroke, a drug called tPA can dissolve the clot, she noted. It needs to be given within a few hours of the initial symptoms.

"Knowing the signs and symptoms of stroke, and calling 911 when they arise, can improve patients' outcomes across the board," Dr. Lisabeth said.

The American Stroke Association has more on preventing a stroke at BrainHealth.StrokeAssociation.org.

Will Certain Foods Bolster Brain Health After Stroke?

Martha Clare Morris, ScD, professor, internal medicine, Rush University Medical Center, Chicago.

Carolyn Brockington, MD, director, Stroke Center, Mount Sinai St. Luke's and Mount Sinai West, New York City.

American Stroke Association annual meeting, Los Angeles.

Stroke survivors who eat plenty of leafy greens, fish and other healthy foods may help preserve their brain function as time goes on, a preliminary study suggests.

Researchers found the benefits among stroke survivors who most closely followed the principles of the so-called "MIND" diet.

It pulls together elements from two eating plans known to improve heart health: the traditional Mediterranean diet and the "DASH" diet, for controlling high blood pressure.

It also makes specific recommendations that are based on research into nutrition and brain health, said senior researcher Martha Clare Morris, ScD, a professor at Rush University Medical Center in Chicago.

For example, she said, the diet puts more value on vegetables—especially leafy greens—than fruit. And when people do eat fruit, the advice is to go heavy on berries, which studies have linked to less cognitive decline.

Stroke and Cognitive Decline

Cognitive decline refers to problems with memory, judgment and other thinking skills that can crop up as people age. Stroke survivors are at heightened risk of that kind of decline, as well as full-blown dementia.

Their risk of dementia is roughly twice the norm, said Carolyn Brockington, MD, who directs the stroke center at Mount Sinai St. Luke's in New York City.

Strokes occur when blood flow to the brain is suddenly reduced, Dr. Brockington explained. That can leave people with brain damage that impairs their thinking. Plus, stroke patients often have underlying conditions, like high blood pressure and heart disease, which are linked to a higher dementia risk.

So it's important to find ways to help preserve their brain function, said Dr. Brockington, who was not involved in the new study.

"This is really a newer area of research," she said. "How can we promote brain health and function as people age?"

Study Findings

For this study, Morris—who created the MIND diet—and her team looked at the relationship between stroke survivors' dietary habits and their odds of mental decline over the next five years.

They tracked 106 survivors, breaking them into three groups based on how well they stuck with MIND-like eating habits. The top one-third were those who most regularly ate foods like leafy greens, berries, nuts, olive oil, fish, whole grains and beans.

In the end, those people had only half the rate of cognitive decline seen in the one-third of survivors whose diets were the least MIND-like. Morris said the foods emphasized in the MIND plan may not only be generally healthy, but specifically good for the brain.

In a recent study, Morris found that older adults who ate one serving of leafy greens each day showed slower brain aging, compared with those who rarely ate them. It was as if they'd shaved 11 years off their age—as far as their brain function was concerned, she said.

Leafy greens (such as spinach, kale and collard greens) contain nutrients that appear to support brain function, Morris explained. They include vitamin K, folate, beta-carotene and lutein.

Expert Advice

For now, Morris said stroke survivors can take heart that it's never too late to eat healthfully.

Dr. Brockington agreed. "We can't establish cause-and-effect from these findings," she said. "But they can show you you're on the right track."

Often, Dr. Brockington noted, people believe that once you suffer a stroke, "that's it."

"But the brain has a great capacity for repair," she said. The healthy brain tissue surrounding the stroke-damaged area can try to make "new connections" to compensate.

The American Stroke Association has more information on nutrition and stroke at StrokeAssociation.org. Search "nutrition after stroke."

Strokes Can Cause Memory Loss, Too

Majid Fotuhi, MD, PhD, a neurologist and medical director at NeuroGrow Brain Fitness Center in McLean, Virginia. He is author of *The Memory Cure* and *Boost Your Brain.*

Alzheimer's disease is the most widely recognized form of dementia. But there's another cause of memory loss that people should know about—but usually don't.

Vascular cognitive impairment (VCI), which is typically caused by multiple small strokes, has been estimated to affect 1% to 4% of adults over age 65. However, because there is no agreement on the exact definition of this condition, the actual number of affected individuals is not known. Most older adults with vascular risk factors—such as high blood pressure (hypertension) and diabetes—may have varying levels of VCI.

Symptoms to Watch for

Specific symptoms of VCI depend on the part of the brain affected. Patients who have suffered multiple mini-strokes may walk or think more slowly than they did before. Some have trouble following directions. Others may feel apathetic or confused.

Some mini-strokes, however, affect only the part of the brain involved in decision-making and judgment. The changes might be so subtle that a patient isn't aware of them—

at least, until subsequent mini-strokes affect larger or different areas of the brain.

Getting the Right Diagnosis

People who exhibit marked cognitive changes usually will be given an MRI or computed tomography (CT) scan. These tests sometimes reveal white, cloudy areas in the brain (infarcts) that have suffered damage from impaired circulation due to mini-strokes.

Often, however, the mini-strokes are too small to be detected. In these cases, patients may be incorrectly diagnosed with Alzheimer's disease. The distinction is important. There is no cure for Alzheimer's disease. In patients with VCI, there are a number of ways to stop the disease's progression and maintain long-term cognitive health.

Better Vascular Health

Brain damage that's caused by mini-strokes can't be reversed. Medication—including cholinesterase inhibitors, such as *donepezil* (Aricept)—may modestly reduce some symptoms in patients with dementia but cannot cure it.

Preventive strategies, however, can be very effective in people with VCI alone. *Most important…*

• **Don't let high blood pressure shrink your brain.** Chronic hypertension is one of the main causes of dementia because the vascular trauma is constant.

My advice: Blood pressure should be no higher than 120/80 mm Hg—and 115/75 mm Hg is better. Most people can achieve good blood pressure control with regular exercise and weight loss, and by limiting sodium and, when necessary, taking one or more blood pressure–lowering drugs, such as diuretics, beta-blockers or ACE inhibitors.

• **Avoid the other "D" word.** By itself, diabetes can double the risk for dementia. The actual risk tends to be higher because many people with diabetes are obese, which is also a dementia risk factor.

Important research: One study found that patients with multiple risk factors, including diabetes and obesity, were up to 16 times more likely to develop dementia than those without these risk factors.

My advice: By adopting strategies that prevent hypertension, including weight loss and regular exercise, you'll also help stabilize your blood sugar—important for preventing or controlling the health complications associated with diabetes.

• **Keep an eye on your waist.** Obesity increases the risk for hypertension and diabetes and has been associated with damage to the hippocampus (the brain's main memory center). Obese patients also have a much higher risk for obstructive sleep apnea, interruptions in breathing during sleep that can increase brain shrinkage (atrophy) by up to 18%.

My advice: Measure your waist. For optimal health, the size of your waist should be no more than half of your height. Someone who's 68 inches tall, for example, should have a waist measurement of 34 inches or less.

• **If you drink, keep it light.** People who drink in moderation (no more than two drinks daily for men or one for women) tend to have higher HDL, so-called "good," cholesterol…less risk for blood clots…and a lower risk for stroke and dementia.

My advice: If you already drink alcohol, be sure that you don't exceed the amounts described above. Drinking too much alcohol increases brain atrophy.

• **Get the right cholesterol-lowering drug.** People with high cholesterol are more likely to develop atherosclerosis (fatty buildup in the arteries) and suffer a mini-stroke or stroke than those with normal cholesterol levels.

My advice: Talk to your doctor about statins, such as *atorvastatin* (Lipitor) and *simvastatin* (Zocor). These drugs not only reduce cholesterol but also may fight blood-vessel inflammation. Other cholesterol-lowering drugs—such as resins, which bind in the intestines with bile acids that contain cholesterol and are then eliminated in the stool—don't provide this dual benefit.

• **Ask your doctor for a vitamin B-12 test.** If your blood level is low, you may benefit from B-12 supplements or injections.

Chapter 5

BRAIN HEALTH

Fit Middle-Aged Women Are Building a Healthy Brain

There's a fitness reward you might not expect: Better memory in your senior years. New research finds that being physically fit around age 50 lowers a woman's risk of developing memory-robbing dementia by almost 90%.

And for those physically fit women who do end up with dementia, they tend to get it much later in life—about 10 years later than others.

"Keeping yourself fit—by exercising and having a healthy diet—may decrease your risk of getting dementia in old age. It will also make you feel better and will reduce your risk of other disorders, [such as heart problems]," said senior study author Ingmar Skoog, MD. He's director of the Center for Ageing and Health at the University of Gothenburg in Sweden.

How does exercise help keep the brain healthy?

"High-fitness is good for your [blood] vessels. Vascular factors have been found to be related to dementia, including Alzheimer's disease," Dr. Skoog explained. He also said that high levels of physical fitness may have a direct effect on nerve cells in the brain.

James Hendrix, PhD, director of global science initiatives for the Alzheimer's Association, agreed that physical fitness is good for the blood vessels.

"We've talked for a while about the heart-head connection. If you've got good oxygenated blood, you'll have healthier organs, and the brain is an organ," Dr. Hendrix said.

The Swedish researchers looked at a group of nearly 200 women between the ages of 38 and 60 in 1968. Their average age was 50.

The women were asked to ride a bicycle until they were exhausted to measure their peak cardiovascular capacity. Forty women had a high-fitness level, while 92 were in the medium-fitness level. Fifty-nine women were in the low-fitness category. Some of the women were placed into the low-fitness category because they couldn't finish the test.

During the next 44 years, the researchers tested the women for memory and thinking problems linked to dementia.

Ingmar Skoog, MD, professor of psychiatry, and director, Center for Ageing and Health, University of Gothenburg, Sweden.

James Hendrix, PhD, director, global science initiatives, Alzheimer's Association.

Neurology, online.

Only 5% of the women who had high physical fitness in middle-age had developed dementia, the findings showed. Twenty-five percent of those in the medium-fitness group went on to have dementia, as did 32% of those who had low physical fitness. Nearly half—45%—of those who couldn't finish the fitness test developed dementia over the years.

But the study wasn't designed to prove a cause-and-effect relationship. It can only show an association, according to Dr. Skoog.

What if someone comes late to exercise, beginning in their 50s or 60s? Could that still help their brain?

Dr. Skoog said he thinks it can, though he expects the effect would likely be smaller.

And, even if someone already has dementia, Dr. Hendrix said that exercise can be beneficial. "Alzheimer's disease isn't just a disease of memory. There's some good evidence that other symptoms, like agitation, can be better managed if someone's active. I know my own sleep is better when I'm exercising," he added.

If you're starting to exercise in middle or late life, Dr. Hendrix said it's a good idea to check in with your doctor first.

"But, in general, it's never too late or too early to start practicing good lifestyle approaches. And, when you try to pick an exercise to do, pick one you enjoy. Whatever exercise you'll continue to do is the best one for you," Dr. Hendrix said.

Findings from the study were published online in the journal *Neurology*.

Hormone Therapy and Your Risk for Alzheimer's Disease

Study titled "Postmenopausal Hormone Therapy and Alzheimer's Disease," by Bushra Imtiaz, MD, MPH, and colleagues, University of Eastern Finland, Kuopio, Finland, published in *Neurology*.

Can hormone therapy (HT) protect you from dementia? After all, estrogen protects neurons in animal studies. Plus, more women than men get Alzheimer's—and some scientists have speculated that naturally falling estrogen levels during and after menopause might increase the risk. If so, replacing that estrogen with HT might be protective against Alzheimer's.

The latest research sheds new light on the issue. The key, it turns out, isn't whether a woman takes HT—but when and for how long.

Background: Results from previous studies have been inconsistent. Some have shown that HT was statistically linked to a reduced risk for Alzheimer's, while other studies have shown increased risk. So researchers from the University of Eastern Finland decided to delve into a robust database to try to get an answer.

New study: All women age 47 to 56 living in Kuopio Province in Finland—more than 13,000—were mailed questionnaires about hormone therapy use every five years for 20 years, from 1989 until 2009. The women were also part of a national medical registry, so researchers could reliably track which ones were diagnosed with Alzheimer's disease over that time.

Results: For most women, HT didn't have an effect on Alzheimer's risk. But for one group of women, the results were striking...

Women who started HT right around the time they stopped menstruating in their early 50s—and who continued HT for more than 10 years—had a decreased risk of developing Alzheimer's. One possible explanation is that there is an "estrogen window" in which hormone therapy may be protective—something already shown for cardiovascular risk.

Bottom line: Studies such as this can find statistically relevant associations but can't prove cause and effect. Only carefully controlled clinical studies can determine whether hormone therapy should be prescribed for the purpose of preventing dementia.

So it's too early to use Alzheimer's risk as a factor in determining whether HT is right for you. But this study does reinforce other evidence that when it comes to hormone therapy, timing is important. For instance, other research cited by the study authors has found an increased risk for Alzheimer's among women who start hormone therapy at an older age (age 64, on average). If you do decide to take HT—for relief of bothersome menopausal symptoms such as hot flashes, for instance—the new research is more evidence that starting earlier may be safer and possibly more beneficial than waiting a decade or more after menopause hits.

Poor Sleep May Predict Alzheimer's

Barbara B. Bendlin, PhD, associate professor of medicine at the University of Wisconsin-Madison. She was an author of "Poor Sleep Is Associated with CSF Biomarkers of Amyloid Pathology in Cognitively Normal Adults," published in an online issue of *Neurology*.

Good sleep can be elusive. Many of us are kept awake by too much caffeine...a stressful lifestyle...or a snoring bed partner.

But lack of sleep is more than just a tiring annoyance. Research shows that regular poor sleep increases your risk of developing diabetes, depression, obesity and cardiovascular disease.

Now: New research has uncovered a link to Alzheimer's disease. Based on this recent analysis, people who don't sleep well may be at greater risk of developing Alzheimer's than sound sleepers. This finding comes on the heels of previous studies also showing that sleep may influence the development (or progression) of Alzheimer's disease.

Recent finding: Researchers at the University of Wisconsin-Madison recruited 101 people (average age 63) with normal cognitive and memory skills, many of whom had risk factors for Alzheimer's—for example, many had a parent with the disease or carried a gene, such as the APOE gene, which can increase one's risk for the disease. Participants answered questions about the quality of their sleep and provided spinal fluid samples that were tested for biological markers of Alzheimer's.

People who reported that they had worse sleep quality, more sleep problems (such as trouble falling asleep, restless sleep or awakening short of breath or with a headache) and daytime sleepiness had more biological markers for Alzheimer's in their spinal fluid than people who did not have sleep problems.

Those biological markers included signs of amyloid and tau proteins that are related to the plaques and tangles found in the brains of people with Alzheimer's disease. The study also looked for other biological markers in the spinal fluid, including signs of brain cell damage and inflammation. The results remained the same when researchers adjusted for other factors such as the use of sleep medication, level of education, depression symptoms and body mass index.

Not every person with sleep problems had abnormalities in his/her spinal fluid. For example, the study found no link between self-reporting of obstructive sleep apnea and biological markers for Alzheimer's.

"Disrupted sleep or lack of sleep may lead to amyloid plaque buildup because the brain's clearance system really seems to kick into action during sleep," explained Barbara B. Bendlin, PhD, the study's lead author. In other words, in the absence of sleep, amyloid may deposit more quickly because it's not being cleared from the brain.

"However, we can't tell from this study if it's the case that disrupted sleep is causing amyloid to build up in the brain, or if it's the other way around, where changes in the brain associated with Alzheimer's are affecting the quality of sleep," she said.

Implications: While more research is needed to further define the relationship between sleep and Alzheimer's, the identification of modifiable risk factors for the disease is important given estimates that suggest delaying the onset of this disease in people by just five years could reduce the number of cases seen in the next 30 years by 5.7 million...and could save $367 billion in health-care spending in the US.

Bottom line: Improved sleep in at-risk people may prevent or delay the onset of Alzheimer's disease. Whether you are at increased risk for Alzheimer's disease or not, if you feel that you need better-quality sleep, be sure to talk to your doctor about strategies that may help.

Is It Normal... Alzheimer's...or Something Else?

Jason Brandt, PhD, professor of psychiatry and behavioral sciences, professor of neurology and director of the division of medical psychology, all at Johns Hopkins University School of Medicine, Baltimore. He also directs the Cortical Function Laboratory at Johns Hopkins Hospital and has developed several widely used neuropsychological tests.

The pot you forgot boiling on the stove. The longtime neighbor whose name you suddenly can't recall. The car keys you think you've lost, only to discover they're...in your pocket.

Chances are you have had a momentary memory lapse like these, often called a "senior moment." Though they happen to everyone on occasion, there's a reason for the moniker—these slipups may reflect the gradual loss of one's mental sharpness with aging.

It's no wonder, then, that repeated lapses can be alarming, especially for those with a family history of Alzheimer's disease or some other form of dementia. The good news is that the minor memory misfires that tend to affect people over age 50 often are caused by normal age-related changes in the brain and nervous system.

But still, memory lapses can be an early marker of Alzheimer's or another type of dementia. So if you have been noticing more of those senior moments, it is perfectly reasonable to see your doctor about it and ask about undergoing a cognitive assessment. These tests can put your mind at ease...or help diagnose a potential problem at the earliest possible stage.

Testing 1, 2, 3

To gauge cognitive function, your physician likely will observe your responses to standardized memory and thinking exercises. Many physicians give patients the Mini-Mental State Examination (MMSE). This exam starts with a set of simple questions that measure orientation—What year is it? What season? What is today's date? What town are we in? Next, the doctor will read a short list of words and ask the patient to repeat them back immediately and then five minutes later.

The doctor also will ask the patient to write a sentence and copy a geometric design. Finally, the doctor will ask the patient to perform a series of actions (such as "touch your left shoulder and then tap your head twice"), which gauges the ability to understand language and follow commands.

Helpful: A perfect MMSE score is 30, and a healthy adult should approach that number (anything above 27 is usually fine).

If your physician is concerned, he/she may refer you to a neuropsychologist for further diagnostic testing. Just as a neurologist and radiologist can decipher the images of a brain MRI scan, this kind of doctor examines patterns of scores on a variety of brain-function tests to try to identify specific disorders.

Among the more commonly used tests for assessing a patient with possible Alzheimer's is the Boston Naming Test. Here, the patient looks at drawings of objects and names them. It begins with common nouns (a dog, a tree) and advances to increasingly obscure ones (a padlock, a zebra) that require the test taker to retrieve rarely used words from memory. This is valuable information, as Alzheimer's patients tend to have trouble recalling the names of objects.

Alzheimer's also diminishes the ability to learn and remember new things. Doctors measure this by reading a brief story and asking the patient to repeat it right away, then 20 minutes later.

Finally, since people in the early stages of Alzheimer's tend to develop spatial confusion, we see whether they have difficulty copying, say, a geometric design or drawing common objects (for example, a daisy) upon request.

Important: Don't look up these tests or "prepare" for them in advance. They are useful only if you don't know exactly what to expect and haven't "practiced."

What a Decline Means

Many patients who visit my clinic have parents or other relatives with Alzheimer's. They're acutely aware of their own periodic memory failures and are understandably worried about how well their minds are working.

Good news: As often as not, after running these tests, I end up telling them, "You're functioning like an average person your age. What you're experiencing looks like typical age-related decline."

That may not sound comforting, but face the facts. Your brain is affected by "wear and tear" as you age. You probably can't run as fast at age 55 as you could at age 35, and your mind isn't quite as efficient as it was two decades ago, either. But if you perform within the average range for your age, there's no cause for concern.

If your results fall below that level, you might be diagnosed with mild cognitive impairment (MCI). If so, your brain function is below the norm for your age even though you don't have dementia.

Keep in mind: MCI is a broad category and encompasses a variety of different things. A patient with MCI who finds it difficult to recall events or the right word to describe an object or who displays spatial confusion, may be in the very earliest stage of Alzheimer's.

In contrast, someone who possesses a solid memory but struggles with executive function (for example, he can't plan well or solve problems effectively) may be at greater risk of developing a frontotemporal dementia—a type of dementia in which personality and language changes are common.

Important: While 10% to 15% of people over age 65 who have MCI will progress to Alzheimer's each year, the diagnosis is not necessarily dire. Many published studies show that patients with cognitive impairment in only one area—just memory or just language or just spatial cognition—have a very strong chance (perhaps as high as 50%) of returning to normal within one year.

How? It could be that the patient who fell into the MCI category was feeling ill the day of assessment...or was sleep-deprived...or drank too much (or not enough) coffee...or even was just in a very bad mood.

Although many factors affect an individual's cognitive performance, these tests are extremely useful when interpreted by an expert neuropsychologist. Recent studies indicate that the brains of patients with Alzheimer's disease undergo changes (observable with special brain-imaging methods) many years before a diagnosis is typically made. So getting a baseline neuropsychological assessment in middle age or a little older may help identify people who should be targeted for more active Alzheimer's prevention.

Your Next Steps

If you do well on the cognitive tests but remain worried about memory decline, work hard to keep what you have.

To achieve this (as well as maintain good overall health), follow these lifestyle choices: Eat a healthful diet...get regular exercise...participate in brain-stimulating activities you enjoy...keep your blood pressure under control...and moderate your alcohol intake.

For a patient who is newly diagnosed with early-stage Alzheimer's, I often recommend that he stop driving as a safety measure, advise him to keep written notes and calendars to aid recall and suggest that he talk with his doctor about whether a prescription Alzheimer's drug might help improve mental function. I also recommend beginning a discussion of future care needs and end-of-life plans with family.

As for people who fall in the middle and display some signs of MCI, I often explain that the "senior moments" they're experiencing might be the beginning of something more serious...or they might mean nothing at all.

Best way forward: Follow the blueprint for patients who tested well cognitively—live a healthful lifestyle, and try to avoid "stressing out." (I frequently recommend mindfulness-based stress reduction programs.) Then I'll reevaluate them in a year and take other measures if needed.

Losing Track of Your Thoughts?

Gurinder Singh Bains, PhD, associate professor, Loma Linda University School of Allied Health Professions, Loma Linda, California. He has researched the effects of laughter on short-term memory.

You're mulling over a problem...and then suddenly, you completely forget what you were thinking about. Are you suffering from short-term memory loss?

This could be a form of short-term memory loss. But don't be too quick to assume the worst. Memory naturally declines as we get older. It becomes a real problem only when such instances become persistent and begin to interfere with your daily functioning—for example, you have difficulties performing at your job because of such memory lapses. In this case, you should definitely see your doctor for an evaluation.

Certain medications, such as sleeping pills and antidepressants, can lead to memory problems. Other causes could be smoking, alcohol and/or drug abuse, a head injury or a stroke. A vitamin B-12 deficiency, which is most common in older people, who tend to have trouble absorbing this vitamin from their food, could also be playing a role.

Other possible causes include lack of sleep and stress. Chronic lack of sleep impairs the brain's ability to consolidate memories. With chronic stress, levels of the so-called "stress hormone" cortisol increase throughout our bodies. When cortisol enters the brain, it can damage the neurons that are needed for learning and memory.

If you think stress is to blame, try some laughter. A recent study found that adults who watched a funny video for 20 minutes had significantly lower cortisol levels than those who did not watch it.

Even better: Those in the study who watched the funny video scored 20% higher on memory tests, including short-term memory, than those in the control group. So get a regular dose of humor, and your memory may kick back into gear!

You Can Lower Your Risk for Alzheimer's

Gayatri Devi, MD, director of New York Memory and Healthy Aging Services and an attending physician at Lenox Hill Hospital, both in New York City, and clinical professor of neurology at SUNY Downstate Medical Center in Brooklyn. A board-certified neurologist, Dr. Devi is author of *The Spectrum of Hope: An Optimistic and New Approach to Alzheimer's Disease.* NYBrain.org

Older adults fear Alzheimer's disease more than cancer. But how worried do you really need to be?

Let's start with the good news...if you have a first-degree relative with the disease (a parent or sibling), you're only at a slightly greater risk than someone who does not have a first-degree relative with Alzheimer's. That's because there are many factors that affect your risk for Alzheimer's...not just your genes (more on this later).

Poor lifestyle choices (such as an unhealthy diet and/or not exercising regularly) also increase your risk—much more so than genetics. That's why one twin in a set of identical twins can get Alzheimer's while the other twin stays healthy.

There's even more good news—a diagnosis of Alzheimer's is not necessarily the disaster you probably imagine it to be. Alzheimer's

Calcium and Dementia

Women over age 70 who had suffered strokes were seven times more likely to develop dementia if they took calcium supplements. Women with no history of stroke or lesions in the brain's white matter had no increased risk for dementia from calcium supplements.

Theory: High calcium levels may damage nerve cells in vulnerable areas of the brain, so consult your doctor before taking calcium supplements.

Note: Calcium from food might be protective against vascular problems.

Silke Kern, MD, PhD, senior researcher, University of Gothenburg, Sweden.

is now viewed by most medical professionals as a so-called "spectrum disorder," rather than a single disease, because different people have different symptoms and different rates of progression.

Most people diagnosed with Alzheimer's are not on the catastrophic end of that spectrum—they are not going to forget who they are or the names of their loved ones. Most will live at home and die at home, particularly if the disease is detected early and symptoms are well-managed with treatments such as medication, a healthy diet and regular exercise.

Bottom line: Even if you are at genetic risk, you can use lifestyle modifications to reduce your risk to below that of someone who has no family history of Alzheimer's.

How to Tweak Your Lifestyle

Most cases of late-onset Alzheimer's disease are preventable—with simple lifestyle changes that reduce one's risk for the disease.

The brain changes of Alzheimer's (the so-called plaques and tangles, which are accumulations of toxic proteins) can start 20 to 30 years before the onset of symptoms. But research shows that preventive measures can stop plaques and tangles as well as symptoms from ever developing...and even prevent symptoms if your brain is riddled with plaques and tangles.

Factors that increase Alzheimer's risk for everyone—regardless of one's genetic predisposition—and how to counteract them...

• **Sedentary lifestyle.** Exercising for 45 minutes, at least three days a week (at an intensity that is 50% higher than your resting heart rate) is a must for reducing your risk for Alzheimer's. It stimulates blood flow to the brain, allowing new neurons to grow. Research shows that it decreases your risk for Alzheimer's by 40%.

Surprising fact: Cognitive abilities such as memory improve by 10% immediately after exercise.

• **Poor diet.** A diet loaded with saturated fats, refined sugar and processed foods increases the risk for Alzheimer's. A Mediterranean-style diet—rich in whole foods such as vegetables, fruits, beans, whole grains and fish—is proven to reduce the risk for Alzheimer's by 50%.

Also helpful: A healthy breakfast, which consists of protein, fiber and fruit. Research shows that if you take in less than 7% of your daily calories at breakfast, your risk for heart disease and Alzheimer's more than doubles.

• **Limited mental stimulation.** Regular mental stimulation reduces Alzheimer's risk—in fact, research shows that even reading a newspaper every day can help prevent the disease.

Best: Engage in a type of mental stimulation that is different from what you do at work, thereby stimulating a different part of your brain.

Example: If you are a computer programmer, learn how to play golf.

• **Social isolation.** Healthy social relationships—with family, friends and in the community—decrease the risk for Alzheimer's disease. Feeling lonely doubles the risk...living alone raises it fivefold.

• **Heart disease.** Circulatory problems cause heart disease and Alzheimer's disease. Medical and lifestyle treatments for cardiovascular issues, including high blood pressure, reduce Alzheimer's risk.

Bottom line: What's good for your heart is good for your brain.

• **Diabetes.** Some experts label Alzheimer's "type 3 diabetes" because of the established link between chronically high blood sugar and the risk for Alzheimer's disease—a person with diabetes has a 57% higher risk of developing the disease. Controlling high blood sugar with medical and lifestyle treatments is crucial for reducing Alzheimer's risk.

Helpful: Keep your glucose level below 100 mg/dL.

• **Insomnia.** Poor sleep increases risk for Alzheimer's, probably because brain plaque is cleared most effectively during sleep. But sleep medications aren't the answer—they also interfere with the clearance of brain plaque.

What works better: Good sleep hygiene, such as going to bed and waking up at the same time every day.

Also helpful: Don't work on your computer in bed or keep your cell phone on your bedside table.

What's Your Genetic Risk?

Genetics is a strong factor when Alzheimer's begins at a young age. The early-onset form is an aggressive familial illness that can occur, in extremely rare cases, as early as in one's 20s, with most people developing the disease in their 50s or 60s. The child of a parent with early-onset Alzheimer's has a 50% chance of developing the disease. Fortunately, early-onset constitutes only 5% of all cases of Alzheimer's disease.

On the other hand, most cases of late-onset Alzheimer's (beginning after age 65) are not inherited. Instead, many medical and lifestyle factors contribute to the development of the illness.

Compelling scientific research: In one of the largest scientific studies that I have ever completed, published in *Archives of Neurology*, I looked at more than 5,500 siblings and parents of patients with Alzheimer's—alongside age-matched adults who did not have the disease.

Presuming (for uniform statistical analysis) that everyone in the study lived to age 90, I found that those with a first-degree relative with Alzheimer's had about a one-in-four chance of developing late-onset Alzheimer's—whereas those without an afflicted relative had a one-in-five chance of doing so.

In other words, if neither your parents nor siblings have (or had) Alzheimer's (and you live to age 90), you still have a 20% chance of getting the disease—while a person whose parent or sibling had Alzheimer's has a 26% chance.

Takeaway: Having a parent or sibling with Alzheimer's puts you at a relatively small increased risk for the disease.

Exception: A person with late-onset Alzheimer's who also has a variant of the apolipoprotein E gene—APOE e4 (the most damaging of the so-called "Alzheimer's genes")—is more likely to have rapid progression of the disease.

Genetic Testing

My take on genetic testing for Alzheimer's: It may be appropriate only for people with a family history of early-onset Alzheimer's disease (before age 65). If a parent has early-onset Alzheimer's, as mentioned earlier, the child has a 50% chance of developing the disease. An estimated 200,000 Americans have the early-onset form of the disease.

If you have this type of family history, consult your doctor and a genetic counselor about genetic testing. Not all the genes that trigger early-onset Alzheimer's are known, but some are. If you decide to have a genetic test—and the test finds that you have one of the genetic mutations for Alzheimer's—you and your family can take that fact into account in various ways.

For example, you would want to create a step-by-step action plan for dealing with the disease, even before symptoms develop, by preparing for the future with advanced directives and financial planning...and perhaps consider entering one of the clinical trials that are testing new drugs to slow Alzheimer's development. (To find such a trial, consult ClinicalTrials.gov and search "early-onset Alzheimer's.")

Important: If you don't have a family history of early-onset Alzheimer's, I typically do not recommend genetic testing. The results would not accurately quantify your risk, and it's crucial that you implement key medical treatments (such as those for high blood pressure or diabetes) and lifestyle changes to reduce your risk for Alzheimer's whether or not you have a genetic variant for late-onset Alzheimer's.

What Your Eyes Say About Your Alzheimer's Risk

Maya Koronyo-Hamaoui, PhD, associate professor in the departments of neurosurgery and biomedical sciences at Cedars-Sinai Medical Center in Los Angeles and senior author of this study.

It's been said that the eyes are the window to the soul...but they may also be a window to the brain!

What's new: Researchers have discovered that a noninvasive, experimental eye scan that examines the back of the eyes (the retinas) may detect signs of Alzheimer's disease that usually appear long before any symptoms occur—and possibly pave the way for earlier treatment approaches that could change the course of the disease.

Background: Traditionally, the only way to officially diagnose Alzheimer's disease was to analyze a person's brain after he/she had died. Even though the use of positron emission tomography (PET) scans for living patients provides evidence of the disease and has recently become more widely used, this test is expensive, involves the use of potentially harmful radiation and requires the patient to be injected with radioactive tracers, which in rare cases cause an allergic reaction.

So what prompted scientists to investigate whether the eyes could provide important clues about Alzheimer's disease?

When brain tissue from deceased Alzheimer's patients is examined under a microscope, two types of protein abnormalities (known as plaques and tangles) appear that are characteristic of the disease. The plaques are made of clumps of a protein called beta-amyloid (believed to be an early sign of the Alzheimer's disease process) that induce inflammation and cause damage to brain cells, while tangles form inside brain cells, where they prevent the transport of nutrients, causing the cells to die.

Based on earlier research suggesting that the eyes may provide important clues about brain health, scientists at Cedars-Sinai Medical Center in Los Angeles decided to further investigate this theory with a carefully designed study.

Study details: Ten patients with symptoms of mild-to-moderate Alzheimer's disease and six younger, cognitively healthy individuals (controls) consumed a solution containing curcumin (a natural component of the spice turmeric) that caused the amyloid plaques in their retinas to "light up" during a high-definition eye scan. When the results were compared, there was a 2.6-fold increase in plaques in the retinas of the Alzheimer's patients compared with the controls.

Implication: Analyzing the retina is a particularly appealing way to detect Alzheimer's early on because an eye scan is relatively easy to repeat, which allows doctors to monitor patients and the progression of their disease to tell whether any treatments are helping.

Note: The scan used in this study captures peripheral retinal regions that are not normally examined in a standard retinal exam.

Bottom line: While more study is needed to determine whether eye scans will ever become widely used to predict Alzheimer's disease, stay tuned! If additional research confirms these findings in larger studies, eye scans could become a simple, inexpensive way to identify signs of Alzheimer's years before symptoms appear.

Questions to Ask If You Are Diagnosed with Alzheimer's Disease

Alzheimer's Association, American Academy of Neurologists, Harvard Medical School, Mayo Clinic.

A diagnosis of Alzheimer's can be terrifying. But the more you know about what to expect, the better off you'll be. *If your doctor tells you that you have Alzheimer's disease, here are important questions to ask...*

• **Are you sure it's Alzheimer's disease?** Doctors can diagnose "probable Alzheimer's disease" with about 90% accuracy. But there's always room for error because many forms of dementia can mimic Alzheimer's. Ask your doctor how he/she will confirm that you actually have Alzheimer's and not another form of dementia that could possibly be more treatable (such as dementia caused by thyroid problems or a vitamin deficiency).

• **What will happen to me first?** With early Alzheimer's, you might notice occasional (and slight) memory lapses. Your cognitive abilities will continue to worsen over time. Some people misplace things, and some make poor decisions or engage in uncharacteristically aggressive behavior. Your doctor can tell you what's typical for each of the three stages of Alzheimer's, but the specific symptoms will vary from person to person.

• **How will my moods change?** You might become suspicious of close friends or family members. You might get angry more than you used to or become increasingly agitated toward the end of each day. If you do notice mood changes, ask your doctor what you can do to cope. In some Alzheimer's patients, certain behavior changes are due to something else altogether—such as depression.

• **What medications are you going to prescribe for me, and why?** Depending on your symptoms and stage, you might be given *donepezil* (Aricept) or *memantine* (Namenda). A newer drug, Namzaric, combines both of these drugs in a one-a-day capsule. The drugs can help improve memory/confusion and delay the worsening of symptoms, although they cannot cure the disease. You might need other drugs—such as antianxiety medications—as well.

• **Could nondrug treatments make a difference in my case?** Preliminary research finds that omega-3 fatty acids may slow cognitive declines in Alzheimer's patients who are missing a particular gene. (The US Food and Drug Administration recommends no more than three grams daily from food and supplement sources combined.) A supplement called huperzine A (a moss extract) has shown some benefit—it has properties that are similar to some Alzheimer's drugs. Check with your doctor before starting (or continuing to take) any supplement.

• **Should I increase my exercise?** There's some evidence that vigorous exercise can slow or temporarily stop cognitive declines in those with an early stage of Alzheimer's disease. But hard exercise isn't safe for everyone—and it might or might not help. Your doctor can help you design the best exercise program for you.

• **Is it safe for me to drive?** Personal safety is always an issue as Alzheimer's progresses. The American Academy of Neurologists says that no one with Alzheimer's (regardless of the stage) should drive a car, though other experts advise deciding case-by-case. Get your doctor's opinion on your situation.

Dance Your Way to a Healthy Brain

Dancing may be good for your brain. The white matter in the brain, which passes messages around the brain, deteriorates as people age. Men and women who were taught increasingly complex country-dancing choreography three times a week for six months had improvement in the denseness of their white matter. But people who did brisk walking or a program of gentle stretching and balance training had declines in their white matter. The cognitive demands of the dancing, which became more and more intricate over time, may have helped strengthen the brain.

Agnieszka Burzynska, PhD, assistant professor of human development and family studies, Colorado State University, Fort Collins, and leader of a study of 174 people in their 60s and 70s, published in *Frontiers in Aging.*

Walk This Way to a Better Brain

Ernest R. Greene, PhD, New Mexico Highlands University, Las Vegas, coauthor of study titled "Acute Effects of Walking on Human Internal Carotid Blood Flow," published in *FASEB Journal.*

For a sharper brain, put your best foot forward. Actually, put either foot forward. Repeatedly.

The physical act of putting your foot on the ground, the impact of your foot, sets in motion a rhythmic response in your cardiovascular system that stimulates beneficial blood flow to the brain, according to a new scientific discovery.

Background: Oxygen is the brain's fuel. Although the brain represents only 2% of an average person's body weight, it uses 20% of the body's oxygen. No wonder optimal brain function relies on robust blood flow—aka, cerebral blood flow (CBF)—to deliver oxygen. Optimal CBF is necessary to meet the brain's metabolic demands and to regulate blood pressure inside the brain. Until recently, CBF was thought to be a constant thing, unrelated to the ups and downs of blood pressure as it changes during, for example, exercise. Then researchers at New Mexico Highlands University in Las Vegas found that vigorous running stimulated CBF. They wondered if everyday walking had a similar effect.

Study: The research team studied 12 healthy young adults, either standing at rest or walking at an easy stride—a little over two miles an hour. They used ultrasound to measure blood flow in the carotid artery, the major conduit of oxygenated blood to the brain.

Finding: Each time the foot hits the ground, it sends a subtle rhythmic pulse upward through the arteries, a kind of blood pressure "wave" that can dynamically increase blood flow to the brain by about 10% to 20%. With walking, the effect isn't as strong as with running—that's 20% to 50%—but it's significant. The retrograde pressure effect doesn't happen at all with nonimpact aerobic exercise (cycling), according to earlier research by the same group.

Bottom line: If you love cycling or swimming or other nonimpact aerobics...by all means keep at it—regular aerobic exercise of any kind is good for the cardiovascular system and brain health, and can help protect against dementia. Strength training is brain-healthy too. But there is something specific to walking and running that helps regulate the brain's blood flow. The rhythmic foot impact, the authors speculate, may optimize blood flow to the brain and thus improve brain function—which may in turn improve one's overall sense of well-being, and could possibly translate into helping to prevent vascular dementia. The next time your mind is foggy, try a walk around the block to get the

Diet Soda and Dementia

Adults who drank one or more artificially sweetened soft drinks daily were almost three times more likely to develop dementia or suffer a stroke, compared with those who did not consume diet drinks, according to a recent 17-year observational study.

Self-defense: Drink water instead of artificially sweetened drinks or sugary beverages, which have been linked in earlier studies to obesity and related chronic conditions.

Matthew P. Pase, PhD, researcher, department of neurology, Boston University School of Medicine.

blood moving to your brain. Wearing thin-soled shoes will give you a stronger pulse—and help increase your bone density! Even better—start a walking book club.

Video Games May Help Protect the Brain

Older adults who played Super Mario 64, a 3-D logic-and-puzzle game, for 30 minutes a day, five days a week, for six months, had increased volume of gray matter in the brain's hippocampus and cerebellum regions—and their short-term memory improved. The effects were not seen in people who took piano lessons for six months or in a control group that did neither activity. Gray matter normally atrophies as people age. Learning new things may help slow the atrophy—but the reason for the specific effectiveness of the video game in this study remains unknown.

Gregory West, PhD, associate professor of psychology, Université de Montréal, Canada, and coauthor of a study published in *PLOS ONE*.

Your Brain Is Hungry!

Drew Ramsey, MD, an assistant clinical professor of psychiatry at Columbia University College of Physicians and Surgeons in New York City, and a leading expert in the use of nutrition for improving mood, brain function and mental health. He produced the Eat to Beat Depression e-course and is the author of *Eat Complete: The 21 Nutrients That Fuel Brainpower, Boost Weight Loss, and Transform Your Health, Fifty Shades of Kale* and *The Happiness Diet.* DrewRamseyMD.com

If you had a doughnut and coffee for breakfast, you probably wouldn't be that surprised if you felt sluggish and even a little blue afterward. Had you started your day with, say, eggs and whole-grain toast or a veggie- and fruit-packed smoothie, you'd expect to feel much better.

While most of us know from our own experience how our diet affects our moods and energy levels, scientific evidence now shows just how crucial food is as "brain fuel."

Latest development: For the first time, high-quality scientific research has confirmed that dietary changes can dramatically improve depression. In fact, diet plays such a fundamental role in mental health that nutritional psychiatry is increasingly being incorporated into evidence-based mental-health practices to help prevent and treat depression and anxiety and even guard against dementia.

To learn more about this important new approach, we spoke with Drew Ramsey, MD, a psychiatrist and leading proponent of the use of dietary changes to improve brain health.

How do the foods we eat affect our brains? Let's begin with the idea that all the molecules in your brain start at the end of your fork. For example, for your brain to produce serotonin, a brain chemical that regulates moods (and sex drive) along with weight, you must consume tryptophan, an amino acid found in higher amounts in some foods such as pumpkin seeds, asparagus, fish and meats.

Other nutrients, such as zinc and omega-3 fatty acids, are key building blocks of the brain and affect neurogenesis (the creation of new brain cells)...levels of brain-derived neurotrophic factor (a hormone that you need to stave off depression)...and chronic inflammation, which is also linked to depression.

Do foods make a big difference or just a little? There isn't a single "superfood" for treating depression or other mood disorders. But dietary changes—eating more plant foods and seafood and cutting out fast food and simple sugars—clearly help, whether they're used alone or in combination with antidepressants or talk therapy.

Haven't we known for a while that nutrition plays a role in brain health? Many studies have suggested that nutritional changes can help patients with mood problems, but there's never been conclusive proof. That changed with the SMILES (Supporting the Modification of Lifestyle Intervention in

Lowered Emotional States) trial, which was published in early 2017 in the journal *BMC Medicine*.

It was the first-ever randomized, controlled clinical study to investigate dietary interventions for treating clinical depression. The study looked at 67 men and women with moderate-to-severe depression, most of whom were taking an antidepressant or receiving regular psychotherapy. Half were put on a Mediterranean-style diet for 12 weeks... the other half continued to follow their usual (and largely unhealthy) diets.

After three months, nearly one-third of those who made dietary changes had improved so much that they no longer met the clinical criteria for clinical depression. In other words, they had full remissions. Those who hadn't improved their diets had only an 8% remission rate.

Can nutrition help with dementia? A healthy diet can help prevent vascular causes of dementia, such as stroke. There's also good evidence that many of the plant-based molecules such as lycopene (found in tomatoes and other red fruits and vegetables) and flavonols (found in onions, wine, chocolate and many other healthy foods) can produce brain changes that reduce the risk for different forms of dementia, including Alzheimer's disease.

What foods do you usually recommend? I focus on overall dietary patterns and categories of brain healthy foods (such as seafood, leafy greens and colorful "rainbow" vegetables)...complex carbohydrates (such as whole grains)...grass-fed meat and dairy...and free-range poultry and eggs.

Important: Seafood is a crucial food category that's missing from most Americans' diets. I advise everyone to eat more salmon, bivalves (such as oysters and mussels), anchovies and other types of seafood.

What about supplements? Several clinical trials have shown that specific supplements—fish oil, zinc, B vitamins, etc.—might be helpful for alleviating depression and other mood problems. Supplements are convenient if you don't eat seafood (a main source of omega-3s), follow a restrictive diet (vegans need to take vitamin B-12) or have a deficiency in need of rapid correction. I tend to emphasize food because no one sits down to a fine meal of vitamins and supplement shakes!

What Are Your Nutrient Levels?

To rule out medical causes of depression, including thyroid disorders, and to check levels of certain nutrients (such as vitamin D and vitamin B-12), psychiatrists routinely order blood tests. A nutritional psychiatry assessment can also be conducted to understand what patients are eating...when they eat... what their favorite snacks are...and so on.

While physicians typically haven't learned much about nutrition in medical school beyond basic biochemistry, this is changing! A culinary medicine curriculum developed by Tulane Medical School is being adopted by 28 medical schools around the country. And the American Psychiatric Association has recently offered the Brain Food Workshop, developed by researchers at Columbia University, at its professional meetings.

Foods That Trash Your Brain

Joel Fuhrman, MD, a board-certified family physician, nutritional researcher and president of Nutritional Research Foundation in Flemington, New Jersey. Dr. Fuhrman has coauthored numerous studies in peer-reviewed medical journals and is author of six books. His most recent book is *Fast Food Genocide: How Processed Food Is Killing Us and What We Can Do About It.* DrFuhrman.com

Most of us know that fast food is bad for us—contributing to obesity, heart disease, stroke and diabetes.

But did you know that fast food can also affect your brain, quickly turning you into a fast-food addict—someone helplessly compelled to overeat this unhealthy fare? Plus, eating fast food can lead to mental issues such as depression, chronic anger, lack of focus and much more due to the toxicity and nutritional deficiencies it causes.

What Exactly Is Fast Food?

"Fast food" doesn't just mean the food you buy at a fast-food restaurant chain. It can be any commercially made, highly processed food that you can get fast, eat fast and digest fast.

Fast food is typically highly flavored and delivers lots of calories but offers few vitamins, minerals and phytochemicals (the active compounds found in plants). It's high in harmful ingredients such as sugar and white flour (which is quickly converted to sugar)... salt...unhealthy oils...artificial ingredients, including artificial color and flavor...preservatives...and thickeners. Plus, it's low in fiber.

Examples of fast food other than a burger and fries: Most deli sandwiches, frozen pizza, many breakfast cereals, a bag of chips, cookies, candy and soda. You might be surprised to know that plenty of organic packaged foods also fall under the fast-food category.

Startling: The majority of Americans get more than half of their calories from fast food.

Fast-Food Addiction

Fast foods can be as addictive as cocaine and other drugs. Food manufacturers design them that way so you'll buy more of their products. *How they hook you...*

• **The low-fiber calories from fast food quickly flood the bloodstream**—a typical fast-food meal is absorbed far faster than a serving of beans. That rush of calories produces a surge of dopamine, the neurotransmitter (brain chemical) that gives us feelings of pleasure. In fact, the amount of pleasure we derive from eating a food directly correlates with the amount of dopamine released in the brain. To repeat and sustain these pleasurable feelings, you desire and eat more fast food.

Additionally, dopamine levels that skyrocket daily quickly lead to dopamine insensitivity—the same amount of dopamine no longer creates the same amount of pleasure.

Upshot: A person who eats a lot of fast food, will crave fast food...overeat fast food ...and become literally addicted to fast food.

• **Trying to break the cycle of overeating fast food is like trying to stop taking drugs.** When you stop eating fast foods, you'll experience withdrawal symptoms as your body starts to detoxify—you may feel shaky, weak, fatigued, headachy, anxious, irritable—and crave more fast food to end those symptoms.

The Malnourished Brain

Modern medical science regularly warns that eating fast food can cause heart disease, fatty liver and kidney failure but ignores the fact that fast food also affects the brain—our most vulnerable organ.

Multiple studies have found a link between an unhealthy diet and impaired brain function and emotional problems. Depression and other mood disorders don't have one specific cause, but research shows that a bad diet can be a major risk factor.

Recent research: A meta-analysis including studies from 10 countries published in 2017 in *Psychiatry Research* found that a diet high in refined grains, sweets and red and/

Go "Green" for Your Brain

People who ate the most leafy greens daily (just over one serving, such as one cup of raw spinach or one-half cup cooked) over a 10-year period had brains that were roughly 11 years "younger" in terms of memory and cognition than people who reported rarely or never eating greens, according to a study of 960 adults ages 58 to 99 without dementia. Whether cooked or raw, spinach, kale and other leafy greens are rich in vitamins E and K, lutein and other substances that may slow cognitive decline.

Martha Clare Morris, ScD, director of nutritional epidemiology, Rush University Medical Center, Chicago.

or processed meat is associated with an increased risk for depression.

Additionally, anger, irritability and aggression...mood swings...poor concentration...brain fog (mental confusion that can include lack of focus, poor memory and reduced mental acuity) and other mental problems can be caused by the toxins in fast food, and/or by the nutritional deficiencies that arise from consuming fast food regularly. Fast food is also linked to Alzheimer's and other forms of dementia.

New research: A study published in *American Journal of Clinical Nutrition* shows that the brains of people who eat a sugary diet that floods the brain with glucose—in other words, a fast-food diet—have much higher levels of beta-amyloid, the toxic protein that accumulates in the brain and is linked to Alzheimer's disease.

That's the bad news. The good news is that there is an easy way out of fast-food addiction and the emotional and intellectual symptoms caused by eating fast food.

Restoring Brain Health

The first step in ending fast-food addiction is to start eating more high-nutrient foods—foods that contain all the vitamins and minerals we require, as well as the phytochemicals and antioxidants that allow brain cells and other cells damaged by fast food to repair themselves. Just cutting back on the fast food you've been eating is not sufficient—people who try to do this almost always fail.

My advice: Eat plenty of Greens, Beans, Onions, Mushrooms, Berries and Seeds, or "G-BOMBS," the superstars of the whole foods menu. To get more of these foods, include them in a big salad every day and add them to whatever you are cooking.

Also: Make a big batch of vegetable-bean soup on Sunday, freeze several servings in pint-size containers, and eat it all week long.

By eating more high-nutrient, high-fiber foods, you'll gradually develop less desire for fast foods.

Try to crowd out all the fast food you've been eating within one week. With this approach, withdrawal symptoms should last no more than three days. After four to six months, the taste buds—dulled by too much sugar and salt—will typically recuperate, allowing you to once again enjoy subtle natural flavors...and you will have lost your emotional attachment to fast foods.

Also: Whenever possible, don't eat alone! Research shows that when people are isolated and lonely, they tend to make bad food choices. When you're experiencing love and connection—and the positive reinforcement and encouragement that go with it—it's much easier to choose healthy food.

Helpful: Join a group (in-person or online) of others interested in eating healthfully so that you can encourage one another. Check with your local health-food store or cooperative, or look online for a Meetup group.

Dirty Air and Dementia

Older women who live in areas where fine-particulate air pollution (emitted by vehicles and power plants) exceeds EPA standards are 92% more likely to develop dementia than those in EPA-compliant areas.

Implication: Based on estimates that 30% of the population reside in areas exceeding EPA standards, fine-particulate air pollution may be responsible for 21% of dementia cases in the US.

Jiu-Chiuan Chen, MD, ScD, associate professor, Keck School of Medicine, University of Southern California, Los Angeles.

Power Up Your Brain!

Concentrated beetroot juice before a workout may boost brainpower.

Recent study: An hour before a 50-minute workout, 26 sedentary adults consumed beetroot juice or a placebo. Over six weeks, beetroot drinkers showed increased brain plasticity, which aids in learning. Beets are rich in nitrates, which help the blood carry oxygen—including to the brain.

Caution: If you are at risk for kidney stones or take medications for heart conditions or erectile dysfunction, consult your doctor before trying the juice.

W. Jack Rejeski, PhD, director, Behavioral Medicine Laboratory, Wake Forest University, Winston-Salem, North Carolina.

Safer Drug to Ease Dementia Psychosis

Clive Ballard, MD, professor of age-related diseases, University of Exeter, England.
Gisele Wolf-Klein, MD, director, geriatric education, Northwell Health, Great Neck, New York.
Gayatri Devi, MD, neurologist, Lenox Hill Hospital, New York City.
University of Exeter, news release.

The "overmedication" of agitated dementia patients—with the use of powerful antipsychotic drugs—is an ongoing issue in US health care.

Now, British researchers say they may have found a medicine that helps ease those symptoms, but in a much safer way.

The newer antipsychotic *pimavanserin* appears to ease psychosis symptoms in people with Alzheimer's disease without the serious side effects caused by current antipsychotics, according to a study funded by the drug's maker.

Background

According to the researchers, psychosis affects up to half of the 45 million Alzheimer's patients worldwide, and that percentage is even higher among patients with other types of dementia.

Currently, there is no approved safe and effective treatment for this common symptom. Standard antipsychotics are widely used, but they can also raise the risk of falls, stroke and even death, and have been linked to a doubling in the rate of brain function decline, according to the study authors.

One study released a few months earlier found that, given these concerns, the percentage of long-term US nursing home residents receiving antipsychotic drugs fell from about 24% in late 2011 to less than 16% in 2017. But advocates for patients say the rate should still be much lower.

"Psychosis is a particularly terrifying symptom of Alzheimer's disease," explained Clive Ballard, MD, the lead author of the current study.

"People may experience paranoia, or see, hear or smell things that are not there. It's distressing both for those experiencing the delusions and for their [caregivers]," said Dr. Ballard, who is professor of age-related diseases at the University of Exeter in England.

The Study

The new phase 2 clinical trial included 180 Alzheimer's patients with psychosis. Ninety of them took pimavanserin and 90 were given a placebo, over a three-month period. The study was funded by Acadia Pharmaceuticals, which markets pimavanserin under the brand name Nuplazid.

Reported in *Lancet Neurology*, the study found that pimavanserin seems to alleviate psychotic symptoms without many of the side effects seen with standard antipsychotics.

"It's particularly encouraging that most benefit was seen in those with the most severe psychotic symptom, as this group is most likely to be prescribed antipsychotics," said Dr. Ballard.

"We are talking about vulnerable elderly, frail people who are suffering terrifying symptoms, being sedated with current antipsychotics even though it's well-known that they cause terrible health issues and even death in people with dementia, and have very little benefit," he said.

How It Works

A prior study found that pimavanserin was effective for people with dementia related to

Parkinson's disease, and it's been approved by the US Food and Drug Administration for this use.

As the researchers explained, the drug works differently from standard antipsychotics, because it blocks a specific nerve receptor (THT2A) in the brain.

Expert Commentary

One geriatrician who's unconnected to the study said pimavanserin does show promise.

The new study "demonstrated that the medication was well-tolerated and did reduce hallucinations at week six," said Gisele Wolf-Klein, MD. She directs geriatric education at Northwell Health in Great Neck, New York.

Dr. Wolf-Klein noted that patients included those "with possible and probable Alzheimer's disease and psychotic symptoms, including visual or auditory hallucinations, delusions or both."

She said that the longer-term effectiveness of pimavanserin remains to be seen, but the drug may be useful for patients experiencing "short term delusions, as seen in acute delirium."

"This option is of particular interest since the safety profile of this drug shows no detrimental effect on cognitive and motor symptoms, contrary to atypical antipsychotics," Dr. Wolf-Klein said.

Gayatri Devi, MD, is a neurologist at Lenox Hill Hospital in New York City who often works with Alzheimer's patients. She stressed that any drug "that is effective for treating psychotic symptoms, which are often more disturbing to caregivers than memory impairment, is very important in allowing patients to function and live at home."

Indeed, Dr. Devi added that "one of the most common reasons for institutionalization is psychotic symptoms, including delusions and hallucinations. Many currently available drugs have serious adverse effects and drugs with fewer side effects are desperately needed."

According to Dr. Ballard's team, the safety and effectiveness of pimavanserin in reducing psychotic symptoms in dementia is now being assessed in a larger clinical trial in the United States.

The National Institute on Aging's website, NIA.nih.gov, has more information about Alzheimer's disease. Search "Alzheimer's."

Even Moderate Drinking Is Bad for the Brain

Over a 30-year period, people who drank as few as four pints of strong beer or five large glasses of wine a week had hippocampal atrophy, a type of brain damage often found in people with Alzheimer's disease. Light drinkers—up to three small glasses of wine or two pints of beer a week—showed no decrease in brain function.

Anya Topiwala, MD, PhD, clinical lecturer in old age psychiatry in the department of psychiatry at University of Oxford, UK.

Women with Parkinson's Receive Less Care

Nabila Dahodwala, MD, associate professor of neurology, University of Pennsylvania School of Medicine, Philadelphia.

University of Pennsylvania, news release.

Women with Parkinson's disease appear to face a disadvantage: They're much less likely than men to have caregivers, a new study finds.

That's probably because women often outlive their most likely potential caregiver—their husband, according to researchers at the University of Pennsylvania School of Medicine.

"Care provided by family and friends to people with Parkinson's disease is an important source of support, and our findings show that women living with Parkinson's are less likely to receive this support than men," said study author Nabila Dahodwala, MD, an associate professor of neurology.

"We need strategies to improve women's access to this support," Dr. Dahodwala said.

About Parkinson's Disease

Parkinson's disease affects 1% of people older than 60, with likelihood increasing with age. It affects certain nerve cells in the brain and interferes with movement. There is no cure, but medications and sometimes surgery can help.

Study Findings

For this study, researchers examined data from more than 7,200 Parkinson's patients in the United States, Canada, the Netherlands and Israel. They found that 79% of female patients reported having a caregiver, compared with 88% of male patients.

Men were also more likely than women to have a caregiver accompany them on their first visit to a study center (61% versus 57%).

Spouses were caregivers for 84% of male patients, compared with just 67% of female patients, according to the study.

Moreover, women were more than twice as likely (3% vs. 1.3%) to have a paid caregiver.

The researchers also found that caregivers of female patients reported much less mental strain than caregivers of male patients.

The study was published in the journal *Neurology.*

Implications

While the study did not examine the reasons for the male/female difference in caregiver support, Dr. Dahodwala noted that women on average tend to live a few years longer than men. Also, women are more likely to take on the role of caregiver.

"Changes in health policy to better support older women with disabilities are urgently needed," Dr. Dahodwala said.

For more information on Parkinson's disease, visit the Parkinson's Foundation at Parkinson.org.

Singing Helps Parkinson's Patients

When 24 Parkinson's patients participated in 60 minutes of vocal drills and singing weekly for eight weeks, their swallowing and respiratory function improved significantly.

The reason: Singing exercises the same muscles as those used for swallowing and breathing, both of which are affected by Parkinson's. Researchers are now studying whether singing is beneficial for others with swallowing issues (due to stroke, for example).

Elizabeth Stegemöller, PhD, assistant professor of kinesiology, Iowa State University, Ames.

How to Stop Your Attention Span from Shrinking

Cynthia Green, PhD, a clinical psychologist, author and one of America's foremost experts on brain health. She is founding director of The Memory Enhancement Program at Icahn School of Medicine at Mount Sinai, New York City, and president and CEO of Total Brain Health and TBH Brands, LLC, in Montclair, New Jersey. CynthiaGreenPhD.com

Admit it—you reach for your smartphone every time you're waiting in a line or even when you wake up at night. We won't even mention that bathroom thing.

When you're home, you're surfing the Internet…or you have the radio or TV on as a constant backdrop…or both. No wonder it's harder to concentrate for any length of time than it used to be. While it's great to connect with old friends on Facebook or be able to look up sports or movie trivia any time, the impact this has on our attention spans is not good…at all.

Why that matters: Cognitive decline is real and can begin as young as age 45 even if you are healthy. We're not talking about dementia, either—smaller problems, such as forgetting someone's name, can be a normal part of aging. Research has shown that continuing to learn is key to minimizing this decline—but to learn, you need to focus.

How Distractions Affect Learning

Say we just met. If I tell you my name at the same time that your phone starts vibrating in your pocket and you glance at the screen, you're not going to hear what I said. Later, you'll think you forgot my name, but you never learned it in the first place!

Constantly switching between activities and attempting to multitask (which no one is really good at) is exhausting for the brain, draining it of the energy needed to focus.

Result: We make mistakes big and small and are less productive, more forgetful and just slower at everything.

So...it's time to rebuild your attention span and your ability to focus. Like any skill, it takes practice. The point isn't only to ward off future cognitive disease but also to improve your ability to accomplish more and feel less stress from perpetual distractions...now.

Concentration Builders

You probably expect me to tell you to stop using technology so much. Sure, that will help. But few of us can resist its lure for long, and these days no one wants to miss that important e-mail or breaking news flash. Instead, you need to exercise better control over the disruptions, put technology to work for you and engage in activities that strengthen attention. *My recommendations...*

• **Stop being so available.** You don't have to answer every call, text or e-mail the minute you receive it—and the truth is, you don't even have to know about every call, text or e-mail the minute you receive it, either. When you're working on a must-do or should-do task, eliminate distractions. Turn off the TV, and quit e-mail, text notifications, Facebook, Twitter and news app notifications until you get your task done. If there are certain people who you feel must be able to reach you instantly, set your phone and other devices to "do not disturb" but program in exceptions for those people.

• **Build up your tolerance.** Digital withdrawal is hard, so take a lesson from behavior-modification therapy and reward yourself for small successes. Set certain times of day when you'll check e-mail, etc., and don't look in between. Start by telling yourself, I'll go for 15 minutes without checking my device, and then when the time is up, give yourself five minutes to glance at e-mail, Facebook, etc. Next, extend your uninterrupted time to 30 minutes before checking, then 45 minutes, then an hour. And experiment with rewards that don't entail going online, such as having a cappuccino.

• **Find a meditative hobby.** I'm not going to tell you that you have to meditate to improve your attention span—although "mindful meditation," including special breathing and visualization exercises, does exactly that by increasing brain volume and density in areas that improve cognitive function such as the hippocampus. But if you're not into meditation, you can get similar benefits from the regular practice of other focused, meditative activities such as gardening...walking in nature...running...swimming laps...drawing or painting...knitting or crocheting...yoga or tai chi.

If you would like to try actual meditation, you don't have to go to a class. Online meditation training (yes, I see the irony of online training!) provides similar benefits to sitting in a meditation class, studies suggest. One

Don't Stop Daydreaming

Daydreaming may be a sign of intelligence. People who reported more frequent daydreaming earned higher scores on measures of intellectual and creative abilities.

Eric Schumacher, PhD, associate professor of psychology, Georgia Tech University, Atlanta, and coauthor of a study of more than 100 people's brain patterns, published in *Neuropsychologia*.

app that I recommend is Headspace, which provides mini-meditations and mindfulness exercises (Apple and Android, $12.99 a month or $7.99 a month if you pay for the year).

• **Get moving.** Regular aerobic exercise also expands the size of the hippocampus. Activity that gets your heart pumping stimulates the release of chemicals that improve the health and survival of brain cells and promotes the growth of new blood vessels in the brain.

Result: You'll think faster and more clearly. Yes, even brisk walking counts!

• **Be social offline.** Social media helps us keep in touch with friends and family and introduces us to new people we might not ever encounter otherwise. But we lose out on the many cognitive benefits of face-to-face social interaction.

Example: Online, you can take time to frame your thoughts before you answer or comment, but you can't pause for five minutes when someone asks you in person, "What's the best mystery you ever read?" By putting yourself in more situations where you have to answer questions and make decisions immediately, you're exercising that ability to think on your feet.

What to do: Get out there with people… and talk!

• **Play timed games.** There are all kinds of purported brain-training and memory-boosting activities, but to rebuild attention span, choose ones that make you beat the clock. Timed word games such as Boggle, in which you have three minutes to choose the right word, are ideal because you have to pay attention and think fast. Sports such as racquetball and tennis, and even dancing, also are great choices because you have to move and react within a certain time.

Tip: Dance lessons, which require you to learn new steps, are especially effective because you're using your body and your brain and socializing all at once.

• **Drink up.** Mild dehydration interferes with the ability to concentrate, but here's the catch—your attention span suffers even if you aren't feeling thirsty yet. So drink water throughout the day whether you think you need it or not.

• **Break out the wiggy music.** Listening to symphonies moves the brain to pay attention as it tries to predict what's coming next in these complex pieces, research has found—and this may train the brain to sustain attention.

• **Use pen and paper.** The very act of writing in longhand engages your brain in ways that promote attention span and new learning.

Example: When students take notes by hand, they listen better and learn more than when they use a laptop, studies show.

• **Good night, phone.** If you don't get enough sleep, you're going to be less focused and make more mistakes, no matter what else you do. Yet how many of us go to bed with a phone or a tablet on our nightstand? If you hear it ping, or even worse, look at the blue light that the screen emits, that disrupts sleep. So turn off message notifications, and leave your devices far enough away that you're not tempted to pick them up as soon as you wake up. If you need an alarm, a traditional clock still can get the job done. Your brain will thank you!

Chapter 6

PHYSICAL INJURY AND BONE HEALTH

4 Balance Exercises to Keep You Steady on Your Feet

When you are young, you can walk confidently just about anywhere without much thought—such as on an uneven sidewalk—or while chatting at the same time. As you get older, just glancing sideways at a store window while strolling can make you wobble—and fall. *Here's what's going on...and some moves that will keep you steadier on your feet...*

Why Falls Occur

One in four Americans over age 65 falls each year. One reason is that older people are more prone to medical conditions that compromise balance—such as vertigo, dizziness, arthritis-related stiffness and weakness, stroke and loss of sensation in the feet from vascular diseases. But even without major health issues, normal physical and vision changes can affect balance.

Your eyes signal the brain where you are in space relative to other objects, which helps keep you stable. Wearing bifocals or progressive lenses requires your focus to change back and forth between lenses, making it harder to notice a loose rug, sidewalk crack or pet.

The natural age-related decline in muscle strength and flexibility also makes it harder to right yourself once your center of gravity is thrown off. That's why the key to staying on your feet is to build your muscle strength and improve your flexibility and agility. *Here's how—work up to doing each move daily to get the most benefit...*

Foot Taps

As we age, our pace typically slows, our step length shortens and our stance widens as shifting from one leg to the other feels less secure. To keep your strides long and confident and avert a shuffling gait, you can do foot taps—an exercise that trains your body to safely shift your center of gravity left and right.

How to do it: Stand in front of a step that is four-to-six-inches high (such as a footstool), feet hip-width apart. Slowly raise one foot to tap the step. Return that foot to the ground and then tap with the other foot. Movement

Caroline DeGroot, MPT, a physical therapist at AthletiCo Physical Therapy in Bannockburn, Illinois. DeGroot founded AthletiCo's Vestibular Program, which focuses on helping people with dizziness, balance disorders and concussions.

should be slow and controlled. Work up to 20 taps for each foot in a session. As your stability improves, try a higher step (six-to-eight inches)...or try tapping the step as lightly as possible to further improve balance and increase muscle control.

Safety note: If needed, you can hold a railing or counter for support. If you use a cane for general walking assistance, hold it in the hand you usually use to hold it throughout the exercise, regardless of which foot you're tapping. If you're using a cane only while recovering from an injury or for a condition that affects your gait, such as arthritis, hold the cane on the side opposite to the injury or painful extremity.

Head Turns

When you turn your head, a response called the vestibular spinal reflex (VSR) causes your brain to send messages to adjust postural muscles to keep you from being pulled in the direction your head turns. Your VSR can become less effective as you age, causing you to often stumble while turning your head. The following exercise helps train your VSR.

How to do it: Stand with your feet hip-width apart. If you need to, you can hold on to a railing, wall, sturdy piece of furniture or counter for support. Now slowly turn your head as far as you comfortably can to the right and then to the left, while maintaining upright posture. Repeat as a continuous movement for 10 repetitions.

Make sure to stay upright without leaning to one side. If you feel dizzy, pause, then continue at a slower pace.

For additional challenge: If you held on to a support, try doing the exercise without holding on to anything. Or try it with your feet only a few inches apart...or with your feet together...or with one foot in front of the other, heel-to-toe. Don't overextend your ability, though—safety first!

Over-the-Shoulder Walks

Try this exercise once you feel comfortable with standing head turns. You will look left and right as you walk—similar to what you might do when scanning shelves while grocery shopping or walking down a hallway while searching for an apartment number.

How to do it: Stand at one end of a long hallway, feet hip-width apart. Turn your head to look over your right shoulder. Maintaining that gaze, take three or four steps forward. Now turn your head to look over your left shoulder while you continue to walk forward another three or four steps. Repeat for a total of five times per side. If you feel dizzy or unsteady, stop turning your head and gaze straight ahead for a few steps. To increase the challenge, increase how quickly you turn your head.

Variation: Try head turns in a store or library. Having a stationary visual target—the items on the shelves—recruits your vision while challenging your VSR.

Ball Handoff

People who worry about falling often are self-conscious about walking—which is counterproductive. The more attention you pay to how you're walking, the more shuffled and fractured your gait becomes. Natural gait needs to be reflexive. This exercise uses a ball for distraction to help your gait become more fluid, increase your walking speed and improve your ability to shift weight left and right.

Safety note: This exercise is not recommended if you need to use a cane to walk.

How to do it: You'll need a partner who is comfortable walking backward and a small ball, such as a tennis ball. Start at one end of a long hallway with your partner facing you and a few feet in front of you, holding the ball. Walk forward while your partner walks backward—handing off or gently tossing the ball back and forth to each other as you go. Perform this exercise for two to three minutes or until you feel tired.

Solo variation: Stand in front of a wall, and march in place while you toss the ball at the wall and catch it as it bounces back.

Repeat for 30 seconds at a time, for a total of three times.

Are You Afraid of Falling? This Can Increase Your Risk

Julie Wetherell, PhD, a board-certified geropsychologist at the VA San Diego Healthcare System and professor of psychiatry at the University of California, San Diego. Dr. Wetherell is also an associate editor of the 2015 edition of the American Psychological Association Handbook of Clinical Geropsychology, and a Fellow of the Behavioral and Social Sciences Section of the Gerontological Society of America.

A loose rug…a tottering gait…a powerful drug…and poor eyesight are all well-known causes of falls. But there's a hidden risk that few people would ever guess.

Latest development: Researchers are now discovering that, paradoxically, the fear of falling significantly increases one's *risk* of falling. In fact, if you're very afraid of falling, you are 34% more likely to fall than someone with the same level of health and fitness who isn't as afraid. Why the difference? It's probably because you slow your walking speed, widen your stance and stiffen your body—changes that worsen balance. *What you need to know about this dangerous risk…*

Why the Fear?

Make no mistake, falls are scary. In adults age 65 and older, falls are the number-one cause of injury-related visits to emergency departments. The most common serious injury that results from a fall is hip fracture, which often leads to permanent disability, loss of independence—or death.

What has surprised even researchers is the degree of harm that can result when people have an unwarranted or excessive fear of falling (which means you're more concerned about falling than you need to be) and how widespread this fear is. Studies show that two out of five older adults are afraid of falling, including many who are reasonably fit and have never taken a spill. In fact, research shows that more seniors are afraid of falling than of robbery, financial troubles or even ill health!

Those who are afraid of falling are also more likely to avoid everyday activities such as walking outside, shopping for groceries or taking a bath…and are far more likely to end up in a nursing home.

Here's a quick rule of thumb: If you've had two or fewer minor falls in the past year…if you don't walk more slowly than other people your age…and if you can stand up from a chair without using your arms, you probably don't need to limit your activities dramatically due to concern about falling. However, if you are more afraid of falling than you need to be, it's important to take steps to reduce your fear.

It helps to see a physical therapist for an evaluation. He/she can assess your need for an assistive device such as a cane or walker and, if needed, give you exercises to improve your balance and strength.

What Else Helps

My colleagues and I conducted a small, preliminary study that reduced fear of falling in eight seniors. Each participant received eight one-hour sessions in his/her home conducted by a physical therapist and psychologist. *Among the approaches we used…*

- **Exposure therapy.** With this type of therapy, you're exposed to what you fear, little by little, in a safe environment, until you're comfortable encountering or doing the thing you fear. In this study, exposure was the most effective technique for reducing fear of falling.

Example: If you avoid taking baths, perhaps because a friend fell in the tub and you think it will happen to you, start by sitting on the side of the tub. When this is no longer fear-provoking, put your legs in the tub. After that, put your legs in the tub with a little bit of water in the bottom. Then do so with four inches of water.

You may need to repeat each of these actions 20 to 30 times over a few weeks until you are certain you can do each one without fear. The final action would be taking a bath.

If you are very concerned about doing this, you might want to start by having a person present while you do these activities—perhaps for a week in the same room, then for a week in the next room, then on a different floor. Eventually, doing these activities alone will reinforce the sense that you can bathe safely.

Note: The risk of falling and fear of falling are two different things. Precautions that reduce the risk of falling can sometimes make fear of falling worse. In the example above, if there's always another person present, it could foster fear, sending you the message that bathing alone is very dangerous.

Caution: If your doctor or physical therapist says that it isn't safe for you to do an activity alone, then your fear is not unwarranted or excessive and you should not do exposure therapy.

What you can do: Gradually expose yourself to the specific situations you fear, or ask a psychologist or physical therapist to help you do so. A friend or family member can do this as well if he gets some training from a psychologist or physical therapist.

• **Home safety.** If you make your home more fall-proof, you'll be less afraid of falling. For example, replace loose floor coverings with mats that have slip-resistant backing...make sure no cords or cables are in walkways...install grab bars in the bathroom...and put a slip-resistant mat in the tub or shower stall. Also, use brighter lights.

• **Cognitive restructuring.** This technique replaces counterproductive, fearful thoughts with helpful, fear-reducing thoughts. To get started, identify thoughts that are unhelpful. Next, when you have such a thought, substitute a helpful thought. For example...

You think: "If I walk on the grass, I'm likely to fall."

Substitute: "I have walked on the grass many times and didn't fall."

• **Exercise.** Balance-improving exercises that the people in my study found enjoyable and effective...

• Walking backward. This strengthens legs, improves balance and builds confidence.

What to do: Find a place where you can walk backward for 10 to 20 feet without looking over your shoulder to avoid obstacles, then reverse direction and walk backward the other way. Try to do this two to three times per day.

Helpful: See how it's done at Eldergym.com/backward-walking-for-increased-balance.

If you are very concerned about doing this exercise, start by doing it with someone else in the room and gradually work up, over a month or so, to doing it alone.

• Sit down in a chair and stand up without using your hands. This exercise is easy to do, builds leg strength and improves balance and confidence. Repeat at least 10 times, once a day.

For additional information on preventing falls, consult the National Council on Aging at NCOA.org (click on "Healthy Living," then on "Falls Prevention").

Surprising Medications That Increase Your Risk of Falling

Jack Fincham, PhD, RPh, professor of pharmaceutical and administrative sciences at Presbyterian College School of Pharmacy in Clinton, South Carolina.

Read the package insert for any medication and you'll likely see dizziness listed as a possible side effect. Still, few of us take dizziness seriously. But we should. Dizziness can lead to a fall...and that could lead to a serious injury.

More Meds, More Risk

More than half of all Americans are taking two prescription medications—20% are taking five or more, according to Mayo Clinic research. So it's important to recognize that side effects, including dizziness, are more pronounced with every drug you take. The increased effects are not additive—they are exponential. After a while, the question is not if you will fall, but when. Falls are one of the leading causes of long-term disability in older adults.

Here are widely used medications that commonly cause dizziness and falls. Chances are you use at least one of the following medications.

Pain Medications

The risks of opioid pain medications (including disorientation and dizziness) are well-known, but there is an increased fall risk even with over-the-counter (OTC) pain relievers. These seemingly benign medications influence many body systems, including the central nervous system (CNS), and can cause dizziness, even at normal doses.

Examples: Nonsteroidal anti-inflammatory drugs (NSAIDs), such as aspirin, *ibuprofen* (Advil) and *naproxen* (Aleve). Surprisingly, aspirin may be the worst offender. In addition to its effects on the CNS, aspirin bombards the vestibular nerve that feeds balance information from the inner ear to the brain. Many people can't take aspirin (even the baby aspirin dose of 81 mg) without experiencing severe dizziness or even vertigo—the nauseating perception that the room is spinning or tilting.

Note: Muscle relaxers are also sometimes prescribed for pain. These drugs cause significant drowsiness.

Examples: *Carisoprodol* (Soma), *cyclobenzaprine* (Flexeril) and *orphenadrine* (Norflex). When paired with a pain reliever, the combination of dizziness and drowsiness is a perfect recipe for a fall.

Sleep Aids and Allergy Drugs

Diphenhydramine is an antihistamine recommended to clear a stuffy nose and induce drowsiness at bedtime.

Examples: Benadryl, Tylenol PM, Advil PM and Aleve PM.

Like aspirin, diphenhydramine affects the CNS and the vestibular system, causing dizziness. It also slows down mental abilities such as thinking and processing information, so you may be less able to recognize side effects.

Because this drug is included in medications as a sleep aid, many people assume that they can sleep away the side effects. But diphenhydramine has a long half-life—in older adults, it can stay in their systems for up to 18 hours. The medication-induced dizziness can cause a fall if you get up during the night, for example, to use the bathroom.

Antidepressants

All antidepressants work at the level of neurotransmitters—the chemical messengers, such as serotonin, norepinephrine and dopamine, that allow us to think, act and experience emotion.

The most widely used antidepressants are selective serotonin reuptake inhibitors (SSRIs), which work by making serotonin more available to the brain, elevating mood and decreasing anxiety.

Examples: *Fluoxetine* (Prozac), *paroxetine* (Paxil) and *sertraline* (Zoloft).

Migraine drugs also work by affecting serotonin availability.

Examples: *Sumatriptan* (Imitrex) and *zolmitriptan* (Zomig).

Serotonin and norepinephrine reuptake inhibitors (SNRIs) are a newer type of antidepressant that makes both serotonin and norepinephrine more available to the brain.

Examples: *Duloxetine* (Cymbalta), *venlafaxine* (Effexor) and *desvenlafaxine* (Pristiq).

Bupropion (Wellbutrin) affects the availability of both norepinephrine and dopamine.

Note: The smoking-cessation medication Zyban also contains bupropion.

Besides affecting mood, these antidepressants carry messages to the brain from the balance centers of the inner ear, so they can affect your equilibrium. In addition, a faulty message can make the communication between brain and body less responsive. When you stand up or move, you may be less able to control your body position, increasing the risk of toppling over.

Blood Pressure Drugs

There are many types of blood pressure medications, including…

- **Diuretics ("water pills"),** such as *furosemide* (Lasix).
- **Beta-blockers,** such as *propranolol* (Inderal) and *atenolol* (Tenormin).
- **Angiotensin-converting enzyme (ACE) inhibitors,** such as *enalapril* (Vasotec) and *lisinopril* (Zestril).
- **Angiotensin II receptor blockers (ARBs),** such as *losartan* (Cozaar) and *olmesartan* (Benicar).
- **Calcium channel blockers,** such as *amlodipine* (Norvasc).

All medications that lower your blood pressure can also diminish your ability to quickly adapt to changing blood pressure needs, such as when you change your body position. Therefore, a common side effect of these drugs is orthostatic hypotension—a sudden spell of light-headed dizziness that happens when you quickly stand up after sitting or lying down.

Anticonvulsants and Neuropathy Drugs

Drugs for epilepsy, fibromyalgia and neuropathy can alleviate pain by putting the brakes on nerve impulse transmission. But this may limit the brain's ability to respond normally and quickly, significantly reducing alertness and increasing dizziness.

Examples: *Gabapentin* (Neurontin), *pregabalin* (Lyrica) and *carbamazepine* (Tegretol), all commonly used to treat diabetic nerve pain and fibromyalgia…and *clonazepam* (Klonopin) and *phenytoin* (Dilantin), both used as antiepileptic drugs.

What to Do

Literally every drug has the potential to cause dizziness and increase your risk of falling. *What to do…*

- **For occasional-use medications**—assess your level of discomfort. If you don't really need a drug, don't take it. If you must take a medication, develop an alternate plan that may include a medication change that is approved after consultation with your healthcare provider.
- **For long-term medications**—never stop taking them without advice from your healthcare provider. Many medications need to be tapered and will create rebound side effects if stopped abruptly.
- **For all new medications**—be alert for signs of dizziness or drowsiness. Are your body and mind as quick and responsive as usual? Do you feel alert? These side effects may be subtle or pronounced, but they should not be ignored. If they occur, avoid any activity that could result in a fall, including using stairs or ladders. If you must use stairs, steady yourself with handrails and move slowly up or down the stairs.

As your body adjusts to a medication, you may be prescribed a higher dosage to get the appropriate therapeutic effect.

Important: Watch for new side effects with each dosage change. They can appear even after the drug has been taken for an extended period.

- **If you experience orthostatic hypotension**—be sure to take your time standing up…and don't immediately start walking. Take a moment to steady yourself. If you become light-headed, sit down immediately. This practice is useful for anyone taking medication.

• **If you feel dizzy or have other troubling side effects while using any medication**—call your doctor...or talk to your pharmacist, who may be more accessible. Ask if there is another treatment that might have fewer side effects and less dizziness.

• **Before driving or exercising**—observe how you are reacting to the medication. Does an effect diminish in intensity after a while? If so, try to drive small distances and exercise carefully with companions to see how you are doing.

Unsteady on Your Feet? A Video Game Can Help

Colin Milner, CEO of the International Council on Active Aging, an organization dedicated to improving fitness and quality-of-life issues in older adults, Vancouver, British Columbia, Canada.

Fact: One in four Americans age 65 and older falls each year, and falls are the leading cause of injuries—both fatal and nonfatal—in this age group.

Staying fit and strong, engaging in exercises that target your "core" abdominal muscles and practicing balance-oriented regimens, such as yoga and tai chi, are key to preventing falls. But another solution may be as near as your TV—active video games that get you on your feet and moving. Dubbed "exergames," they're great for everyone—from healthy older adults who want to stay that way to those challenged by chronic conditions that impair balance.

Before the Fall

Changes that often come with aging can make you more wobbly on your feet. The biggest contributor for otherwise healthy people is general physical decline—loss of strength and power, poor balance and slower reaction time. Vision problems, foot-health issues, such as peripheral neuropathy, and medication side effects also can contribute to balance issues, as can certain medical conditions, such as Parkinson's disease.

Staying active and fit is the best way to maintain the muscle strength and quick reaction time needed for good balance. But even if you haven't been particularly active, exergames can help you improve balance in a short period of time.

Get in the Game

Exergames are video games that involve "whole-body motion." You can see an animated version of yourself (your "avatar") on screen, which makes it easier to make the right moves. When it comes to balance research, most of the studies use the Nintendo Wii Balance Board, which you stand on for some of the games in Nintendo Wii Fit. It relays your movements to the screen and lets you adjust your stance in real time. *Exergames...*

• **Help healthy older people who live independently improve balance.**

Example: One 2015 study of retired Australian men and women published in *Journal of Aging and Physical Activity* found that 30-minute unsupervised sessions of Wii balance gaming three times a week over six weeks significantly improved balance as measured by tasks such as standing on one leg...compared with a similar group that was encouraged to simply keep exercising in their normal way. Their enjoyment in playing also increased over the six weeks.

• **Are safe.** A recent review of 60 studies looking at the effectiveness of gaming technology for adults age 65 and older published in *International Journal of Medical Informatics* concluded that "exergames show promise as an intervention to improve physical function in older adults, with few reported adverse events."

• **Are great for people with chronic conditions that affect mobility and balance.**

Example: A recent Northwestern University study of patients with Parkinson's disease found that eight weeks of playing Wii Balance Board (the games included marble tracking, skiing and bubble rafting) three times per week significantly improved measures of gait and balance. Other research has found that exergames help stroke patients recover muscle function and balance.

Ready to play, but not sure where to start? Exergames range from light activity to a real workout. It's definitely an investment—you'll need to buy a Nintendo Wii (about $600) and a Wii Balance Board ($39). *Once you're set up, here are some popular games to try…*

• DanceDanceRevolution, which has you two-stepping on a sensored pad to match the dance moves shown on a screen. It features 30 dance tracks and three levels of fitness. ($49)

• Wii Ski. Use the balance board to hit the slopes on any of 14 breath-taking courses including races, freestyle, moguls and slaloms at beginner, intermediate and black diamond levels. ($20)

• Wii Sports. This suite of games uses a handheld remote to let you play tennis, baseball, golf, bowling and boxing. ($38)

What about other types of exergames? There's been some research on using Xbox Kinect games to improve balance, so that's one alternative. One benefit to using Xbox Kinect—you do not have to hold the remote, which can cause arm fatigue. Instead, the Xbox's sensor tracks your body as you move.

If you haven't been active for a while, or have physical limitations or a chronic health condition, talk with your doctor before trying exergaming. Research from University of Washington also finds that combining exergaming with regular sessions with a physical therapist is a particularly effective way to improve balance quickly.

Exercise In, Vitamin D Out for Preventing Falls

Alex Krist, MD, MPH., US Preventive Service Task Force vice chair, and professor, family medicine, Virginia Commonwealth University, Richmond.

JoAnn Manson, MD, DrPH, professor, medicine, Harvard School of Medicine, and chief, preventive medicine, Brigham and Women's Hospital, Boston.

With aging often comes worry about falls and the bone fractures they cause. Now, a panel of US experts has new advice on what helps and what doesn't when it comes to staying upright.

For starters, get off the sofa. And don't rely on vitamin D to keep you from falling.

In a change from its 2012 recommendations, the US Preventive Services Task Force (USPSTF) is recommending against vitamin D supplements for "community-dwelling" (those living at home) adults over 65 for preventing falls. A review of existing research showed insufficient evidence to recommend a supplement.

The task force also recommended against daily supplementation of 400 international units of vitamin D and 1,000 milligrams (mg) or less of calcium to prevent fractures in postmenopausal women living at home.

It wasn't clear, however, if higher doses might provide a benefit, according to the new USPSTF recommendations. There also wasn't enough evidence for the task force to determine whether vitamin D and calcium supplements could help men or premenopausal women avoid fractures.

The USPSTF is a volunteer panel of national experts. They develop recommendations for disease and injury prevention after a rigorous review of scientific evidence.

Closest Thing to a Magic Pill for Falls

So what does help people prevent falls? Exercise, the task force said.

"The strongest evidence is for exercise. If you're at risk of falling, you should think about exercise," said the task force's vice chair, Alex

Krist, MD, from Virginia Commonwealth University in Richmond. He added that about 20% of Americans over 65 have a fall each year.

The review and recommendations were published in the *Journal of the American Medical Association*.

An author of an editorial that accompanies the new recommendations agreed exercise can be beneficial.

"These recommendations are suggesting that we need to go beyond popping pills in order to have a major impact in preventing falls and fractures," said JoAnn Manson, MD, chief of preventive medicine at Brigham and Women's Hospital in Boston.

"Regular exercise can reduce falls with injury and it can also reduce heart disease, stroke, type 2 diabetes, dementia and some forms of cancer," Dr. Manson said.

"Physical activity is as close to a magic bullet as there is. And it doesn't take that much—just 30 or 40 minutes three times a week can make a difference," she added.

What Kind of Exercise Is Best?

Both Drs. Krist and Manson advocated for a variety of exercises. They said for someone healthy enough, the general physical activity guidelines of 30 minutes of aerobic activity most days of the week, and strength training twice a week, are a good place to start.

But not everyone over 65 can achieve that goal. Dr. Krist said to start with your doctor to get a better idea of what exercise might be right for you. For some people, the supervision that comes with physical therapy is helpful. For others, a class such as tai chi might work best. And for others, more vigorous activity may be fine.

Doctors Should Review Other Causes of Falls with Patients

The new recommendations suggest that doctors should selectively offer multifaceted interventions to seniors at a high risk of falling.

These might include: group or individual exercise, psychological therapy, nutrition therapy, education, medication management, urinary incontinence management, environmental modification, and physical or occupational therapy. Social services and referral to specialists such as an ophthalmologist, neurologist or cardiologist are other options.

Referrals can be important because some issues may be reversible. For example, sometimes addressing problems with vision can aid in fall prevention.

"Often, older individuals assume vision loss is inevitable and a normal part of the aging process. Very often, though, problems such as cataracts or glaucoma are treatable," Dr. Manson said.

Avoid the Double Whammy

"Falling is a major concern for older adults, and some are afraid to go outdoors because they're afraid of falling," she said. That leads to a double whammy as they stay inside, their muscles may atrophy, they don't get any sunlight and may develop a vitamin D deficiency, and they're losing out on important social interactions, Dr. Manson explained.

"I recommend at least doing strength training inside the home, or getting a treadmill to use at home. Or find a friend or family member that can go out for a walk, or start a walking club in your neighborhood," she suggested.

Learn more about preventing falls from the U.S. National Institute on Aging visit NIA.NIH.gov and search "preventing falls."

How to Cope When Only One Hand Is Working

Jeanine Beasley, EdD, OTR, CHT, FAOTA, an occupational therapist, certified hand therapist and past board member of the American Society of Hand Therapists. Dr. Beasley is a professor at Grand Valley State University's occupational science and therapy department and a hand therapist at Mary Free Bed Rehabilitation Hospital, both in Grand Rapids, Michigan.

It would take far more than 10 fingers to count all the tasks we use our hands to accomplish each day. From eating to typing to driving to combing our hair, we rely on our hands nearly every waking moment. But what if one hand is out of commission—either temporarily from a broken wrist, torn tendon or other injury...or permanently, because of a bigger setback such as a stroke, rheumatoid arthritis or an auto accident?

When you lose the use of one of your hands, it becomes difficult or impossible to button a shirt, for example, tie your shoes, wash a glass or cut your food...in other words, to function normally.

Good news: There are several effective—and simple—ways to fight back and regain your independence.

2 Questions to Answer

When only one hand is working properly, answering two key questions will give you the best possible combination of coping tips for your particular needs…

Is your dominant hand affected? As you might expect, it's generally a much larger problem when your dominant hand—whether you're a righty or a lefty—is the one that's out of commission.

Is your hand problem temporary or permanent? Before buying any adaptive equipment, consider how long you may need it. Someone with a wrist fracture may be one-handed for only a few weeks. Those who've suffered a stroke or traumatic brain injury may be challenged long-term. Some insurers may cover the cost of certain assistive products if they are considered a medical necessity. Check with your insurer.

Tricks and Products

Tricks and products (widely available online) for one-handed tasks…*

*An occupational therapist or hand therapist can also help with exercises and strategies. To find one near you, ask your doctor for a referral or contact The American Occupational Therapy Association at AOTA.org or the American Society of Hand Therapists at ASHT.org.

• **Typing, texting or writing.** Speech-to-text tools, such as voice-recognition computer software or smartphone options, can reduce the need for bilateral hand involvement when typing or texting.

Or you can try the one-handed Matias Half-QWERTY Keyboard ($575). With this keyboard, your functional hand does traditional touch-typing. Letters that would ordinarily be typed with the nonfunctioning hand are accessible by holding down the space bar with your working thumb so you can then use the same finger movements you would normally use with the other hand.

For people with wrist fractures, a "fat pen" is easier to grip while your wrist is in a cast. These pens can be found for just a few dollars.

Another option: You can make a pen "fatter" by taping pipe insulation or layers of tape around it. Find out by trial and error the thickness that is most comfortable for your limited grip.

• **Cutting food.** A pizza cutter can help stabilize meat as you cut it.

Another option: "Rocker knives," such as the Ronco Rocker knife ($8.99).

If you're chopping vegetables, a nonskid polyurethane cutting board with aluminum spikes that secure the food can be found for about $40. And when eating out, ask to have the chef cut your meat before it leaves the kitchen.

• **Cooking.** Dycem makes a non-slip mat (starting at $14) that stabilizes mixing bowls while stirring.

• **Opening jars.** A variety of one-handed jar openers are available for less than $10.

You can also try this: If you have a stable drawer, place the jar in it and lean into the drawer to stabilize the jar, then open the lid with one hand.

• **Playing cards.** One-handed cardholders (starting at less than $10) make it easy to play your favorite card game. For do-it-yourselfers, cardholders can be made from a block of wood or even a trimmed, flattened pool foam noodle with a narrow slit cut out for the cards.

- **Washing dishes.** A brush with a suction cup that can be secured to the sink (starting at just a few dollars) allows you to wash dishes with one hand. If you'll be one-handed only temporarily, you may prefer to use paper plates/cups and plastic utensils…or order in so you won't need to worry about washing pots and pans.

- **Bathing.** A long-handled brush can help you wash under your arms and reach farther. You can find an 18-inch-long brush with natural bristles starting at about $10.

When it comes time to dry off your back, slip on a cotton terry cloth bathrobe (put the weaker arm in the robe first). Use a towel on the floor to dry off your feet and a reacher or dressing stick to pull the towel up onto your legs. A dressing stick is made by securing a rubber-coated hook on the end of a dowel rod. Dressing sticks are also available online.

- **Hair drying.** Mount your hair dryer on a wall. With a hands-free hair-dryer holder that's mounted with suction cups, you don't need to hold the dryer at all. Models are available for less than $10.

- **Dressing.** Always dress the weak arm first. A good way to remember this is "in first" and "out last" when dressing the weaker extremity.

Fastening a bra can be challenging, so donning a sports bra instead can help, especially if you place the weaker arm in first. When removing the bra, take the stronger arm out first. This makes it easier to remove the bra from the weaker arm. Or you could try the Buckingham Bra Angel Dressing Aid (available online for about $38) to help stabilize one end of the bra fastener.

Slip-on shoes or those with Velcro fasteners eliminate the need to tie shoes.

When putting on socks, insert all the fingers of your stronger hand into the open end of the sock and spread to enlarge the sock opening. Then slip the sock over your toes and pull up with your stronger hand. Or you can try a "pull-on sock aid," available for around $20.

Pants and skirts with elastic waists can ease dressing.

Buttons or zippers on your clothes can be replaced with Velcro. You can also try a zipper pull and button hook, available for less than $10.

You Could Have a Spinal Fracture and Not Know It

Vinil Shah, MD, assistant professor of clinical radiology and associate program director of the neuroradiology fellowship program at University of California, San Francisco. Dr. Shah's areas of academic interest include assessing clinical outcomes of spine intervention.

Did you know that you can get a spinal fracture from simply stepping off a curb, sneezing, lifting a small pet or even just getting out of bed?

Fractures due to osteoporosis are much more common than many people realize. In fact, after age 50, one in two women and one in five men will have an osteoporosis-related fracture in their lifetimes.

The most common type of fracture linked to osteoporosis is a vertebral compression fracture (VCF)—a break in a vertebra of the spine. VCFs are more common than hip or wrist fractures…often are painful…and can lead to loss of height and a stooped back. So why do a shocking two-thirds of VCFs go undiagnosed and untreated?

Osteoporosis can weaken the bones so much that even routine activities or seemingly innocuous movements can cause a spinal fracture. Sudden, nonradiating pain ranging from mild to severe is typically the first sign. But the pain is often mistaken for arthritis or a pinched nerve. And because many people with osteoporosis don't even know they have it, VCFs simply aren't on their radar.

Quick Action Is Vital

An undiagnosed VCF will often heal on its own, with the pain diminishing in six to eight weeks. But you don't want this fracture to go undiagnosed! One VCF increases the risk for a subsequent VCF fivefold. And multiple fractures result in a loss of height and stooped posture. With each additional untreated VCF, the spine can get a few millimeters shorter. If the vertebrae in the upper back fracture and become wedge-shaped, the spine curves abnormally causing kyphosis, a rounding of the back better known as a dowager's hump.

If you're a woman or man over age 50 or a postmenopausal woman under age 50 who is experiencing new, unexplained mild-to-severe midline back pain that doesn't go away in a day or two, you need to see a doctor. Your primary care physician will perform a physical exam to check for back tenderness and will likely order an X-ray to confirm the diagnosis, following up with a CT scan or MRI to evaluate the problem further. Your doctor will then advise you on the best treatment for your specific situation.

Treating the Fracture

If the pain and loss of function from a VCF are mild, conservative treatments are usually recommended...

- **A few days of bed rest.** VCF pain tends to worsen when sitting or standing and improves when lying down.
- **Pain relievers.** Over-the-counter pain relievers, such as ibuprofen (Advil) or acetaminophen (Tylenol), help reduce mild pain.
- **A hyperextension back brace.** Wearing a rigid hyperextension back brace for a few weeks can help relieve pain and improve function in some patients. Ask your doctor for guidance.
- **Physical therapy (PT).** PT helps strengthen back muscles and can improve posture and prevent the development of chronic pain. It also has a beneficial effect on bone mineral density in osteoporosis patients and may prevent future fractures.

Note: PT can be started once the patient's pain is under control.

Conservative treatment of a VCF is not recommended for more than a few weeks or for those with more severe pain or limited function. Prolonged bed rest may lead to loss of bone mass (up to 1% loss each week) and muscle strength (10% to 15% loss each week). Bed rest can also increase risk for blood clots and bed sores, and painkillers should only be used short term.

Other Treatments

Patients whose pain doesn't resolve in two to three weeks with the treatments above may be candidates for a minimally invasive procedure called vertebroplasty. Guided by computed tomography and/or fluoroscopy (a continuous X-ray "movie"), the doctor injects bone cement into the fracture. The outpatient procedure takes about 45 minutes while the patient is typically conscious but sedated. The cement not only stabilizes the fractured vertebra, it also prevents nearby nerve endings from causing pain.

Studies show that 75% to 100% of patients enjoy good-to-moderate pain relief and increased mobility quickly after vertebroplasty, often the next day. The procedure usually doesn't restore much height loss, but it can prevent further height loss and additional fractures.

With *kyphoplasty*, a modification of vertebroplasty, a balloon is inflated in the fractured vertebra to create a cavity that is then filled with cement. This procedure may offer a better chance of restoring height loss. However, kyphoplasty is more expensive than vertebroplasty, and there is mixed data on its benefit over vertebroplasty.

In general, vertebroplasty and kyphoplasty are safe when done by an experienced doctor. Interventional radiologists and neuroradiologists often do these procedures. Look for a doctor who has experience in using image guidance for spine procedures. Like all invasive medical procedures, these treatments do have risks—such as infection or bleeding. And in rare cases, the cement can leak into the spinal canal, causing nerve compression, or travel into adjacent veins, which can lead to blood clots in the lungs or heart.

The best candidates for these procedures are patients who have pain of at least moderate intensity (rated a five or greater out of 10) that impacts their mobility and daily quality of life. Additionally, those who have fractures that have occurred recently (within a few months prior to the procedure) tend to have more success with vertebroplasty and kyphoplasty than those who have older fractures. The age of a fracture can be determined by an MRI.

Preventing Future Fractures

Treating the underlying osteoporosis to help prevent future fractures is crucial. Ask your doctor for a bone mineral density test called a DXA (or DEXA)—this low-dose X-ray measures bone density in the hip and spine and can guide your physician in choosing the best course of action for your case. Options include prescription medications such as bisphosphonates (patients should weigh the risks versus benefits of these drugs with their doctors)...calcium and vitamin D supplementation...and weight-bearing exercise to improve bone strength and other exercises to build core strength. Multiple clinical trials have shown that early treatment of osteoporosis can increase bone mineral density by 5% to 15%, reducing vertebral fracture rates by 40% to 70%.

Yogurt May Help Keep Bones Healthy

Older adults who ate yogurt daily had a 3% to 4% higher bone-mineral density measurement compared with those who did not eat yogurt. Daily yogurt consumption also was linked to lower risk for osteoporosis—39% lower in women and 52% lower in men. The study showed association but not cause and effect. Daily yogurt eaters may live a more healthful lifestyle. Other dairy products did not produce a similar effect on bone strength.

Eamon J. Laird, PhD, research fellow, Trinity College Dublin, Ireland, and leader of a study of 4,310 Irish adults, ages 60 and older, published in *Osteoporosis International.*

Do You Need Bone Meds?

Emily M. Stein, MD, endocrinologist and associate research scientist, Hospital for Special Surgery, and assistant professor of medicine, Weill Cornell Medical College, both in New York City.

If you've been diagnosed with osteopenia, your doctor might prescribe Fosamax even if you have no history of fractures. Do you really need to take bone medicine?

That depends. A diagnosis of osteopenia means your bone density is low but not as low as the more severe diagnosis of osteoporosis. While low bone density is one reason to recommend medications that preserve bone, it is critical to ask your physician why the treatment is recommended. There may be other factors in your medical history that are placing you at high risk for osteoporosis. While a prior fracture that occurred without major trauma is the most significant, other factors—taking glucocorticoids (Prednisone) for a long time, for example—affect bone quality without making bone density particularly low. Therefore, when deciding whether to begin treatment, it is important to take all risk factors into account, not just the bone density test.

Osteoporosis medications, such as *alendronate* (Fosamax), are typically very effective and can reduce the risk for fracture by half. However, the medications can cause side effects, such as severe heartburn, ulcers, muscle aches and difficulty swallowing. For patients who are at low fracture risk, medication is typically not prescribed because the risk for a side effect outweighs the risk for fracture. For patients at high risk for fracture, treatment is recommended because the consequences of a serious osteoporotic fracture can be very serious. For example, major osteoporotic fractures can greatly interfere with quality of life, and the ability to care for yourself and live alone. In the first year following a hip fracture, 25% of people will die from complications. Many more people are unable to walk or get about unassisted after a major fracture.

Talk to your doctor about other things that you may do to improve your bone health, such as engaging in weight-bearing exercise, consuming adequate amounts of calcium and vitamin D and quitting smoking. These are helpful things for everyone to do. However, it is important to realize that for patients who are at high risk, these can be helpful in addition to medication but are not sufficient on their own.

You might also consider a consultation with a metabolic bone specialist to understand your fracture risk and to clarify the specific risks and benefits of treatment. A metabolic bone specialist is typically an endocrinologist or rheumatologist who has specific expertise taking care of patients with osteoporosis or other bone problems. You can ask your primary care doctor or gynecologist for a recommendation or look for a metabolic bone center affiliated with a major medical center in your area.

Birth Control Pills May Protect Women's Knees

Female athletes using birth control pills are less likely to need surgery for anterior cruciate ligament (ACL) injuries than those not taking the pills. Those with the highest rates of ACL surgery were 22% less likely to be taking the pills than those who did not have an ACL injury.

Female athletes are twice as likely as males to injure the ACL, which connects the top and bottom parts of the knee. The female hormone estrogen is thought to make women more vulnerable to ACL injury, possibly by weakening the ligament—and birth control pills help maintain estrogen at lower and more consistent levels.

Study of 23,438 women, ages 15 to 19, by researchers at University of Texas Medical Branch, Galveston, published in *Medicine & Science in Sports & Exercise.*

New MRI Danger

Emanuel Kanal, MD, professor of radiology and neuroradiology and director of magnetic resonance services at University of Pittsburgh Medical Center. He serves as a consultant to the FDA on magnetic resonance safety issues and is lead author of the American College of Radiology's Guidance Document on Magnetic Resonance Safe Practices.

Actor Chuck Norris recently claimed that his wife, Gena, endured ongoing weakness and bouts of pain due to an injection she received as part of an MRI scan—is he right?

If you have an MRI, you might first be given an injection of gadolinium, a metal element that serves as a component of a "contrast agent" that makes tumors and inflammation easier to spot. But gadolinium can be toxic, and recent studies have found that traces of gadolinium can linger in patients' brains, bones or other tissues for years, rather than

Better Bones in 60 Seconds

Just one or two minutes daily of high-intensity weight-bearing exercise was associated with 4% and 6% better bone health, respectively. This degree of improvement can be enough to decrease fracture risk. Exercise intensity levels were the equivalent of medium-paced running for younger women or a slow jog for older ones.

Takeaway: For better bones, pick up your pace for at least a minute when you're out walking.

Victoria H. Stiles, PhD, senior lecturer, sport and health sciences, University of Exeter, UK.

be flushed away by the kidneys in a few hours as previously believed.

Medical science cannot yet say even if gadolinium is responsible for Gena Norris's symptoms or whether it is dangerous in the small concentrations that linger after an MRI—research is ongoing. But it is reasonable to not want even a tiny amount of an unneeded and potentially harmful metal in your body.

What to do: If your physician recommends that you get an MRI, ask whether he/she requested that a contrast agent be used. If the answer is yes, ask your doctor to speak with the radiologist to confirm that using the contrast agent is necessary with your specific MRI. In many MRIs where the referring physician requests a contrast agent, it may not actually be needed. Only digital radiologists are trained in the complex subject.

If you do not have kidney disease and if the radiologist confirms that using a contrast agent is crucial to your MRI, the benefits of undergoing an MRI examination in which a contrast agent is used likely dwarfs any potential risk from the gadolinium itself.

Natural Rx for Stronger Bones

Jamison Starbuck, ND, a naturopathic physician in family practice and writer and producer of Dr. Starbuck's Health Tips for Kids, a weekly program on Montana Public Radio, MTPR.org, both in Missoula. She is a past president of the American Association of Naturopathic Physicians and a contributing editor to *The Alternative Advisor: The Complete Guide to Natural Therapies and Alternative Treatments.* DrJamisonStarbuck.com

Osteoporosis, a condition marked by weak and brittle bones, can't be felt and it isn't fatal by itself, but if you have it, you're much more likely to fracture a bone if you fall. And recent research points to greater risk for premature death following an osteoporosis-related fracture. Osteoporosis can't be seen either, but one possible tip-off is a loss of height. The condition affects both men and women, but most often postmenopausal women.

Conventional doctors often treat osteoporosis with calcium supplements and perhaps prescription drugs such as *alendronic acid* (Fosamax) or *raloxifene* (Evista). These medications can have side effects that range from joint pain to weakening of the jawbone with Fosamax...and hot flashes to chest pain with Evista.

Note: People with moderate-to-severe osteoporosis and/or a strong family history of osteoporosis may need medication.

I recommend calcium as well but prefer that patients get it from food. Although more research is needed, studies have indicated that getting too much calcium from supplements may increase risk for heart disease. Excess calcium can also cause constipation and lead to kidney stones. So if I do recommend a calcium supplement, I advise a calcium/magnesium combination (the magnesium reduces risk for constipation) along with 400 international units (IU) of vitamin D to aid absorption.

Many of my patients choose my protocol as their only treatment for osteoporosis, but it can be used in conjunction with prescription medication.

Important: It's also crucial for patients to not smoke (smoking increases risk for osteoporosis). *My osteoporosis prevention and treatment plan...*

- **Improve diet.** Studies show that people who eat foods that are low in minerals and vitamins are more likely to develop osteoporosis and experience a fracture than those who eat a diet emphasizing leafy greens, nuts, beans, whole grains, dairy and oily fish like salmon and sardines. That's because these foods contain lots of the nutrients necessary for healthy bone growth—calcium, magnesium and vitamins D and K. Get plenty of these foods in your daily diet.

Beware: Frequent alcohol consumption, diets high in meat protein and salt and drinking carbonated beverages daily all will increase your odds of osteoporosis.

• **Enhance digestion.** In addition to eating healthy foods, you have to be able to digest them effectively to get all of their benefits. Minerals and fat- soluble vitamins like D and K need plenty of stomach acid to be broken down and absorbed. Acids like fresh lemon juice and vinegar help speed up the breakdown of minerals and vitamins in your stomach so that they get absorbed into your bloodstream quickly. Just sprinkle some vinegar or fresh lemon juice (or any fresh citrus juice) on vegetables, fish and meat, and be sure to choose a vinaigrette salad dressing.

• **Optimize strength and balance.** Weight-bearing exercise helps build bone strength and stem bone loss.

Good options: Walking, dancing, lifting free weights and using resistance bands. Try to do weight-bearing exercise for 30 minutes, five times a week. Wearing a weighted vest when at home or when walking helps, too. Practicing yoga (even for just 15 minutes three times a week) gently develops muscles and balance.

Also: Practice walking on slightly uneven ground, like a footpath or dirt road—it will improve your balance and make you less likely to fall.

Yes! You Can Stop Bunions from Forming

Dr. Mitchell Yass, DPT, creator of The Yass Method, which uniquely diagnoses and treats the cause of chronic pain through the interpretation of the body's presentation of symptoms. Dr. Yass is the author of two books, *Overpower Pain: The Strength Training Program That Stops Pain Without Drugs or Surgery*, and *The Pain Cure Rx: The Yass Method for Resolving The Cause of Chronic Pain*.

Are bunions keeping you from wearing your favorite sandals in public?

Bunions occur when excess bone develops at the base of the first toe (known as the first metarsal head). That excessive bone can make weight-bearing on the foot severely painful and almost impossible—as many of you likely already know.

People will try bunion pads or other bunion correctors to alleviate some of the force being absorbed at the base of the first toe. Bunion correctors are "Band-aids." They fix nothing and do not address the cause (which I explain below).

Some people will try to alter how they walk so they don't elicit pain from the bunion. (This tactic ultimately can lead to pain at another location because the altered weight-bearing designed to limit pressure on the bunion is now causing excess force somewhere else.)

Some people will try going to a podiatrist to have the bunion scraped or shaved.

Once the pain becomes so excessive and no other alternative relieves the pain, surgery typically becomes the last option. Sometimes the surgery is just to remove the bunion. Other times the surgery is more involved to correct the bunion as well as a misalignment of the first toe.

For most people, the development of a bunion and the symptoms and treatment of the bunion appear to be out of their control. It is all part of the existing medical quandary that most people find themselves stuck in—a medical system there to help address symptoms that develop, but no guidance on how to prevent these problems in the first place.

Well, I am going to blow your minds and present the idea that bunions—and their associated pain—not only can be limited in severity, but they can be completely prevented from ever occurring!

What Really Causes Bunions?

First, you need to understand the mechanism that develops the bunion in the first place.

When you stand on your foot, the goal of proper weight-bearing is to feel pressure through the entire foot. This means that you should feel as much weight-bearing going through the fifth metatarsal head as the first (the metatarsal heads are the balls of your feet)—i.e., that your body weight is being distributed evenly over five points of contact to the floor.

What can happen, and in fact happens often, is that a person's gluteus medius muscle will strain and weaken. This muscle, which sits at the side of the pelvis and attaches to the hip joint, is responsible for creating stability and balance. And it's this muscle that is critical to keeping the pelvis level when single-leg standing, such as when walking. When the pelvis stays level, then a person will be weight-bearing through the whole foot and distribute body weight evenly through all five balls of the feet when she or he walks.

If the gluteus medius muscle is strained and weakened, the pelvis cannot be held level. The side of the pelvis opposite from the one being stood upon will start to drop. In dropping, it causes a person to weight-bear through the inside of the foot rather than the midline. The person ends up weight-bearing on the first and second balls of the feet, or sometimes strictly on the first metatarsal head only.

This means that five points worth of force is now only being applied to one or two points of contact. When excessive force is applied to a bone, the body responds by making more bone at the first ball of the foot—i.e., a bunion.

To stop the continued development of an existing bunion or to prevent a bunion from developing at all, the process is quite simple. You need to make sure you are weight-bearing through all five balls of the feet.

To accomplish this goal, you need to make sure that the gluteus medius muscle is strong, as well as two muscles that support the inside of the foot and the ankle. By strengthening these muscles, the pelvis will be able to stay level when single-leg standing and you will find it easy to weight-bear through the whole foot. This ends any excessive load being applied to the first ball of the foot and therefore traumatic bone growth will be inhibited from developing.

You probably have never heard of information like this before, and certainly the existing medical model of treating bunions is designed to simply minimize your symptoms until you are directed toward a surgery that will temporarily remove the bunion. But my responsibility is to explain why things happen so you can be more preemptive in your ability to stop problems like this from happening in the first place.

Self-Test: Is Your Glutueus Medius Weak?

To test your gluteus medius muscles, simply stand on the foot with the bunion and see how long you can stand with the other foot off the floor. Then try it with the unaffected side.

If the gluteus medius muscle is weak on the affected side, you will find it more difficult to single-leg stand on that side and you will have a tendency to fall toward the opposite side (and likely have to put the opposite foot down to prevent you from falling).

Also notice whether your foot and ankle have a tendency to collapse to the inside. If that is the case, it shows that the excessive force is being developed at the foot and ankle, causing a loss of support at the inner foot and ankle. This is what leads to the excessive loading of the first ball of the foot...and, ultimately, to bunions.

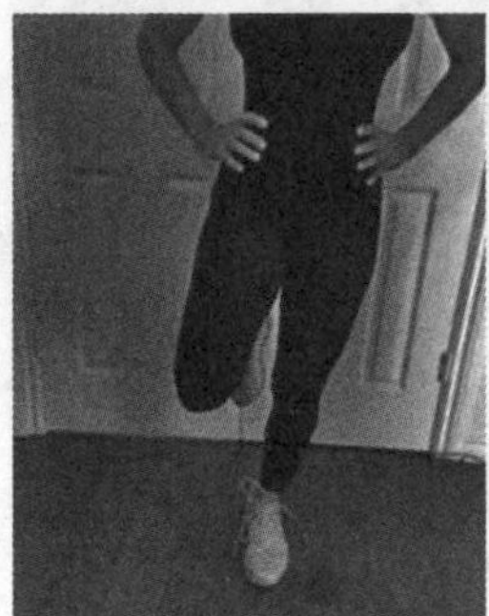

Pelvis level

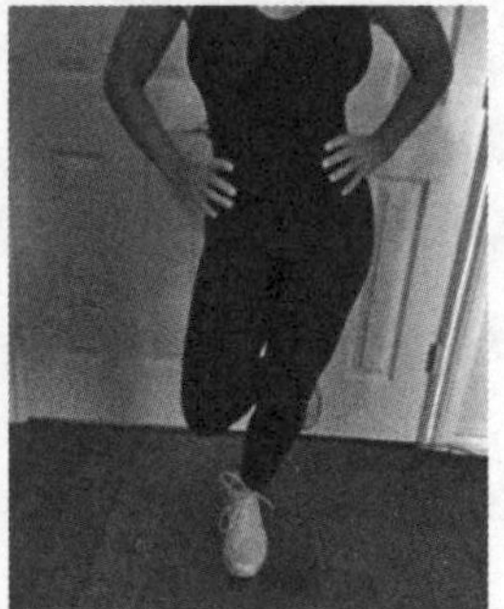

Pelvis drops on opposite side

Strengthening Exercises to Stop Bunions

• **Hip Abduction (gluteus medius).** This exercise can be performed either lying on your side or standing. To do it correctly, make sure you do not go too far when moving your leg outward. People falsely believe that more range of motion is better, but in this case too much range of motion means you are using the lower back muscle to create the motion, not the gluteus medius (hip muscle). The gluteus medius muscle can only move the leg out to the point where it is parallel with the hip joint. Any outward motion beyond that is created by the lower back muscle.

To do the exercise lying down, lie on your side with the knee of the bottom leg bent and the top leg straight. The top leg should run in a continuous line from the torso—if the leg is angled in front of the torso, you would use the wrong muscle. Start to raise the top leg off the supporting leg until your top leg is parallel with the floor. As you lift, try to turn the leg in slightly so the heel is the first part of the foot that is moving. This puts the gluteus medius in the optimal position to raise the leg. Once your leg reaches parallel to the floor, begin to lower it back onto the supporting leg.

If you prefer to stand, the outward movement is similar to when lying down—lead with the heel, and don't move your leg too far to keep the exercise focused on the gluteus medius. Holding on to a sturdy table or chair while you perform the exercise will make it easier to use proper form.

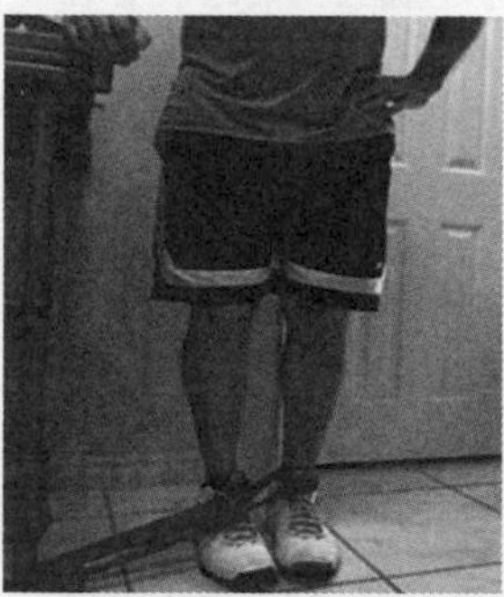

Start

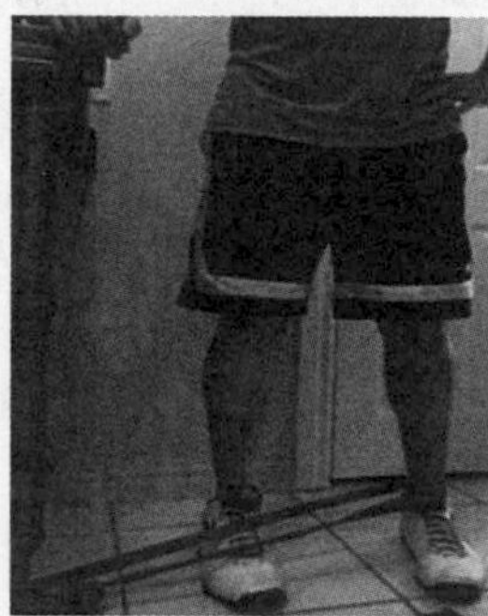

Finish

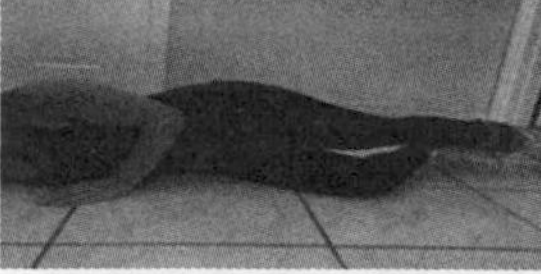

Start

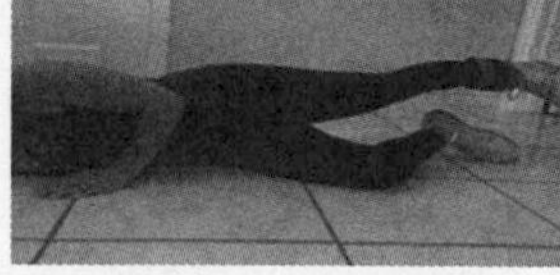

Finish

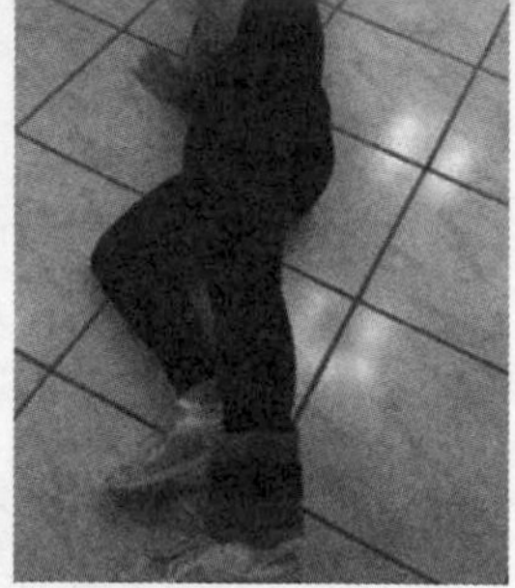

Side View

• **Dorsiflexion (anterior tibialis).** I've also advised this exercise for relieving plantar fasciitis, knee pain and even for symptoms of diabetic neuropathy.

Secure a resistance band under a sturdy table or knot one end and put the knot behind a closed door. Sit on the floor and extend your weak leg but keep your knee bent. Slip the end of the resistance band over your foot so that it is supported on the front of the foot in the mid-foot region. Start with the ankle angled about 30 degrees forward. Next flex your foot, pulling it toward you about 10 degrees beyond perpendicular. Return to the start position.

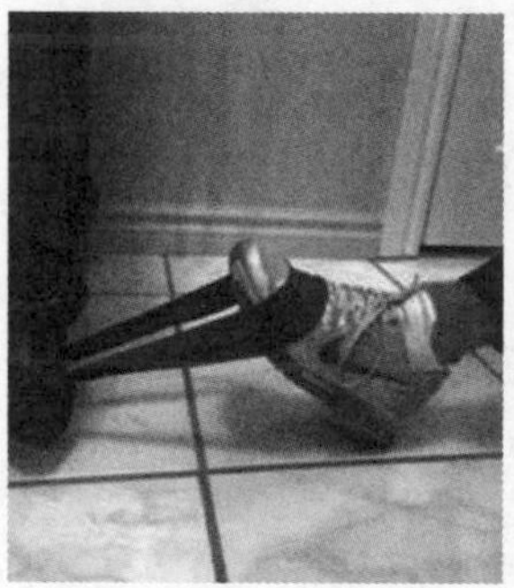

Start

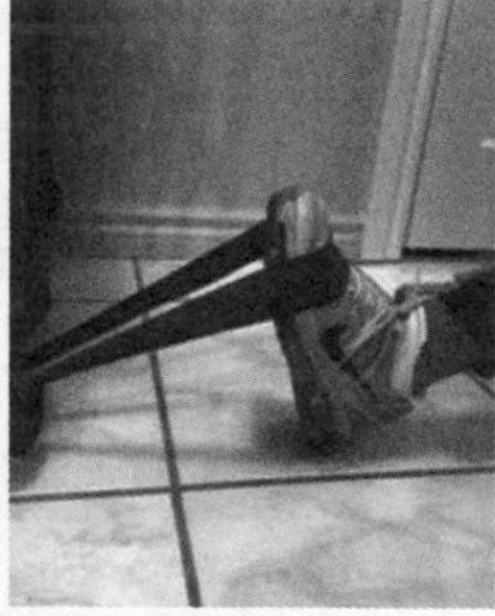

Finish

• **Inversion (posterior tibialis).** Secure a resistance band as described above. Sit in a chair placed parallel to the door or table. The resistance needs to come from the side of the leg to be exercised—so if it's your right food, the band should be secured from the outside of the right foot at about the same level as your foot. Place the resistance band around your instep and sit with your working leg at a 90-degree angle so that your heel is under the knee. Keeping your heel touching the ground, raise the rest of your foot and place the toes outside the line of the ankle. Slowly pull the toes inward until they are inside the line of the ankle. (The foot will turn upward slightly as the foot is moved inward at the end of the range.) Place your hand on the side of the knee of the working leg to make sure it does not move. You do not want any movement or rotation of the working leg. The only motion should be at the ankle. Return to the start position.

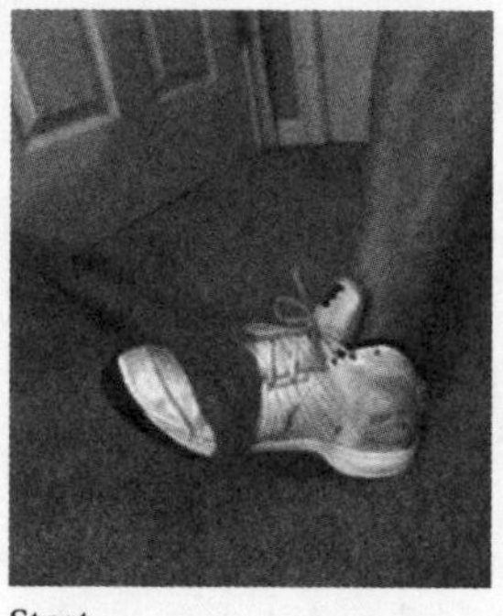
Start

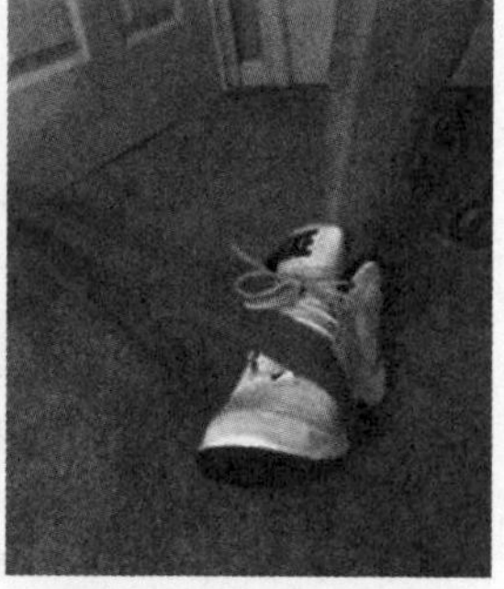
Finish

Perform these exercises three times a week. For each, do three sets of 10 repetitions with a one-minute break between sets. Continually increase the resistance used until the muscles involved are strong enough to perform your functional activities without straining and emitting symptoms.

Good news/bad news: If a bunion began, doing these exercises can stop its progression. If it did not begin, you can prevent it from initiating by keeping these three muscles strong. But—you cannot reverse a bunion once it has started; it is actually traumatic bone growth.

Yoga Can Be Dangerous

Timothy McCall, MD, a board-certified internist and medical editor at *Yoga Journal*...coeditor of the 2016 medical textbook *The Principles and Practice of Yoga in Health Care*...and author of the best-selling *Yoga as Medicine*. Dr. McCall lectures and teaches yoga therapy seminars worldwide. DrMcCall.com

---

Yoga is good for you, right? Not always. *Troubling recent finding:* For one year, researchers tracked more than 350 people who took yoga classes. Nearly 11% of the participants developed a new pain problem, often lasting a few months. And 21% reported that yoga had aggravated existing injuries.

What I tell my patients and clients: As a medical doctor and yoga instructor for more than 20 years, I know that the risk for injury from practicing yoga can be much lower than from many other forms of exercise such as running or tennis—if you avoid making common mistakes. And by staying injury-free, you will enjoy the many benefits of regular yoga practice—relaxation and stress relief...pain relief...a stronger, more flexible body...and a more peaceful mind.

Here's how to bypass the injury-causing errors people often make when they practice yoga...

Wrong Type of Class

There are many different styles and types of yoga—from the gentle and restorative to the intense and aerobic. Some of the styles investigated in the new study were intense types in which participants move quickly from pose to pose without stopping. (*Examples*: Vinyasa Flow, Power Yoga and Ashtanga Yoga.)

In my experience, most yoga injuries happen to people doing more vigorous and acrobatic styles of yoga. Vigorous, flowing styles of yoga such as Vinyasa can be challenging and invigorating and therefore appealing. But it is not always a safe choice for anyone middle-aged or older because it's too fast and demanding, making injury more likely. Also, because the sequence of poses is quick, participants often do the poses incorrectly, with muscles and bones improperly aligned, increasing the risk for injury. The teacher may not notice these mistakes in alignment because students move so quickly from pose to pose.

My advice: If you are fit and under age 50, more athletically demanding yoga may be fine for you. If you are over age 50 and already practice flowing yoga without problems, you may be fine to continue, but the older you get, the riskier it becomes. If you are not fit or if you have a chronic health problem such as rheumatoid arthritis, poorly controlled high blood pressure or a degenerative disease of the nervous system such as Parkinson's, choose a gentler style of yoga. Examples may be called gentle yoga, restorative yoga or yoga for seniors. Other good choices include Yin Yoga and beginning Iyengar Yoga classes.

Helpful: If you want to practice a fast-paced Vinyasa-style yoga, first take a few classes in which you learn to do the poses slowly and correctly—and then speed up.

Red flag: Anyone who is pregnant, has multiple sclerosis or a chronic inflammatory condition such as lupus or inflammatory bowel disease should avoid hot yoga, including a type of hot yoga called Bikram Yoga—in which the room may be heated to 105°F. The intense heat can aggravate inflammatory conditions or harm a growing fetus.

Undertrained Teacher

All the yoga teachers in the new study had at least 200 hours of training—the amount required by the Yoga Alliance, a nonprofit association of yoga teachers and schools.

That might sound like a lot of training, but it's nowhere near enough to ensure quality instruction. In some instances, much of that training happens online without direct supervision by a qualified teacher.

Bottom line: You are more likely to be injured in a class conducted by a teacher who is undertrained.

My advice: If possible, find a teacher who has more training, say, 500 hours, or one who has many years of experience. To check the teacher's qualifications, you can call a yoga studio, check online or ask the teacher directly.

If you have a serious medical condition, consider consulting a yoga therapist, a yoga teacher trained to work with students with a wide variety of illnesses. To be certified in yoga therapy by the International Association of Yoga Therapists (IAYT), a teacher needs at least 1,000 hours of training. The IAYT website (IAYT.org) has a search function for finding IAYT members in a growing number of locations.

Strained Breathing

In a good yoga class, you are taught to pay attention to your breath. And if you do that, the breath becomes an indicator of whether you are about to make a mistake and hurt yourself.

Often the first sign of an imminent mistake is strained breathing—gasping or holding your breath. If you maintain a discipline of breathing slowly and deeply, it's much less likely that you will hurt yourself. Added benefits of attending to your breathing include a greater sense of calm and mindfulness (steady focus in the present).

My advice: Tune into the breath throughout your yoga practice. If it becomes strained or uneven, make an adjustment that corrects the problem or come out of the pose.

Trying Too Hard

A common cause of injury in yoga is what I call "over-efforting"—trying to stretch more deeply into a pose when your breath and body are telling you that the extra stretch is not a good idea. Sharp pain and/or strained breathing are sure signs that the deeper stretch is a mistake. Over-efforting often happens because of peer pressure—almost everyone else in class is doing the pose in a certain way, so you want to keep up, too.

My advice: A yoga pose should be a balance of effort and ease. If the pose is more effort than ease—get out of it. If you get a sharp pain, particularly one in a joint such as the knee—get out of it. Even if the rest of the class is doing the pose…and even if the yoga teacher is telling the class to stay in the pose…if your body is telling you to get out of the pose, get out of it.

Riskier Poses

There are several common yoga poses that are the most likely to cause injury, and they should be avoided by beginners and many people with chronic medical conditions. *These poses include…*

- **Headstands,** which can damage the neck. When I attend a general yoga class, it often is the case that about half the class should not be doing a headstand—ever. While doing the pose, their faces are red and strained, and they obviously can't wait for the teacher to tell them to come out of the pose. Upside-down poses also can be risky for those with eye problems caused by glaucoma, retinal disease or diabetes.

• **Shoulder stands and Plow pose.** These poses can overstretch the back of the neck. If your neck feels tight or uncomfortable, you probably should not be doing the pose.

My advice: It may help to put folded blankets under your shoulders (but not under your head and neck) to take the strain off your neck.

• **Lotus pose,** a sitting pose in which you put the right foot over the top of the left thigh and vice versa. This pose is only for people with flexible hips. If you use your hands to force your legs into this position, you create tremendous torque on your knee joint and you could rip or otherwise injure a knee ligament.

• **Chaturanga (yoga push-ups).** In many athletic yoga classes, students cycle through a series of 12 poses known as a sun salutation. One element is Chaturanga, where you lower your body from Plank pose to a low push-up position. Doing this repeatedly can be murder on your shoulder—particularly if you allow the top of your upper-arm bones to jut forward in the shoulder joint.

My advice: If you can't maintain good shoulder alignment, drop both knees to the ground in Plank pose, which takes some weight off, then descend the upper body to Chaturanga.

• **Deep back bends,** twists or forward bends. When in doubt, favor less extreme versions of these poses. *Surprising*: Less demanding versions of poses confer most or all the health benefits of the deeper versions.

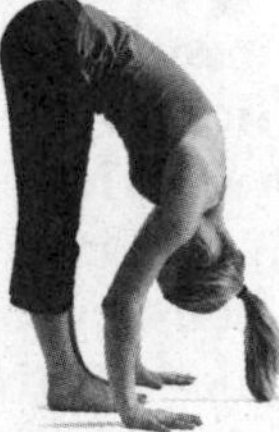

Aggressive Adjustment

Another potential cause of serious yoga injuries is when a teacher aggressively pushes on your body to take you more deeply into a pose (light touching to indicate how or where to move is fine).

My advice: Do not allow an instructor to manually force your body into any yoga position. If you are in a class with an instructor who does that, find a new instructor.

Better Care for Broken Bones

Adults over age 60 with ankle fractures underwent a new treatment called *close contact casting*, in which a surgeon applies a molded, below-the-knee cast with minimal padding while the patient is under anesthesia.

Result: Those who wore fitted casts for six weeks had similar mobility and discomfort as those who had open surgery involving plates and screws. Plaster casts (another traditional treatment) are linked to increased risk for misaligned bones.

Keith Willett, MBBS, professor of orthopaedic trauma surgery, University of Oxford, UK.

How You Can Protect Yourself from Danger the Way a Spy Does

Jason Hanson, a former CIA officer who twice won the CIA's Exceptional Performance Award. He is founder of Spy Escape & Evasion, a Cedar City, Utah–based company that offers advanced safety training. He is author of *Spy Secrets That Can Save Your Life* and the forthcoming *Survive Like a Spy*. SpyEscapeAnd Evasion.com

It probably will never happen to you. You probably never will be kidnapped or carjacked. You probably never will be targeted by a home invader or a mugger or caught in the middle of an "active-shooter" situation. But no doubt the people who find themselves in these terrible situations did not expect that these things would happen to them either. Sometimes the worst does happen. When it does, it's the people who are prepared with the right tools and techniques who have the best chance of surviving. *Here's what an experienced spy says you should know and do now...*

How to Spot Danger

If you pay attention to your surroundings, you often can spot would-be muggers, rapists, terrorists and other dangerous people before they strike. Their faces and body language might betray out-of-place emotions—perhaps they look tense in a location where everyone else is calm and happy. Their movements might be unusual, too—if you are walking slowly and window-shopping, why hasn't this person passed you?

If you do spot a potential threat, these strategies can help you assess and deter the danger...

• **Pick a pointless path.** If you think someone might be following you, travel along a route that does not make much sense. Walk or drive through point C on your way from A to B. If this person takes the same route, the odds are high that you're being followed. In spycraft, this is called a "surveillance-detection route."

Example: A woman shopping in a department store thought a man might be watching her. She walked from the shoe department across the store to the housewares department—where she spent a few minutes—and then back across the store to women's apparel. She saw the man lurking at each stop, so she pointed him out to a security guard. The man immediately ran away, and the guard walked the woman to her car.

Warning: A good surveillance-detection route does not take you through anywhere secluded, particularly if you are on foot. If someone does mean you harm, seclusion could give him/her an opportunity to strike.

• **Make extended eye contact...followed by verbal contact.** Your instinct when you feel the eyes of a predator upon you might be to avoid eye contact or scurry away. But that would only reinforce this predator's conclusion that you are a perfect passive victim—someone who won't fight back if attacked.

Instead, if you think a stranger is watching you, watch him back. Turn to face him and make strong, extended eye contact. This sends the message, *I know you're there, and I'm not intimidated.* That's enough to convince most bad guys that you're not a suitable target after all. If this person does not quickly break eye contact, make verbal contact as well. If you are confident that this person is up to no good, you could speak aggressively. If you are less certain, you could just speak in an ordinary fashion because that may be enough to fluster a predator who had expected to be in total control of the situation.

Example: A man followed a married couple down a quiet street, switching sides of the road to get behind them. The husband turned, made steady eye contact and asked this potential mugger if he knew what time it was. The man appeared flustered, told him the time and then turned and walked the other way.

If someone whom you suspect has targeted you reverses his direction after you make eye contact and/or verbal contact, it is likely that he did have bad intentions.

• **Ask a lie-detector question.**

Scenario: The man at your door offers a potentially legitimate reason for being there. Maybe he's selling vacuums, or he needs your signature for a delivery. Should you remove the door's security chain and open it? First, ask a question that should be easy for this person to answer, such as, "So, how many vacuums have you sold today?" or "Where did you park your delivery van? I don't see it." If this is a real salesman or delivery person, your question will sound like relatively normal conversation and he should answer without missing a beat. If this person is a criminal, there likely will be a pause as he tries to think up a plausible lie...and you might see a look of confusion or anxiety on his face.

Best Self-Defense Tools

Guns are effective self-defense tools only if you know how to use them safely and it's legal to carry them where you live. Fixed-blade knives can be effective as well, but these, too, can attract odd looks. *Two weapons—and one additional self-defense item—that you can bring almost everywhere without causing raised eyebrows...*

- **Folding knife.** Knives can serve as weapons if you are attacked...or as cutting or prying tools if you become trapped. Folding knives can fit in a pocket or purse, but unfortunately, most of them are not made well enough to be reliable self-defense tools. Companies that make high-quality folding knives that won't let you down in an emergency include Spyderco (Spyderco.com, folding knife prices start at around $60 for a 5.8-inch knife with a 2.25-inch blade) and Benchmade (Benchmade.com, folding knife prices start at around $110 for a 6.8-inch knife with a 2.9-inch blade).

- **Tactical pen.** A tactical pen is an actual working pen, an item so harmless in appearance that you even can carry it onto an airplane. But it has a pointed end and is made of a strong material, typically steel, titanium or aircraft-grade aluminum. In an emergency, you can use it as a weapon—hold the pen in your fist and jab with it as you would an ice pick.

Example: A Florida woman used her tactical pen to fight off two men who apparently meant to abduct her.

Type "tactical pen" into Amazon.com to find numerous well-reviewed examples for less than $25.

Helpful: If you are grabbed by someone larger or stronger than you and you have no weapon or martial arts training, the easiest and most effective self-defense strategy is to gouge the attacker's eyes with your thumbs.

- **Bulletproof panel.** This is a lightweight sheet of Kevlar that slips into a laptop bag, briefcase or even a three-ring binder. In an active-shooter situation, hold the bag, briefcase or binder containing the panel in front of your chest to significantly reduce the odds that you will be hit by a fatal bullet.

Example: BulletBlocker (BulletBlocker.com) offers a range of Kevlar panels, most for $100 to $220. They typically weigh 10 to 20 ounces.

How to Ward Off Danger

Home invaders and burglars generally do not target houses randomly—they case neighborhoods and select properties that seem particularly vulnerable. You probably can guess what would make your home seem unappealing to bad guys—security cameras and an alarm system, a dog and exterior motion-detector lights. *What surprises many home owners is how easy and inexpensive it is to take advantage of these deterrents...*

- **If you don't want the dog, get dog toys.** Spread a few brightly colored dog toys around your yard, and put a dog bowl on your porch. Pick toys and a bowl meant for big dogs. That should be enough to convince someone casing the neighborhood that there's a big dog waiting inside. Crooks avoid messing with big dogs even more than they avoid home-security systems—dogs don't take 10 minutes to respond to break-ins.

- **If you don't want the security system,** get fake security cameras. Type "fake cameras" into Amazon.com, and you'll find convincing examples that cost less than $10 apiece. Mount one on every side of your home. Criminals know that getting captured on video greatly increases their chances of getting captured in real life.

- **If you don't want to pay an electrician to wire motion-activated exterior lights,** install solar-powered motion-activated lights. Solar lights typically do not require any external electrical connections. They actually are a more reliable deterrent than wired lights, too, because they won't stop working during widespread power failures, a common time for break-ins. They are available for around $40 apiece in home stores and online.

Chapter 7

DIABETES AND BLOOD SUGAR BREAKTHROUGHS

That Dip in Estrogen Contributes to Increased Risk for Diabetes

You're perimenopausal and healthy—ideal weight, don't drink or smoke, exercise every day—but your insulin levels are nearly at prediabetes levels. Can approaching menopause possibly increase your risk for diabetes?

Yes, menopause and an increased risk for type 2 diabetes are connected.

One reason is that estrogen, which of course drops as a woman approaches menopause, helps to move excess blood sugar out of your bloodstream, where it can do damage, and into your muscles, where it can be used more quickly. With less estrogen, more sugar stays in the blood. Estrogen also helps more evenly distribute fat around your body so that it doesn't accumulate in your belly—your "love handle" area. With less estrogen, fat may gather in the abdomen—and excess abdominal fat is associated with an elevated risk for diabetes and heart disease.

How much estrogen is in your bloodstream is also partly regulated by the bacteria in your gut—which are affected by what you eat and how active you are. Taking antibiotics can alter your gut bacteria as well—and not in a good way.

If you're already taking some smart steps to stay healthy, you may just need to fine-tune your diet and lifestyle a bit more. Even if you aren't overweight, make sure you're limiting (or eliminating) soda, cutting back on packaged foods that contain lots of added sugars and eating plenty of vegetables, fruits and legumes. A dietitian can evaluate your diet and advise you on other changes that can help. *Meanwhile, keep these recommendations in mind…*

- **Avoid taking antibiotics unless your doctor says that it's absolutely necessary.**
- **Add fermented foods such as pickles, kimchi, sauerkraut and kefir to your diet.** These can improve gut bacteria, which can help reduce belly fat. (For more on menopause and diabetes, see page 271.)

Mache Seibel, MD, member of the faculty at Beth Israel Beth Israel Deaconess Medical Center and Harvard Medical School, both in Boston, and an expert in women's health and menopause. He is editor of *The Hot Years: My Menopause Magazine* and author of *The Estrogen Window: The Breakthrough Guide to Being Healthy, Energized and Hormonally Balanced—Through Perimenopause, Menopause, and Beyond.* He is the past editor-in-chief of the medical journal *Sexuality, Reproduction & Menopause.*

Got Prediabetes?

Gerald Bernstein, MD, an internist and endocrinologist, who is program director of the Friedman Diabetes Institute at Lenox Hill Hospital in New York City. Dr. Bernstein was president of the American Diabetes Association and has served on its national board of directors and on the editorial board of *Clinical Diabetes*.

If you're over age 45 and you get regular checkups, your doctor will probably test you for diabetes. But only about half of doctors, according to recent research, raise the alarm when those same tests indicate prediabetes, characterized by slightly elevated blood sugar that hasn't yet progressed to full-blown clinical diabetes.

Why that's a dangerous omission…

• **Prediabetes now affects 38% of American adults.** The risk increases substantially over age 60.

• **Unless you treat prediabetes as a wake-up call to change your lifestyle,** your chance of progressing to clinical diabetes is a whopping 70%.

• **Prediabetes hurts your health now—**even if it doesn't progress to clinical diabetes. Years of higher-than-normal blood sugar can cause some of the same damage as full-fledged diabetes.

• **It's much easier to reverse prediabetes than full-blown diabetes.** In prediabetes, your body is developing insulin resistance so that you need more insulin to regulate blood sugar. But if producing that extra insulin overtaxes your pancreas so that you can't keep up with the demand for insulin, you've got type 2 diabetes—and reversal is much harder to achieve.

• **America's doctors are missing the boat on treatment of prediabetes, too.** Even when patients are diagnosed with prediabetes, only 33% get counseling about nutrition…only 32% get counseling about exercise...and a mere 26% about both.

My advice: As a patient, you need to take prediabetes seriously. *Here's how…*

Get Tested

Prediabetes is a stage between a normal blood glucose level and one that's so high that it triggers the "big" diagnosis. It's measured with the same blood tests that doctors use to identify diabetes.

My advice: Given the enormous number of people who develop prediabetes, every adult should get tested—without exception.

There are three common tests—any one of which is sufficient to diagnose prediabetes, so you'll need only one…

• **Fasting plasma glucose (FPG).** This is the standard blood test for diagnosing both diabetes and prediabetes. Take the test first thing in the morning (since you have to fast for at least eight hours). A reading of less than 100 milligrams per deciliter (mg/dL) is normal…100 mg/dL to 125 mg/dL is prediabetes…and 126 mg/dL or higher means you already have diabetes.

• **A1C (glycated hemoglobin).** This blood test measures the percentage of glucose that's attached to the hemoglobin in blood. It indicates your average blood sugar level over the last two or three months. I recommend this test because it's fast, inexpensive and doesn't require fasting. A normal reading is below 5.7%. A reading between 5.7% and 6.4% indicates prediabetes. A reading of 6.5% or higher means diabetes.

• **Glucose tolerance test.** This test is more cumbersome but more accurate. Instead of eating a meal, you consume a standard amount of glucose, and then your blood glucose is measured at 30 minutes and at least one hour and two hours afterward. If your blood sugar tests high (between 140 mg/dL and 199 mg/dL) two hours after drinking the glucose solution, it means that you have prediabetes. If your blood sugar tests 200 mg/dL or higher, then you have diabetes.

How often should you get tested? If your result is normal but you also have two or more diabetes risk factors (such as being overweight and sedentary), get tested annually…otherwise, every three years is fine. But if the test shows prediabetes, you should embark on a program to reverse it—and make sure your doctor retests you more frequently, such as every six months, to see if your changes are working.

How to Reverse Prediabetes

Most people with slightly high blood sugar can lower it with basic lifestyle changes, along with medication in some cases. Make sure you discuss various interventions with your physician, and, if possible, work with a diabetes educator, especially one associated with a diabetes program. *The basics...*

• **Start with weight loss.** Not everyone with prediabetes is overweight—but most patients are. Often, losing just 10 pounds is enough to improve insulin sensitivity and bring blood sugar into the healthy range.

• **Take a daily walk.** A daily 30-minute walk reduces your risk of developing diabetes by 30%, according to the Harvard School of Public Health's Nurses' Health Study and the Health Professionals Follow-Up Study. Exercise increases insulin sensitivity. It also increases metabolism and muscle mass, which lower glucose even more.

• **Eat whole grains.** Research has shown that people who eat two to three servings of whole grains daily, compared with those who eat little or none, are 30% less likely to develop type 2 diabetes. Processed grains—such as white rice and most breakfast cereals, etc.—are digested quickly and cause a faster rise in glucose.

• **Minimize red meat.** Red meat (especially fatty cuts) is high in saturated fat, which can increase diabetes risk. Be especially sparing with processed red meats, such as bacon and bologna. In one large Harvard study, people who ate as little as two ounces of processed red meat daily had a 19% increased risk of developing diabetes.

• **Say no to sugary soft drinks.** A Harvard study found that women who drank one or more of these beverages a day, compared with those who drank them rarely, had an 83% higher risk of developing diabetes. Beware of any sugar-sweetened drink, including sugar-sweetened teas and sports drinks.

My advice: Sugary drinks should be avoided altogether.

What About Medication?

Nearly 10 years ago, the American Diabetes Association updated its guidelines to include *metformin* (Glucophage) for treating high-risk patients with prediabetes. Research shows that it cuts the risk of developing diabetes by 31%. Yet it's still prescribed for only a small fraction of these patients. The drug can cause diarrhea and gas, but the side effects usually go away within a week or two. It can also diminish appetite, which is sometimes a benefit for people trying to lose weight. I recommend it for people who can't get their blood sugar under control with lifestyle measures alone. If you tolerate it well, you can stay on it indefinitely.

How a Healthy-Cooking Expert Was Diagnosed with Prediabetes

Alma Schneider, LCSW, licensed clinical social worker, creator of Take Back the Kitchen, LLC, and author of *Take Back the Kitchen: Identify and Own Your Cooking Personality Type and Get Cooking!*

Gerald Bernstein, MD, FACP, coordinator of the Friedman Diabetes Program, department of endocrinology, Lenox Hill Hospital, New York City.

Prediabetes was never on Alma Schneider's radar. Why would she worry about a condition that can lead to type 2 diabetes when her life's work is teaching people how to create healthy home-cooked meals? Not to mention that she diligently practices what she preaches in her own kitchen...she's not overweight...and she exercises.

That's why she was thrown for a loop when her doctor called last year with the results from a routine checkup. Her blood showed that she was very close to having prediabetes...then things got worse and she was prediabetic.

Her story has lessons for nearly all of us. After all, 86 million Americans have prediabetes. So there's plenty of worry to go around. What appeared to be Alma Schneider's losing battle with her rising blood sugar highlights an important debate in the medical community. Does getting a prediabetes diagnosis really help—or is it just another medical label that makes people feel bad about themselves? Does one size really fit all? Check out Alma's story—and the lessons one respected diabetes expert draws from it.

Alma's Story

A cooking coach and author of *Take Back the Kitchen: Identify and Own Your Cooking Personality Type and Get Cooking!*, Alma Schneider is a clinical social worker and creator of Take Back the Kitchen, a lifestyle program that helps people overcome obstacles to cooking healthy meals at home.

Forty-seven at the time, Schneider was shocked at her blood test results but also frustrated with her doctor's seemingly automatic advice to clean up her diet and increase her activity. She already cooked most of her meals from scratch with whole "real" ingredients. She already avoided added sugar. And she already worked out three times a week.

There wasn't much more she could change, but she did what she could. No more dried fruit (it's got a lot of concentrated natural sugar). She limited even healthy carbs, including whole grains, such as brown rice, and sweet potatoes, which are high in fiber. Instead of bananas, which contain a fair amount of natural sugar, she switched to berries, which contain less. She started eating more foods that are low on the glycemic index—meaning they cause only a gradual, modest increase in blood sugar—such as lentils.

As it happened, three months later Schneider had an appointment with her endocrinologist (whom she saw regularly, having had thyroid cancer a decade earlier). She insisted he do a repeat blood test.

The result: Her blood sugar had risen further, with her A1C, a score that indicates blood sugar over the previous three months, edging up from 5.5 to 5.7—officially prediabetic, albeit at the lowest end of the blood sugar range for that label. She chronicled her struggles in a series of humorous blog posts with titles such as *How My Body Betrayed Me Following My Carb Revenge* and *Could I Belly Dance My Way Out of Prediabetes?*

Was she overreacting? How important is prediabetes anyway?

The Prediabetes Debate

The definition of prediabetes is straightforward. The American Diabetes Association defines the condition as having levels of blood glucose—aka blood sugar—that are higher than normal but not quite high enough to qualify as full-blown diabetes. That translates to an A1C between 5.7 and 6.4. Above that level, it's type 2 diabetes. Most of the time, prediabetes has no symptoms.

Here's why it matters: Without lifestyle changes, as many as 70% of people with prediabetes will develop full-blown diabetes within a decade. But lifestyle changes can upend those odds. A not-very-difficult structured lifestyle program can cut the risk by 58%—and that goes up to 71% in people over age 60. Losing even a small amount of weight—5% to 7% of body weight or 10 to 14 pounds for someone who weighs 200 pounds—is a key part of that approach.

But not everyone is happy with diagnosing so many millions of people—including 80% of Americans over age 60—with prediabetes. Some bloggers, citing arguments in the medical community, write that it just makes people feel bad about themselves, "medicalizes" and labels them, and doesn't really help them change. Instead, they argue, we should focus as a society on encouraging healthier eating and more exercise for everyone. Alma Schneider certainly had a strong emotional reaction to learning that she now fit into the high-risk group of "prediabetics"—it challenged her self-image.

Yet while the "prediabetic" label may be controversial—since most of us already know we should be eating better and exercising more and watching our weight—it serves an important purpose, says Gerald Bernstein, MD, coordinator of the Friedman Diabetes Program at Lenox Hill Hospital in New York. Why? By reinforcing the need to be vigilant about trying to prevent type 2 diabetes—and by giving patients a measure of their progress on the path to prevention.

If a patient falls into a prediabetes range for whatever reason, she and her doctor must figure out what to do from there. For most people, lifestyle modifications are a good first line of defense. (Sometimes the drug *metformin* is also prescribed to reduce the risk for progression to type 2 diabetes.) An A1C test result in the prediabetes range, Dr. Bernstein notes, does not mean that diabetes is inevitable.

Indeed, a rise in A1C from 5.5 to 5.7 is not particularly concerning, notes Dr. Bernstein—unless it continues to go up every few months. In Alma's case, it didn't. Now more than a year later, it's still 5.7—and her endocrinologist now checks it only once a year. Still, he applauds Schneider for taking this seriously and searching for ways to tweak her lifestyle to reduce her blood sugar.

There's another lesson to be learned here, too—your health is not defined by any one number. While Dr. Bernstein thinks a prediabetes diagnosis is a wake-up call for anyone, he emphasizes that everyone's case is individual. Clearly, the numbers Schneider got from her A1C test weren't the whole picture. Her healthy habits put her ahead of the game. Her other numbers, such as blood pressure and cholesterol, were just fine. Indeed, her own primary care doctor reassured her that it was unlikely she'd develop diabetes as long she kept up those habits.

Alma's Kitchen Tips to Manage Prediabetes

Alma was shocked by her diagnosis of prediabetes...then she worked extra hard to eat more healthfully...and then she rebelled against that stringency by eating an excess of carbs. Eventually, she figured out a balance that works for her physically and emotionally.

Now she is comfortably in a regular, healthy-eating-and-exercise routine. She realizes she's living a healthy life and that she will most likely be just fine. She's kept some of the changes she made when she first got the diagnosis—less dried fruit, moderate carb portions—and she feels good about her healthy lifestyle. And she has some culinary advice to share. *If you're looking to avoid a prediabetes diagnosis—or reverse one—here are her tips...*

- **Rely on fresh whole foods as much as possible.** There's so much added sugar in prepared and restaurant food it's hard to know what's in your meals unless you start from scratch as often as you can.
- **Fill your kitchen and pantry with healthy staples.** Rely mostly on vegetables, low-sugar fruits such as berries, lean protein and complex high-fiber carbs such as brown rice rather than white.
- **Head off hunger.** To avoid mindlessly reaching for high-calorie, high-fat, low-nutrition items when you get hungry for a snack, keep easily accessible, ready-to-eat whole foods on hand. Try hard-boiled eggs, cut-up veggies, hummus, edamame dip. Put together little bags of nuts to keep in your car so you don't stop at a gas station and pick up something unhealthy if you get hungry on the road.
- **Make your own healthier chips.** Are you in a "can't eat just one" state of mind? Instead of reaching for commercial potato chips or other snacks, make your own kale chips. Toss five cups of kale pieces with enough olive oil to lightly coat them, sprinkle with salt, spread on a wire rack set atop a baking sheet, and bake in a 350-degree oven until crisp (about 15 minutes).
- **Use low-carb flours.** If you're craving something baked, experiment with using almond or coconut flour, which are lower in carbs than wheat flour. They also make a tasty breading for chicken cutlets and fish fillets.

- **Satisfy a sweet tooth by creating desserts that include fresh fruit flavored with coconut milk or cinnamon,** both of which are naturally sweet with little or no added sugar.

Most important, forget trying to be perfect. What Alma Schneider learned from her prediabetes saga is to relax and accept that she's a pretty healthy person—and she doesn't need to hit the perfection mark every moment.

Don't Fear Diabetes! Straight Talk for the Newly Diagnosed

Theresa Garnero, RN, MS (nursing), a member of Bottom Line's Diabetes Resource Center expert panel and an advanced-practice registered nurse (APRN), board-certified in advanced diabetes management (BC-ADM), certified diabetes educator (CDE) and instructional designer in the Family Health Care Nursing division at University of California, San Francisco. She is the author of *Your First Year with Diabetes: What to Do, Month by Month.*

If you've recently been diagnosed with diabetes, you may be in shock for a bit…that's normal. But if you're afraid or panicked, try not to give in to those feelings or let your imagination run wild. It's easy to jump to conclusions based on the worst outcomes you've heard about or seen within your family or friends, such as amputation and blindness—but the reality, with today's know-how, is usually nothing like that.

Key insight: For most people with well-managed diabetes, the most common complication is…no complication at all! And even though you will have to make some lifestyle changes, you're not doomed to a lifetime diet of no treats and no carbs.

As a diabetes educator, the first thing I do with new patients is to help them face their fears. Doing so not only helps them feel better but may motivate them to take the manageable small steps that will help in so many ways. *Let's get started…*

What's Good About a Diagnosis

Think of a diagnosis of type 2 diabetes as a bit of good fortune in one way. As many as 40% of people with type 2 diabetes are walking around unaware that they have it, which means the disease is doing damage to their bodies unchecked. With a diagnosis in hand, you're a step ahead—and you can stay ahead by employing some smart management strategies.

Can you look at the glass-half-full side of your diagnosis?

Here's the first benefit: You can take action. I see people every day who amaze me in their ability to take control of their condition rather than the other way around.

This means managing your blood glucose…which in turn reduces your risk of getting many diabetes-related complications. And if you do have complications, taking action means tackling those problems head-on and early so they don't progress. Your diagnosis also can be the inspiration you need to tweak some habits that may have needed it anyway, such as eating a healthier diet and exercising.

Though it's normal to be overwhelmed at first, remember…knowledge is power. It's also the best way to counter anxiety and remain in control. Ready to face your fears, one by one? Here are the top five worries that people newly diagnosed with diabetes ask me about, the reality behind them—and how you can take action.

Five Common Diabetes Fears

- **I'll need amputation.** The thought of losing a foot or leg is terrifying. But there's typically a long chain of events that would have to happen before you'd need an amputation, and most of them are avoidable. First, blood glucose would have to be very high for a number of years…think, a wildfire burning out of control. Next, you would need to injure your foot and not notice it and not get it treated. Finally, a rip-roaring infection would have to take hold.

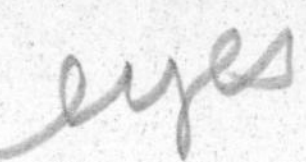

Take action: The key to avoiding all diabetes complications, including the prospect of amputation, is doing your best to monitor and manage your blood glucose, blood pressure and cholesterol or "lipid" (blood fat) profile.

Why are all three important? Think of your blood vessels as like the plumbing in your house—it is a closed circuit. The water should stay in the pipes. If your water pressure is high (the analogy being high blood pressure) or filled with years of debris (think fat deposits built up along the inside of your arteries), then the water flow changes (think of blood circulation with less flow). Now add uncontrolled high levels of blood glucose, which can block the mechanisms that the body enlists to fight infections. If your blood is "sweet" and doesn't flow well because it is under a constricted, high-pressure system and full of debris, that all combines to increase your risk for foot infections after an initial injury or small skin cut occurs.

Uncontrolled high glucose, blood pressure and cholesterol can also lead to a decreased sensitivity in your feet. If left unchecked, it can lead to damage of the nerves, called neuropathy. This is a significant factor for people with diabetes who are faced with an amputation. You might not even realize your foot has a cut if you can't feel it. That is why you need to take good care of your feet! Check your tootsies daily for any cuts or scrapes, and protect them by wearing closed shoes. See a podiatrist if you have a problem, such as an ingrown toenail...don't attempt "bathroom surgery." If you get a pedicure, bring your own tools to avoid being exposed to bacteria from the shop's tools.

• **I'll go blind.** While it's true that the risk for blindness is higher in people with diabetes than in people who don't have the disease, most people with diabetes don't go blind... and even more modest vision loss, when it does occur, doesn't happen overnight. It's usually the result of a trifecta—unchecked high blood glucose, high blood pressure and high cholesterol.

Here's what happens: High blood glucose causes damage to the blood vessels in the retina. That in turn makes the tiny vessels in the eye prone to bleeding or leaking fluid. It is the tiny hemorrhages in the eye that over time can block vision. Unhealthy levels of cholesterol in your blood further gum up the works. And high blood pressure puts a lot of strain on the vessels in the back of the eye. Over time, and unchecked, these factors may lead to vision loss.

Take action: Schedule an eye exam with dilation at least once a year to check for problems. If it is discovered that you have retinopathy, several treatments exist including injections in the early stages (Anti-VEGF therapy or corticosteroids) or laser surgery in the late stages.

• **Taking insulin is scary or dangerous.** Plenty of people hate the very idea of sticking themselves with a needle, and that's natural. Most believe, wrongly however, that insulin itself is somehow harmful. Insulin is simply a hormone your body is missing and that needs to be replaced. Some believe that going on insulin is a sign their disease has just become serious. The truth is that by the time most people get a type 2 diabetes diagnosis, they've already lost 50% to 80% of the function of insulin-producing beta cells, as well as some of the cells, in the pancreas.

Take action: Remember that diabetes is a progressive disease...nearly everyone who lives long enough with the disease eventually needs insulin. You might need it now, or you might not for a few years or even decades. Don't think of it as a punishment or a sign of failure but as another step in managing your condition and living your life to the fullest. You haven't failed—your pancreas has. Many patients end up saying, "I wish I had started insulin earlier because I feel so much better." And if you fear needles...take heart. If you participate in a diabetes-management program, you'll learn about the latest and greatest equipment, including insulin pens. These needles are really tiny—I can't tell you how many times people trying them have said, "I didn't even feel that."

• **I'll need dialysis.** Dialysis is necessary when your kidneys can no longer do the job of filtering waste from your blood. While kidney problems are a known complication of diabetes, dialysis is not a given by any means. As long as you get the recommended screening tests, you'll be warned of any potential kidney problems so you can take lifestyle steps—and if needed get appropriate medications—to help protect your kidneys.

Take action: All of the things that are good for your health in general—such as focusing on whole, fresh foods...watching your blood pressure and cholesterol...not smoking or being around second-hand smoke—are also good for your kidneys. The tiny blood vessels in the kidneys, just like the ones in your eyes, don't do well if your blood glucose or blood pressure is high. Exposure to tobacco smoke also constricts vessels.

- **I won't be able to eat anything fun.** Hold on! The key to managing diabetes isn't cutting out entire categories of foods, such as fat or carbs. It's eating more mindfully and with more planning. You can still have some bread, pasta—even sugar. While no one food is "forbidden," though, you do have to think about the timing of meals and snacks and how much you eat. You'll also learn how to balance out carbs with protein and to figure out which foods have the biggest impact on your blood sugar.

Take action: Follow some basic rules, such as relying more on fresh, whole foods and less on packaged or processed items. Do a "food inventory" of your kitchen to see how you can better stock your fridge and cupboard for success. Discover what inspires you. Get the help of a registered dietitian who specializes in people with diabetes. You can ask your local hospital or search the website of the American Association of Diabetes Educators. With that expert help, you'll learn diet strategies that work for you.

Notes for the Journey

Taking small steps is the best advice for conquering any fears you have when you're first diagnosed with diabetes. Letting yourself be consumed by stress can lead to burnout or fatalism. Start by realizing that this is a journey, not a destination, and that there are measures you'll be taking daily to remain healthy. Get ready for bumps in the road—and for successes and opportunities.

A few final thoughts...

- **Pay attention to your numbers**—blood glucose, cholesterol, blood pressure and others. Knowing these stats helps you stack the deck in your own favor and avoid complications.

- **Focus on overall health.** If other health issues come up as a result of your diabetes, there are many things that can be done to minimize or stop their progression. It all starts with being aware, engaged and involved.

- **Don't rely only on one doctor.** People with diabetes have better results with a health-care team that includes (ideally) an endocrinologist... and if that's not possible, a primary care provider with a focus on diabetes. Your team should also include a diabetes educator, who may be a nurse or a registered dietitian, to whom you can turn with questions. You'll also need an eye specialist, podiatrist and dentist—all part of ongoing maintenance to keep you tuned up.

- **Don't go it alone.** You might also want to find a support group, either online or in person, to get and share tips from others in your shoes. That may be more meaningful than what the person in the white coat says! People with diabetes who participate in support groups have lower glucose levels, on average. You can find a community to connect with by searching the American Diabetes Association support community or the Diabetes Hands Foundation. You may also find it helpful to use an app for your phone like MySugr, which has more than a million users worldwide, or a new app called KingFit that offers free diabetes education from national experts.

- **Most important...try to focus on the positive.** Swap negative thoughts (about what you have to stop doing) for positive ones (about changes that will be good for you). Having diabetes is a challenge, and your efforts are worth the energy it takes to maintain your health. You've got this!

8 Tips for Living Alone with Diabetes

Judith H. McQuown, a patient advocate with first-hand diabetes experience and the author of 12 books. The tips here come from her book *1,137 Secrets for Living Well with Diabetes* (Bottom Line Books).

It's easy to feel vulnerable when you have diabetes and live alone. I know—I've had type 1 diabetes for more than 30 years, and I've lived alone for most of that time. Taking steps to feel safer, especially in an emergency, can reduce your stress. And when you're less stressed, your blood glucose levels stay more even. *So here are my favorite tips for living alone with diabetes—they are helpful whether you have type 1 or type 2 diabetes...*

• **Have a buddy system.** You should have someone to check in with every morning. Your buddy doesn't have to have diabetes—anyone who lives alone and might need help will benefit from this arrangement, and so will you.

Your call or text can be brief: "Hi, it's me. Are you OK? I'm OK. Do you need anything?" What counts is that you and your friend have made sure that each of you is alive and well.

• **Make blood sugar checkpoints easier with a vibrating watch.** Self-care for your diabetes is your responsibility, but living alone makes it that much more important to remember all the checkpoints in your day.

A subtle helper: A vibrating watch. Rather than sounding an alarm, it gives the wearer an unmistakable (but silent) reminder. Originally created for people with hearing loss, a vibrating watch can keep us on schedule, too. You'll find many brands and prices to choose from online. A smartwatch may also have this function.

• **Post medical emergency information.** Put this information on two sheets of paper on which you have drawn big red borders and written MEDICAL EMERGENCY INFORMATION. Include the same information on each paper—your name, medical problems, the drugs you are taking, any allergies or drug reactions, the name and phone number of your contact person and your blood type if you know it. Stick one of the pages onto the inside of your front door, and display the other page prominently on your refrigerator door.

• **Protect yourself from falls against sharp-edged furniture.** Why do we fall against sharp-edged furniture, especially at 3 am when our blood glucose is dropping? Because it's there! To prevent or minimize black-and-blue marks and potential fractures, pad everything. Use folded towels or movers' pads. Doorknobs can also do major damage—they are just the right height for you to hit your head on if you fall in a hypoglycemic swoon. For an easy fix, cover doorknobs with Bubble Wrap and secure with rubber bands.

• **Prepare for a power outage.** Between blizzards and hurricanes and anything else that might cause power blackouts, you must keep emergency supplies on hand, especially if you live alone. Besides extra drugs and equipment, you should have several flashlights and lots of extra batteries, a few transistor radios (one may fade out after a week of continuous use), a first-aid kit, at least five gallons of water and lots of candles with sturdy candleholders and matches. Also, keep a week's supply of canned food that you can eat cold in an emergency. My favorites are mostly 100% protein—canned chicken breast, salmon and tuna. But I also include some canned ravioli and chili in case I need some carbohydrates. And make sure you have a hand-operated can opener.

If your fuse box or circuit breakers are in your basement, paint the edge of every step with luminous white or Day-Glo paint. Then if your power goes out, you can get safely down the basement stairs to change the fuse or reset the circuit breakers. And always take a flashlight!

• **Designate a spot for important items.** One of the toughest aspects of living alone is misplacing something vital. Designate a spot in your home—the bottom of your underwear drawer, a kitchen shelf or a table in your front hallway—to be "home base" for possessions that you absolutely can't lose. When you can't find your car keys, they'll be in your "spot." You may want another space—near your bed?—for your glucose meter, test strips, lancet and glucose tablets.

• **Stay motivated with photos.** When living alone, it can be hard to stay motivated about blood glucose control and to keep your spirits up during difficult times. Keep photos of loved ones, pets and even heroes in full view. They will serve as reminders of love and courage during bad or just lonely times.

• **Dawdle over dinner.** Too many people who live alone race through their meals in front of the TV. Make your dinner last at least 45 minutes and try listening to relaxing classical music instead of watching TV. This turns eating into a pleasurable experience...and gives your body the opportunity to start feeling full, a process that takes 20 to 30 minutes, which means there's less chance that you'll overeat.

Can Whole-Body Vibrations Help Prevent Diabetes?

Meghan E. McGee-Lawrence, PhD, department of cellular biology and anatomy, Medical College of Georgia, Augusta University, and lead author of the study titled, *"Whole-body Vibration Mimics the Metabolic Effects of Exercise in Male Leptin Receptor Deficient Mice,"* published in *Endocrinology.*

Standing still—or better yet, lying down—in a gym or at home on a machine that does all the work for you seems like a cheater's vision of exercise. But for many people who are obese and/or have a lack of stamina or other issues that make it difficult to exercise, it may be a realistic vision.

Good news: These folks may be able to get many of the benefits of exercise—including reduced blood sugar and increased insulin sensitivity—in a different way. It's called whole-body vibration.

Background: Whole-body vibration (WBV)—standing, sitting or lying on a machine with a vibrating platform—causes muscles to contract and relax repetitively, placing a "biomechanical load" on the body that is similar, in some ways, to what exercise does. Although it's been around for decades, new technology has revived interest in it. But does WBV provide the same protective effects on the body—including preventing diabetes—as traditional physical exercise? Researchers from the Medical College of Georgia decided to find out.

Study: This was an animal study, but it sheds light on basic physiology. Researchers used obese mice with diabetes. Half of the mice exercised for 45 minutes a day on a treadmill. The other half were given whole-body vibration for 20 minutes a day.

Results: After 12 weeks, the two groups showed similar improvements. Muscle fiber increased 24% in the vibration group compared to 29% in the treadmill exercisers. The size of fat cells went down by 15% (vibration) versus 21% (treadmill). Both groups had similar improvements in insulin sensitivity, which reduces the severity of diabetes, and similar reductions in fat deposits in their livers—a risk factor for both fatty liver disease and for diabetes. Overall, treadmill exercise was more effective than whole-body vibration at improving blood sugar control and reducing weight—but only slightly.

Early Menopause Linked to Diabetes

Early menopause is tied to type 2 diabetes. Researchers found that women who experience menopause before age 40 are almost four times as likely to develop type 2 diabetes as women whose menopause occurs later—at age 55 or older.

Study of nearly 4,000 women by researchers at Erasmus University Medical Center, Rotterdam, the Netherlands, published in *Diabetologia.*

Surprising finding: The whole-body vibration mice experienced a mild bone benefit, too. Just like the treadmill exercisers, they had small increases in blood levels of osteocalcin, a marker for bone formation.

Bottom line: Whole-body vibration does indeed provide some of the same physical and metabolic benefits as more strenuous physical exercise. To be sure, this study doesn't prove that standing on a vibrating platform is as good at preventing or controlling diabetes as running, swimming or riding a bike. But the findings are encouraging—and other research on people has found that whole body vibration can improve muscle strength and coordination while improving the flexibility of blood vessels and reducing high blood pressure. You can find whole-body vibration machines (often referred to as vibration trainers) at some gyms. They are also available in stores that sell fitness equipment, as well as on online. If you know someone who just can't or just won't exercise, these "good vibes" may be a good alternative.

Diabetes from Your Mouthwash?

Marvin Fier, DDS, Pomona, New York, about a study titled, "Over-the-counter mouthwash use and risk of pre-diabetes/diabetes," published in *Nitric Oxide.* SmileRockland.com

Using mouthwash twice or more a day may keep your breath "minty fresh," but it also may increase your risk of developing type 2 diabetes.

A recent study observed 945 adults for three years. The people studied, ages 40 to 65, were overweight or obese, so they already were at increased risk for diabetes—but the results may be important even for people who are not overweight.

Findings: Participants who used a mouthwash twice or more a day typically had 55% higher risk for prediabetes or diabetes than those who used mouthwash less frequently or not at all.

This kind of study can't show cause and effect, and it leaves many questions open—especially about the kind of mouthwash people used. But there are reasons to avoid excessive use. Most mouthwashes contain alcohol or other ingredients, either synthetic or essential oils, that kill microbes indiscriminately—including beneficial ones that help the body make nitric oxide. But you need nitric oxide—it's a remarkable compound that is important for everyone's health, protecting against not only obesity and insulin resistance but also high blood pressure.

The truth is, you don't need to use mouthwash at all. It's not particularly effective at improving oral health anyway. For example, brushing and flossing are much better at disrupting plaque, the biofilm that sticks to teeth and causes cavities, gum disease—and, often, bad breath.

Tip: Thin, unwaxed floss is best at physically dislodging plaque. (If you still love the mouthwash habit, choose alcohol-free products to avoid drying the delicate mucous membranes of the mouth.)

Finally, don't ignore persistent bad breath. It could point to a health problem. If you are using mouthwash several times each day to get rid of bad breath or a bad taste, speak with your dentist or other health-care provider.

For Better Blood Sugar, You Can't Beat Beets

Christopher Bell, PhD, department of health and exercise science, Colorado State University, Fort Collins, and coauthor of the research article "Concurrent Beet Juice and Carbohydrate Ingestion: Influence on Glucose Tolerance in Obese and Nonobese Adults," published in *Journal of Nutrition and Metabolism,* "10 Best Juicing Recipes for Diabetics," iFocusHealth.com.

If your blood sugar is too high and you're fighting the battle of the bulge, there's an easy way to enhance your insulin sensitivity and better regulate your blood sugar.

Drink a long cool glass of beet juice before a meal.

Background: The idea that drinking beet juice has a positive effect on general health is hardly new. Beet juice is rich in dietary nitrate, which the body uses to make nitric oxide, a compound that helps widen blood vessels, improving circulation. Drinking beetroot juice has been shown to reduce blood pressure, improve blood flow to the brain, improve athletic performance and even prevent altitude sickness. Improving circulation also helps the body deliver glucose to the tissues more efficiently so that the body needs to produce less insulin to metabolize food and control blood sugar. But obese people tend to have low nitric oxide levels. Could beets help boost their nitric oxide and improve their insulin sensitivity? To find out, researchers gave people beet juice and a large amount of sugar to digest. It's a way to simulate the effects of a meal in a lab.

Study: Twelve nonobese men and women and 10 obese men and women took part. Being obese is a significant risk factor for developing diabetes, although none of the participants actually had diabetes. They all were asked to not eat any nitrate-rich foods such as beets or greens the day before. They were also asked to not brush their teeth, floss or use mouthwash for 18 hours before the test. On the day of the study, they each drank a 17-ounce glass of beet juice and then were given a large amount of glucose sugar to consume.

On another day, they rinsed with mouthwash—which prevents the body from turning beet's nitrates into nitric oxide—before consuming the beet juice and sugar. It may seem odd to study this—after all, who rinses with mouthwash before a meal? But the researchers had a reason. They knew that the healthful bacteria in the mouth are needed to convert beet's nitrates into nitrites, the first step for the body to make nitric oxide. When you kill the bacteria in your mouth with mouthwash, they aren't around to do the necessary work.

Result: For the obese beet-juice drinkers, insulin resistance was improved and blood sugar didn't go up as much in the 60 to 90 minutes after consuming the sugar—compared to when they rinsed with mouthwash first. Their insulin resistance and blood sugar still were slightly higher than in their nonobese counterparts—but it was a big improvement for them. That's a key benefit, since elevated insulin resistance plus high blood sugar, over time, increase the risk of developing type 2 diabetes. For the obese, who likely started with low nitric oxide levels, drinking beet juice apparently boosted nitric oxide levels high enough to help them better metabolize sugar.

But the beet juice didn't have the same effect on participants who weren't obese—their insulin sensitivity and blood sugar response to eating sugar was normal when they drank beet juice and when they negated the benefits of beet juice by rinsing with mouthwash. Why? One probable reason is that their nitric oxide levels were already sufficient to help their bodies metabolize sugar, so boosting it a little extra with beet juice didn't have any practical effect.

Bottom line: Obese adults at risk of developing insulin resistance may benefit from adding healthful nitrate-rich foods—including a glass of beet juice—to their meals.

What about the sugar naturally contained in beet juice itself? It's true that there's a lot of sugar in beets—and even more in beet juice. But evidence suggests that the physiological benefits outweigh the sugar—just make sure you skip less healthy sources of sugar such as soda, candy and other sweets. You can also experiment with other nitrate-rich foods, such as spinach.

Try this nitrate-rich homemade beet/apple/celery/spinach juice at breakfast: The night before, cut up one medium-sized beet into cubes and freeze it. The next morning, put the cubes in your juicer along with one sliced and cored apple, two chopped celery stalks, one-half cup of spinach and the juice of one small lemon. Like your beets at lunch or dinner instead? Nothing beats roasted beets!

Caution: Before consuming beet juice regularly, ask your doctor whether there's any reason you should avoid or limit foods such as beets, beet juice and spinach. These foods may not be safe for people who are at risk for kidney stones or who are taking certain medications for heart conditions or erectile dysfunction.

Fish Oil May Raise Women's Diabetes Risk

Fish oil may raise women's diabetes risk. In a study, the group of women who took the most fish oil—1.6 grams of fatty acids daily—had a 26% higher risk of developing type 2 diabetes than women who took in less than 1.3 grams a day. The biggest risk increase was in women of normal weight, with BMIs less than 25—their risk rose 38%.

Study of 71,334 women led by researchers at INSERM Centre for Research in Epidemiology and Population Health, Villejuif, France, published in *Diabetologia.*

Beware: Artificial Sweeteners Are Not a Safe Alternative to Sugar

John La Puma, MD, a member of Bottom Line's Diabetes Resource Center panel of experts, is a board-certified specialist in internal medicine, a professionally trained chef and culinary medicine pioneer. He is cofounder of the popular video recipe series "ChefMD" and *The New York Times* best-selling author of *Refuel: A 24-Day Eating Plan to Shed Fat, Boost Testosterone and Pump Up Strength and Stamina.* DrJohnLaPuma.com

If you're borderline diabetic, you may have started using artificial sweeteners to help cut back on sugar.

Not so fast.

If you're borderline diabetic—aka, you have prediabetes—you should cut back not just on sugar and starches but also on artificial sweeteners. Use them rarely—no more than once a month.

Why? Since the 1950s, when tiny tablets of saccharin became available to shake into your morning coffee, artificial sweeteners have promised dulce...but for people with blood sugar concerns they are more likely diablo.

Recent evidence: An 18-year study of 61,440 women showed that those who "always or almost always" used artificial sweeteners of any kind had an increased risk of developing type 2 diabetes. The link was not based on the likelihood that people who are overweight may be using artificial sweeteners. It was independent of body weight.

New research is uncovering just how artificial sweeteners may contribute to diabetes—or make it worse if you already have it.

Example: Aspartame (NutraSweet, Equal) can alter the activity and composition of the microbes in your intestine, creating glucose intolerance. It may also increase levels of the stress hormone cortisol and increase systemic oxidative stress—both contributors to metabolic diseases including diabetes. Aspartame may also interfere with the N-methyl D-aspartate (NMDA) receptor in nerves, which can cause insulin deficiency or resistance. It's not the only artificial sweetener that's troubling—Sucralose (Splenda), although considered safe for most people, has been reported to raise blood sugar levels in people with diabetes.

The truth is, artificial sweeteners are bad for everybody, not just for people with prediabetes or diabetes. Healthy people who drink more diet soda, compared with those who drink little or no soda, are more likely to become obese...and have big bellies. That, too, may have something to do with interference with a healthy gut microbiome. Plus, by tricking your palate into thinking that you are eating something with calories (sugar) when there are no calories, you may stimulate your appetite, making it easier to overeat. A recent review of 37 studies found that long-term use of artificial sweeteners was associated with weight gain, diabetes, high blood sugar and heart disease.

Small amounts of stevia, a natural sweetener derived from a South American plant, are likely safe for daily use. But I wouldn't use large amounts of stevia extracts, which may disrupt hormones in large doses according to some reports. Extracts are different from the whole unprocessed leaf, which is likely the safest choice—you can boil the leaves in water and then keep the sweetened water in the refrigerator to use by the teaspoon.

You can also reeducate your sweet tooth. Gradually cut back on natural sweeteners such as sugar, honey and maple syrup to reprogram your "sugar meter" so you crave sweetness less. Fruit, which is naturally sweet, has a place in a balanced diet. Dried fruit is often high in sugar, but you can learn to use small amounts to sweeten dishes. For cooking, especially whole grains and whole-grain salads, I like "sweet" herbs and spices such as cinnamon, anise, clove, fennel and allspice. And you know what? Your gut bacteria will come back in balance shortly after you stop the synthetics.

New Natural Sweeteners Can Help You Cut Back on Sugar

Janet Bond Brill, PhD, RDN, FAND, a registered dietitian nutritionist, a fellow of the Academy of Nutrition and Dietetics and a nationally recognized nutrition, health and fitness expert who specializes in cardiovascular disease prevention. Based in Allentown, Pennsylvania, Dr. Brill is the author of *Blood Pressure DOWN*, *Cholesterol DOWN* and *Prevent a Second Heart Attack*. DrJanet.com

It's not news that consumption of refined sugar in the US has skyrocketed—the average American now consumes an incredible 23.5 teaspoons a day, almost double what the average American consumed 100 years ago! But why are we doing this to ourselves? Refined sugar not only contributes to weight gain but also has been linked to increased risk for diabetes, heart disease, anxiety, depression and other health conditions. What's more, the desire for sugar can be addictive, making it extremely difficult to cut back.

Luckily, there's an ever-growing number of natural sugar alternatives that can be a big help if you'd rather not use an artificial sweetener or go cold turkey, which is very difficult to do. All can satisfy the craving for sugar and provide lower calories than table sugar. *Some of the newest and best natural sweeteners on the market...*

- **Lite & Sweet is a blend of xylitol and erythritol,** sugar alcohols derived from berries and other fruits. It comes in bulk and packet form—one teaspoon has four calories (there's 16 calories in a teaspoon of table sugar). Lite & Sweet looks like regular sugar—and when using it for baking and cooking, it can be substituted for regular sugar teaspoon for teaspoon.

Both xylitol and erythritol are considered safe for human consumption if consumed in small doses. However, if you have too much of them, they can have a laxative effect.

- **Nature Sweet is a combination erythritol, fructose, chicory root fiber and two plant-derived sweeteners.** The first is stevia, which comes from the leaves of the stevia plant and has up to 200 times the sweetness of table sugar. The second plant-derived sweetener comes from monk fruit, a subtropical melonlike gourd, and is about 150 to 200 times sweeter than regular sugar. The new kid on the block at Starbucks, one packet of Nature Sweet (it comes in a green packet) has zero calories. In addition to using it in beverages, Nature Sweet can be used in recipes where the primary role of sugar is to sweeten, not to add bulk or tenderness, such as in sauces, salad dressings, fruit pies and cheesecake.

All sweeteners in Nature Sweet have been approved by the FDA for use in the US and do not appear to pose any health risks when used in moderation.

•**Just Like Sugar is made primarily from chicory root fiber.** Chicory root offers a high concentration of the prebiotic inulin, which supports the growth of "friendly" bacteria that are associated with improved bowel function and better general health. Sold in bulk form, it has zero calories per serving. It can be used like table sugar to sweeten beverages, etc. Plus, there is a version that can be used specifically for baking.

Caution: Some people experience bloating, gas, stomach cramping and/or diarrhea when consuming excess fiber, and individuals sensitive to pollen and other related plants may have an allergic reaction to the chicory in this product.

Substituting a natural sweetener in your favorite daily beverage, instead of using refined sugar or drinking a presweetened beverage, can be a great first step in cutting back on sugar and put you on the road to better health!

Are You Gluten-Free? Watch Your Blood Sugar

Gluten-free pasta may raise blood sugar. *Recent study:* Researchers gave 13 healthy adults either regular wheat-based pasta or one of three gluten-free varieties. All the gluten-free pastas raised blood sugar levels over the next two hours more than wheat pasta. Rice/corn brought blood sugar levels 47% higher, brown rice pasta 18% higher and corn/quinoa 14% higher. Over time, elevated post-meal blood sugar levels increase one's risk of developing type 2 diabetes.

Carol Johnston, PhD, RD, professor and associate director, nutrition and health sciences, Arizona State University, Phoenix.

Yogurt...Not Butter!

When it comes to diabetes risk, food choice is crucial. In a four-year study of nearly 3,500 middle-aged and older women and men at high cardiovascular risk, those who ate an additional three pats of butter a day more than doubled their risk for type 2 diabetes, and each ounce of cheese increased risk by about one-third.

However: Whole milk didn't budge the needle, and each daily 4.5-ounce serving of full-fat yogurt (compared with no yogurt) cut risk by 35%.

What to do: Favor plant-based sources of fat, such as olive oil and nuts, over butter and cheese. Whole milk is fine, and full-fat yogurt is healthy.

Marta Guasch-Ferré, PhD, research fellow, department of nutrition, Harvard T.H. Chan School of Public Health, Boston.

The Gut Bug That Protects Against Diabetes

Study titled "Indolepropionic acid and novel lipid metabolites are associated with a lower risk of type 2 diabetes in the Finnish Diabetes Prevention Study" by researchers at University of Eastern Finland et al., published in *Scientific Reports*.

Andrew Rubman, ND, naturopathic physician, Southbury Clinic for Traditional Medicines. SouthburyClinic.com

Here's a diabetes paradox. While most people who get type 2 diabetes are overweight or obese, some overweight/obese people never get diabetes—even those with elevated blood sugar levels and prediabetes!

What's protecting them? One possibility is the beneficial bacteria living in their guts. Ironically, the best way to foster these good-for-you bugs may be to eat foods that you may be trying to avoid in the search for diabetes prevention!

Background: There is growing evidence that the "gut microbiome"—the collection of helpful organisms living in the gut that play a key role in digestion—influences type 2 diabetes risk.

Study: Researchers from Finland and Sweden compared two groups of people who had participated in the Finnish Diabetes Prevention Study, which began in the 1990s with more than 500 adults who were at high risk of developing diabetes because they were overweight and had high blood sugar. Like the American Diabetes Prevention Program, the Finnish program focused on lifestyle change to stop progression to diabetes. Fifteen years later, 52% of the participants remained free of the disease.

The researchers compared 104 individuals who remained diabetes free for 15 years with 96 individuals who developed diabetes within the first five years of the study. They looked closely at levels of various metabolites—by-products of digestion—to see whether there were big differences between the two groups. They compared diets, too.

Results: In participants who had not developed diabetes, there were much higher blood levels of indolepropionic acid. This compound, produced by beneficial bacteria in the gut, is known to protect the ability of beta cells in the pancreas to secrete insulin. The compound also improves insulin sensitivity—making insulin more effective. Both reduced insulin sensitivity and flagging insulin production are linked to developing type 2 diabetes.

Surprising finding: Higher levels of indolepropionic acid were also associated with lower levels of C-reactive protein, a marker of inflammation throughout the body. High levels of C-reactive protein can signal an increased risk for heart disease.

Diet connection: When the researchers looked at the participants' diets, they found that higher levels of indolepropionic acid were associated with high fiber intake...particularly from whole grains, especially rye. And, as it turns out, whole grains' fiber stimulates gut bacteria that convert the amino acid tryptophan from protein-rich foods into...indolepropionic acid.

These results not only back up the observation that people who have high-fiber diets are less likely to develop diabetes, but they also help explain why high-fiber diets are protective against diabetes.

Bottom line: Weight loss and exercise remain the cornerstones of diabetes prevention. But a healthy diet that supports "good bugs" is important, too.

Many people, when they find out they're at risk for diabetes, cut way back on carbohydrates—often as a way to lose weight. That can backfire by cutting out sources of gut-friendly high-fiber foods. A diet rich in fiber and whole grains, such as whole-grain rye and steel-cut oatmeal, is good for everyone, but it may be especially protective if you're at high risk for diabetes.

For a healthy microbiome, according to Andrew Rubman, ND, you'll also want to include plenty of fresh fiber-rich fruits and vegetables—both raw and cooked—as well as beans.

You Might Have Type 1

More than 40% of people with type 1 diabetes first develop it after age 30. It's an autoimmune disease. But adults in their 30s, 40s, 50s and beyond often are misdiagnosed with the more common type 2 diabetes. If you were diagnosed with type 2 but have trouble controlling your blood sugar with oral medications, especially if you're thin, talk to your doctor about type 1 testing. It's treated differently.

Gerald Bernstein, MD, coordinator of the Friedman Diabetes Program, department of endocrinology, Lenox Hill Hospital, New York City.

Glucose Dips Are Common

People with a history of heart disease who are hospitalized for any reason have a greater likelihood of hypoglycemia (low blood sugar) episodes—even if they are not known to have diabetes, a review of 1.2 million hospital patients has found.

Details: Patients developing hypoglycemia had almost four times the risk for death as those who did not develop hypoglycemia.

Takeaway: Blood sugar should be monitored daily in heart disease patients who are hospitalized (more often if the patient has diabetes).

Shuyang Fang, MD, endocrinology resident, Mount Sinai St. Luke's and Mount Sinai West, New York City.

Vinegar Can Do Wonders for Your Blood Sugar

Carol Johnston, RD, PhD, professor and assistant director of the School of Nutrition and Health Promotion at Arizona State University, Phoenix. Dr. Johnston has published nine papers on the medical use of vinegar in leading medical journals.

Apple cider vinegar is a classic home remedy with traditional uses ranging from reducing age spots to easing arthritis. Only one use is scientifically proven—a specific effect on blood sugar that is beneficial for anyone with diabetes or prediabetes. *Here's what you need to know...*

- **The scientific evidence of vinegar's blood sugar benefits is strong and consistent.** A recent statistical analysis of the 11 best studies concluded that consuming vinegar with a meal, compared with having the same meal without vinegar, reduced postmeal blood sugar spikes by an average of 40%.

Why this matters: Much of the metabolic damage caused by diabetes—and prediabetes—is caused by these spikes.

- **Any vinegar works.** Sorry, apple cider vinegar enthusiasts. It's the acetic acid—in every vinegar—that blocks absorption of carbohydrates and helps clear blood sugar from the bloodstream.
- **Raw vinegar is best.** Cooking can break down acetic acid.
- **You don't need much.** Studies suggest that two tablespoons of vinegar is a good "dose." Less isn't as effective—and more doesn't add any benefit.
- **Timing matters.** For the best effect on blood sugar, consume vinegar at or near the start of a meal.
- **Consider a premeal drink.** For the most reliable effect, dilute two tablespoons of vinegar in a glass of water and drink it with the first bites of the meal. You can sweeten it with a non-nutritive sweetener such as stevia. Or try a commercial flavored apple-cider-vinegar drink made by Bragg.
- **Make your own vinaigrette** if you'd rather incorporate vinegar into a salad or vegetable dish (after the vegetables are cooked). Why? Store-bought vinaigrettes often have more oil than vinegar. Mix your own using two parts vinegar to one part oil. Try red wine vinegar—it delivers acetic acid plus a healthy dose of cell-protecting polyphenols. Mustard counts, too—most mustards are rich in vinegar.

Start your next meal with a dish dressed with vinegar. And while you don't want to be eating a lot of bread, if you do have a slice, instead of slathering it in butter, dip it in vinaigrette.

The 4 Best Nondrug Remedies for Diabetic Nerve Pain

Michael Murray, ND, naturopathic physician and educator, based in Scottsdale, Arizona. He serves on the Board of Regents of Bastyr University in Seattle, and is author of more than 30 books, including *How to Prevent and Treat Diabetes with Natural Medicine* and *The Encyclopedia of Natural Medicine*. DoctorMurray.com

If you have diabetes, there's a seven-in-10 chance that you will eventually develop diabetic nerve damage, or neuropathy. It's just one of the many consequences of poorly controlled blood sugar, which is why controlling your blood sugar through diet and exercise is the best way to prevent—or at least slow—the often painful condition.

While neuropathy doesn't always cause symptoms, over time most people who have it will develop uncomfortable tingling, numbness and even chronic pain in the extremities—feet, legs, hands, arms. Other symptoms of neuropathy can include nausea, indigestion, constipation and dizziness. Unfortunately, there's no medical treatment that can cure diabetic neuropathy, only medications, including antiseizure drugs and some antidepressants, that help the pain.

But if you have diabetes, or even prediabetes, you don't have to accept that neuropathy is inevitable—and if you have diabetic neuropathy, you don't have to just live with its variety of terrible symptoms. Besides diet and exercise, there are certain supplements and one proven topical treatment that can help prevent, delay and even possibly reverse the cascade that ultimately causes neuropathy.

Here are four remedies—three supplements and one topical pain treatment—for diabetic neuropathy that I recommend. With the supplements especially, it's important to talk with your doctor before you start them.

Alpha-lipoic Acid

My top recommendation for people with diabetic neuropathy is alpha-lipoic acid (ALA). It's a powerful antioxidant, a natural compound produced by our cells that helps convert blood glucose into energy. Yet it's often deficient within the nerve cells in patients with diabetes. By improving nerve blood flow and nerve conduction velocity, ALA is associated with improvements in pain, tingling, numbness, sensory deficits and muscle strength.

Scientific studies back this up. The strongest evidence is for intravenous ALA, which has been shown to provide substantial short-term relief from pain and numbness. But oral supplements have also had positive effects. In a randomized, double-blind study of 181 patients with diabetic neuropathy, those who took 600 mg of ALA once daily for five weeks had a 51% reduction in their "total symptom score," which measured symptoms such as stabbing pain, burning pain, a prickling sensation and foot numbness, compared with 32% in the placebo group. In a very small (45 participants) randomized study, those who took 600 mg of ALA for four weeks had a similar reduction in painful symptoms. For those who continued ALA for a total of 16 weeks, there was a further reduction in symptom severity. For those who stopped taking ALA after four weeks, however, symptoms showed no further improvement—and they wound up taking more pain medications than those treated with ALA.

In the longest trial to date, four-year treatment with oral ALA in mild-to-moderate diabetic retinopathy resulted in a clinically meaningful improvement and prevention of progression of impairment in nerve function and was well-tolerated.

The typical oral dosage of ALA is 400 mg to 600 mg daily. There are no known complications or drug interactions with the use of ALA, although at higher doses (e.g., greater than 1,200 mg per day), some people may experience nausea and dizziness. Since ALA also may lower blood sugar, if you are taking a diabetic medication, discuss taking ALA with your doctor.

Animal studies suggest that oral ALA may be even more effective when combined with GLA (see below).

Benfotiamine

Another way enhance the effectiveness of ALA supplementation is to combine it with 600 mg of benfotiamine, a synthetic form of vitamin B-1 that is fat-soluble and easily absorbed and may have a beneficial effect on several biological pathways that contribute to diabetic neuropathy. It has been shown in preliminary trials to be helpful in some cases of diabetic neuropathy, and one clinical trial suggests that use with ALA is an effective combination.

Gamma-linolenic Acid

Another supplement that I recommend for diabetic peripheral neuropathy is gamma-linolenic acid (GLA), one of the omega-6 fatty acids. Normally, most of the GLA that we need to maintain nerve function and other functions comes from vegetable oils that contain an essential fatty acid that the body converts to GLA. But diabetes is known to substantially disturb fatty acid metabolism. A key part of that disturbance is impairment in the ability to convert this fatty acid to GLA.

Supplementing with GLA can help bypass that disturbance.

Example: In a randomized, double-blind study of 111 people with diabetic neuropathy, those who took 480 mg a day of GLA had a statistically significant improvement in 13 out of 16 measures of diabetic neuropathy severity after one year, compared with the placebo group that didn't get GLA. Participants who had good glucose control had bigger improvements than those with poor glucose control.

GLA is found in some plant-based foods and herbs, including oils of borage, evening primrose and black currant seed. Most GLA supplements are derived from these oils. Just remember that the dosage is based upon the level of GLA, not the amount of the source oil. The GLA content of these oils is usually stated on the label—look for a GLA dose between 360 mg and 480 mg.

Important: If you are taking a supplement or medication that thins the blood or that may affect bleeding time (ginkgo biloba, aspirin, *warfarin*, *clopidogrel*, etc.), talk to your doctor before taking GLA. It may increase the risk of bleeding, so the combination can be dangerous. Don't take GLA if you have a seizure disorder, as there have been case reports of the supplement contributing to seizures in people with such disorders. It can interact with other prescription medications as well, so be sure to talk with your doctor before taking GLA.

Topical Capsaicin

You may already know that hot peppers can provide pain relief—you can find pepper-based topical pain creams on the shelves of any drugstore. And in fact, I recommend topical capsaicin, the active component of cayenne pepper, for many patients with diabetic neuropathy. When applied to the skin, capsaicin works by stimulating and, ultimately, desensitizing, the small nerve fibers that transmit the pain impulse. Numerous double-blind studies have shown capsaicin to be of considerable benefit in relieving the pain of diabetic neuropathy. In those studies, roughly 80% of participants experienced significant—often tremendous—pain relief.

Topical capsaicin is available in both prescription and over-the-counter forms. Prescription patches with 8% capsaicin can provide surprisingly long-term relief—studies find that a single 60-minute application can reduce pain for weeks. This high-dose capsaicin works just as well at reducing pain as *pregabalin* (brand name Lyrica), the commonly used oral medication for nerve pain, and it avoids the systemic adverse effects associated with oral nerve-pain medications, including drowsiness, blurry vision, constipation and an increased risk for infection.

Capsaicin is also available over-the-counter as a cream and a patch. My recommendation is to use the cream so that it can be applied more liberally. Look for a concentration of 0.075% capsaicin, and apply it twice daily on the affected area. (Be sure to cover your hand with plastic wrap to prevent cap-

Socks for Neuropathy

Neuropathy—the tingling, burning pain or numbness that's often a side effect of diabetes, medications or autoimmune disease—is caused by nerve damage. Foot-warming socks can help soothe this type of nerve pain. Some foot-warming socks are heated in the microwave, while others are battery-powered. Prices range from $20 to $40.

To prevent burns: Test microwaved socks before putting them on, and do not sleep in battery-powered socks.

Janice F. Wiesman, MD, FAAN, associate clinical professor of neurology at New York University School of Medicine, New York City.

saicin from later coming in contact with your eyes, nose, mouth or lips, where it can be especially irritating.) It takes a few days for the nerve fibers to become desensitized, so the capsaicin cream can produce a tingling or burning sensation initially. After a few days, however, the nerve fibers will no longer transmit the pain signal. At these lower doses—as compared with the prescription patches—capsaicin works only with regular application. Capsaicin does not interfere with normal nerve function—it only affects the perception of pain.

Above all else: Although the nondrug remedies in this article can help with neuropathy, the primary goal for everyone with diabetes is to keep blood sugar in the healthy range. Reducing excess blood sugar—with a healthy diet, weight loss, regular exercise and managing stress—improves many of the consequences of diabetes, including neuropathy.

Chapter 8

INFLUENZA, PNEUMONIA AND OTHER INFECTIOUS DISEASES

Don't Let the Flu Turn Into Pneumonia

The flu lands hundreds of thousands of people in the hospital each year and kills tens of thousands. But flu that leads to pneumonia is even deadlier.

Startling statistic: Flu-plus-pneumonia ranks eighth in leading causes of death in the US.

The Flu/Pneumonia Combo

Every year, pneumonia affects more than one million Americans—and about 50,000 die. People most susceptible to pneumonia include the elderly, especially nursing home residents and individuals who have chronic health conditions such as heart or lung disease. The flu-to-pneumonia progression isn't the only cause of pneumonia, of course, but since the combo is so deadly—and often so preventable—it's worth special attention.

Here's what happens: You get the flu, a contagious respiratory illness caused by an influenza virus. You get the typical symptoms—sore throat, cough, body aches, fever, headaches and chills. But the flu also makes your lungs more susceptible to a bacterial infection caused by *Streptococcus pneumoniae* (S. pneumoniae), the most common cause of pneumonia in adults.

When that happens, air sacs fill with pus and other liquid, making it harder for oxygen to reach the bloodstream and making it difficult to breathe. Death can come from organs that are starved of oxygen—or from a blood infection (sepsis).

Here's how to protect yourself...

Step One: Get a Flu Shot

If you don't get the flu, you won't be at risk for that combination of flu virus/S. pneumoniae that is so dangerous to susceptible people. Getting a flu shot is the best way to protect yourself. It is recommended for everyone over the age of six months. While not 100% effective, it does offer substantial protection.

Why a flu shot is so important: A bad flu year means that pneumonia cases could potentially soar. The 2019 flu shot should be a good match for the kinds of flu viruses coming our way, which, according to the World

William Schaffner, MD, an infectious disease specialist at Vanderbilt University Medical Center in Nashville and medical director of the National Foundation for Infectious Diseases. NFID.org MyFluVaccine.com

Health Organization (WHO), includes two new strains.

Step Two: Make Sure You're Up-to-Date on Pneumonia Vaccination

Effective vaccines exist against S. pneumoniae, which, as described earlier, causes the vast majority of pneumonia cases in adults. Everyone age 65 and older should be vaccinated—yet only about 50% of healthy adults in this age group are. Some adults need protection before they turn 65—smokers and anyone with a chronic health condition (heart or lung disease, diabetes, asthma, etc.). For the best protection, you'll need two different vaccines, spaced out over a year or more…

- **Start with a onetime-only dose of the pneumococcal conjugate vaccine called PCV13 (Prevnar 13),** which protects against 13 types of pneumococcal bacteria.
- **One year later, get a dose of pneumococcal polysaccharide vaccine PPSV23 (Pneumovax),** which protects against 23 strains of pneumococcal bacteria. Prevnar 13 primes your immune system so that Pneumovax works better than it would if you took it by itself.
- **Based on your age and health,** your doctor may advise another dose of Pneumovax five years later.

Step Three: Watch Your Meds

Certain health conditions and medications can affect your susceptibility to pneumonia…

- **Steroids and other immunosuppressive drugs can make you more susceptible to pneumonia.** These drugs interfere with the immune response, so your body can't fight off infection as easily.

Low-dose steroids, even taken long-term, may not increase pneumonia risk, but higher doses (such as 20 mg a day) can do so in as little as two weeks. If you need a high-dose steroid to control your condition, be especially vigilant during flu season—get vaccinated, wash your hands frequently, stay away from crowds, and call your doctor at the first sign of illness such as a sore throat.

- **Acid-suppressive medications,** such as proton pump inhibitors including *omeprazole* (Prilosec), as well as histamine-2 receptor antagonists including *ranitidine* (Zantac), inhibit the production of stomach acids. But these acids help keep harmful gut bacteria in check.

Less acid means more potential for harmful bacteria to colonize and eventually enter the lungs. Unless your doctor prescribes these on a long-term basis (a rare occurrence), use them only for short periods of time—no more than four weeks for heartburn/gastroesophageal reflux disease (GERD), for example.

- **Pneumonia occurs less often in adults who get routine dental checkups.** Routine dental visits can help decrease the overall amount of bacteria in your mouth, including those that can cause pneumonia in susceptible people.

Bonus: A healthy mouth reduces heart disease risk, too.

If You Do Get the Flu…

Since the flu shot doesn't always prevent infection, be on the lookout for symptoms including feeling feverish, chills, body aches, sore throat and fatigue. If you suspect that you have the flu, call your doctor. You may be a candidate for prescription antiviral medication such as *oseltamivir* (Tamiflu), which can shorten your illness duration and possibly decrease the odds of it progressing to pneumonia. But you need to take it within a day or two of the first symptoms for it to be effective.

More from William Schaffner, MD

Pneumonia and Your Heart

Adults hospitalized with pneumonia have a heightened risk for cardiovascular problems including sudden heart attack, often with no warning signs.

What happens: Oxygen deprivation from a bout of pneumonia can starve cardiac muscle cells so that they function less well or even die off. One study found that within the first month of pneumonia diagnosis, the risk for stroke, heart attack or death due to heart disease grew by as much as fourfold...and remained elevated for years. Patients recovering from pneumonia also are predisposed to developing it again—another good reason to prevent it in the first place.

More Effective Flu Shot

For most people, flu shots can be injected into the muscle or the skin.

New study: Eczema patients who got the shot in a muscle were four times more likely to develop protection against the flu than those in the skin group.

Why: Staphylococcus aureus, which thrives on the skin of up to 90% of people with eczema, can hamper the body's immune response, making the vaccine less effective.

Donald Y.M. Leung, PhD, MD, Edelstein chair of pediatric allergy and immunology, National Jewish Health, Denver.

Is Your Arthritis Really an Infection?

David Lans, DO, FACP, a clinical assistant professor of medicine at New York Medical College in Valhalla, New York, chief of rheumatology at NewYork-Presbyterian/Lawrence Hospital in Bronxville, New York, and an internist and a rheumatologist in private practice at Integrative Rheumatology of Westchester in New Rochelle, New York. Dr. Lans is board-certified in rheumatology, internal medicine and allergy and immunology.

When you think of arthritis, what probably comes to mind is osteoarthritis, the wear-and-tear disease that affects more than 30 million Americans.

What you may not realize: Other types of arthritis can ravage joints, including arthritis caused by infection. For example, a recent study published in *Arthritis Care & Research* found that more than 16,000 people go to the emergency room every year with septic arthritis, an infection that can cause irreversible damage and deformity to joints.

Infections play a role in many cases of arthritis, both acute and chronic. Because these types of arthritis are less common than osteoarthritis, they are often misdiagnosed or overlooked. *What you need to know about...*

• **Septic arthritis.** Triggered by bacteria in the bloodstream that settle in a joint, this is the most serious form of infectious arthritis. Without prompt treatment, deep bone infections may occur and take months to resolve. One-third of people with septic arthritis suffer joint damage—and 10% die.

About half the time, the infection is in the knee, and pain and swelling are so severe that walking is difficult. The joint will also be red and hot. And you'll have a fever and chills and feel very sick. The knee is a common site for septic arthritis because of its large size and location.

People who have weakened immune systems, including adults over age 65 and children, are the most common victims of septic arthritis. You're also at higher risk if you already have a joint problem, such as osteoarthritis, gout or rheumatoid arthritis, which is an autoimmune disease...if you're taking medications for rheumatoid arthritis, which suppress the immune system...if you have an immune-weakening disease, such as diabetes or cancer...or if you have fragile skin that is easily injured and heals poorly (a fairly common problem among older adults and those with diabetes), allowing bacteria ready access into your bloodstream.

Many types of bacteria can cause septic arthritis. The most common bacterial culprits are Staph and Streptococcal species. If the infection isn't stopped, bacteria can destroy cartilage, causing permanent damage.

What to watch out for: Sudden, severe pain in a knee or other joint, and flulike symptoms, including fever and chills.

Treatment: Go to the emergency room or see a doctor—immediately. The joint will be drained with a needle or tube (arthroscopy), and the fluid will be cultured to identify the bacteria. It's likely you'll also get blood tests to help pinpoint the infection and X-rays to see if the joint has been damaged.

If you're diagnosed with septic arthritis, you'll receive IV antibiotics, followed by oral antibiotics. The usual antibiotic treatment duration is about six weeks. If antibiotics aren't effective, you may need surgery to drain the infection.

• **Reactive arthritis.** This type of arthritis can plague joints for weeks to years. Doctors aren't certain if reactive arthritis is an infection of the joint...or a joint-centered inflammation triggered by an infection elsewhere in the body. Either way, the arthritis is typically caused by either a sexually transmitted bacterial infection, such as chlamydia or gonorrhea, or a gastrointestinal infection, such as C. difficile or salmonella. Food poisoning is a common trigger.

What to watch out for: Joint pain that develops a few weeks or months after a sexually transmitted or gastrointestinal infection.

Treatment: A blood test will be given to detect the bacteria. If it's positive, you'll take antibiotics that target the organism. Nonsteroidal anti-inflammatory drugs (NSAIDs), such as *ibuprofen* (Motrin)...corticosteroids... or antirheumatic drugs, such as *methotrexate* (Trexall), may also be prescribed.

• **Lyme arthritis.** Lyme disease, a bacterial infection from a tick bite, is found throughout the US, but mainly in the Northeast, from Maine to Virginia, and in Minnesota, Wisconsin, Michigan and northern California. Some people never overcome the infection and develop chronic Lyme disease. Among those, more than half develop Lyme arthritis—one or more swollen joints (usually a knee), with pain (typically mild) that is intermittent or constant.

What to watch out for: Lyme arthritis usually develops several months after the tick bite. As with all types of arthritis, joint swelling and pain can occur.

Treatment: Lyme arthritis often resembles reactive arthritis. To make a definitive diagnosis, your doctor will order a blood test to detect antibodies to *B. burgdorferi,* the bacterium transmitted from the tick bite. The doctor may also remove fluid from your joint for a polymerase chain reaction (PCR) test, which detects the presence of DNA from B. burgdorferi.

If one or both of these tests are positive, your doctor will probably prescribe oral or intravenous antibiotics for one to three months. In most cases, this treatment cures Lyme arthritis, especially if it's initiated early on.

However, in some patients, the treatment fails, and chronic arthritis, as well as other symptoms (such as fatigue, headache and difficulty concentrating), may persist. If the disease isn't controlled, a drug used for rheumatoid arthritis—a disease modifying antirheumatic drug, or DMARD—often helps control the Lyme arthritis. Some patients require long-term treatment, while others improve over a period of months.

• **Viral joint infections.** Many viruses can trigger acute arthritis, but the joint pain that results is usually mild and goes away on its own after a few weeks. *Viral infections that can cause arthritis include...*

• Zika virus, from mosquitoes that carry it.

• Epstein-Barr, the virus that causes mononucleosis.

• Hepatitis A and B, the liver-infecting viruses that cause about one-third of virus-triggered arthritis.

• Parvovirus, a respiratory infection common in adults who are routinely exposed to children, the primary carriers of this infection, which causes a distinctive face rash.

What to watch out for: Sudden, mild joint pain (viral arthritis can affect almost any joint).

Treatment: Your physician will order a blood test for antibodies to specific viruses that can cause acute arthritis. Pain control is the goal, typically with an over-the-counter NSAID, such as *ibuprofen* or *naproxen* (Aleve).

HPV Vaccine Safe for Adult Women

Anders Hviid, MSc, PhD, senior investigator, department of epidemiology research, Statens Serum Institute, Copenhagen, Denmark.
Benjamin Schwartz, MD, chairman, department of obstetrics and gynecology, Southside Hospital, Bay Shore, New York.
Mitchell Kramer, MD, chairman, obstetrics and gynecology, Huntington Hospital, Huntington, New York.
Journal of Internal Medicine.

Vaccines that ward off the cancer-linked human papillomavirus (HPV) are safe for adult women, according to a study of more than three million Scandinavians.

The researchers, who used Danish and Swedish hospital data to track the incidence of 44 different illnesses over 10 years, found no "serious safety concerns" for women who'd gotten the HPV vaccine to reduce their odds for cervical cancer.

The vast majority of cervical cancers are thought to be caused by infection with HPV.

The Study

Diseases or conditions studied in the new analysis included epilepsy, paralysis, lupus, psoriasis, type 1 diabetes, rheumatoid arthritis, thyroid issues and Crohn's disease, among others.

The study did find slightly higher odds for celiac disease among vaccinated women, but this was seen only in Denmark. The authors noted that celiac disease is "markedly underdiagnosed" in the Danish population, so that could account for that finding. Celiac disease is an autoimmune disease that is triggered by eating gluten, a protein found in wheat and grain products.

The study was published in the *Journal of Internal Medicine*.

Implications

Because HPV is sexually transmitted, the US Centers for Disease Control and Prevention recommends vaccination before the start of sexual activity. Ideally, that is between the ages of nine and 12.

But adult women may wish to get the shot, so this study should reassure them about the vaccine's safety, said the team led by Anders Hviid, MSc, PhD, of the Statens Serum Institute in Denmark.

Two US obstetrician/gynecologists agreed.

"Since the vaccine is typically given to young girls to try to protect them before they are sexually active, few studies have explored the side effects and risks of the vaccine in women that are more mature," said Benjamin Schwartz, MD, chair of obstetrics and gynecology at Southside Hospital, in Bay Shore, New York.

"This is a very important strength of the study, because it further explores the safety of the vaccine in adults," he said.

Dr. Schwartz stressed, however, that because of a minority of vaccine skeptics in the United States, actual rates of use of the HPV vaccine are still "quite disappointing." But the new findings "further demonstrate the lack of evidence of adverse risks of the HPV vaccine," he said.

Expert Recommendation

Mitchell Kramer, MD, is chair of obstetrics and gynecology at Huntington Hospital in Huntington, New York. He agreed that the study shows "no connections between the administration of the HPV vaccine among adult women and the development of serious, chronic disease." He added that "the celiac issue described in the article is insignificant."

Prevention of HPV-linked cancers is "a tremendously important public health issue, and hopefully [this study] will encourage more women to get vaccinated against HPV," Dr. Kramer said.

Find out more about the HPV vaccine at the Centers for Disease Control and Prevention website, CDC.gov. Search "HPV vaccine."

Reasons to Get Screened for Hepatitis C

Talk to your doctor if you had a blood transfusion or organ transplant before 1992, when blood-supply screening began...shared needles to inject drugs, even once...had a sex partner who had hepatitis C...have evidence of liver disease, such as abnormal liver tests. Of the roughly three million Americans known to have hepatitis C, 75% are baby boomers. But only 14% of boomers had been screened as of 2015 (latest data available).

AARP Bulletin.

C. Diff. Infections Linked to Dental Care

Stacy Holzbauer, DVM, MPH, lead author of the study and career epidemiology field officer for the Centers for Disease Control and Prevention and the Minnesota Department of Health.

The next time your dentist recommends that you take an antibiotic, ask your dentist if it is really needed.

Background: Dentists write more than 24.5 million prescriptions for antibiotics a year. Why do they do this? If you've got, say, an infection from a tooth abscess, that would be a good reason—bacteria from the abscess can get into the bloodstream and cause a life-threatening infection.

However, some dentists still prescribe antibiotics when it's no longer recommended by the American Dental Association (ADA) that they do so. For example, prior to a routine dental procedure such as filling a cavity, a dentist might prescribe an antibiotic to prevent a heart infection in people with heart conditions...or to prevent an infection in patients with an artificial joint, such as a hip or knee replacement. In those cases, the risk of taking an antibiotic (see next column) is greater than the risk for an infection to the heart or joint.

Despite ADA guidelines, medical providers may also ask dentists to prescribe antibiotics prior to invasive dental procedures, especially for patients with joint replacements or a history of congenital heart disease. Dentists have often been overlooked as major partners in programs that promote appropriate antibiotic use, but it is crucial that dentists are included in efforts to improve the prescribing practices of these drugs.

When dentists prescribe antibiotics unnecessarily, they may be unknowingly contributing to an uptick in dangerous infections caused by the bacterium *Clostridium difficile* (C. diff.), which can sometimes cause a deadly diarrhea, according to recent research conducted by the Minnesota Department of Health.

Important finding: In a recent six-year study of 1,626 people with community-acquired C. diff., 57% reported that they had been prescribed antibiotics and 15% of those for dental procedures.

Note: When a C. diff. infection is labeled "community-acquired," it means that the person who got sick had not stayed overnight in a hospital or nursing home, where the illness tends to develop most often.

The study, which was presented at the 2017 annual meeting of the Infectious Diseases Society of America, found that patients who were prescribed antibiotics for dental procedures tended to be older and were more likely to receive *clindamycin*, an antibiotic that is commonly prescribed for C. diff. infection.

Of those patients who had received antibiotics from their dentists, 34% had no mention of it in their medical charts, which means that there's a lack of communication between dentists and medical doctors that may play a role in the overprescribing of antibiotics. Diagnosis of C. diff. may be delayed because doctors are not aware of the antibiotic prescription. Also, many times, dentists are not aware when complications develop from antibiotic use. Patients tend not to go to their dentist when they develop diarrhea.

What this means: A C. diff. infection can develop after just one dose of an antibiotic—the drug can wipe out protective bacteria in the patient's gastrointestinal system, allowing the C. diff. bacteria to thrive.

The situation is complicated by the fact that the C. diff. germ is easily spread from person to person (via the feces of an infected person who doesn't wash his/her hands adequately and then touches food or objects) or by contact with improperly cleaned medical equipment such as commodes or rectal thermometers. In a single year, C. diff. caused nearly a half million infections and led to 15,000 deaths in the US, according to research published in 2015.

Bottom line: During routine medical appointments, be sure to inform your doctor of any medications, including antibiotics prescribed by your dentist (or other medical professional), since your last visit.

And if your dentist or doctor offers to prescribe an antibiotic for you, be sure to ask, "Do I really need it?" Health-care providers sometimes prescribe an antibiotic even when you don't need one, out of fear that you will be unhappy without the prescription. You're less likely to get an antibiotic you don't need if you make it clear to your doctors that you would prefer not to take the medication unless it is really necessary.

Do You Have a C. Diff. Infection?

If you've taken an antibiotic recently (most patients develop C. diff. within two weeks of starting antibiotics, but the times vary greatly) and have any of the following symptoms, call your doctor immediately...

- **Severe, watery diarrhea.**
- **Abdominal (belly) pain/tenderness.**
- **Fever.**
- **Nausea.**
- **Loss of appetite.**

What's Really Causing That "Stomach Bug"

Deborah A. Fisher, MD, associate professor of medicine in the division of gastroenterology at Duke University School of Medicine, associate director of gastroenterology research at Duke Clinical Research Institute and director of social and digital media accounts for Duke's GI division, all in Durham, North Carolina. Dr. Fisher's research has been published in many professional journals. Twitter: @DrDeborahFisher.

When stomach upset hits, if you're like most people you blame that awful cramping, diarrhea, nausea and other gastrointestinal (GI) distress on something you ate. It's true that one in six US adults do experience a bout of food poisoning every year (see page 153). *But there are other culprits that are less recognized...*

- **Medications.** *Certain prescription and over-the-counter medications can cause GI distress...*
  - Nonsteroidal anti-inflammatory drugs (NSAIDs). *Ibuprofen* (Advil, Motrin), *naproxen* (Aleve) and other NSAIDs are known to cause dyspepsia. Dyspepsia, better known as indigestion, is marked by pain and burning in the upper abdomen, below the breastbone, and queasiness without vomiting. Dyspepsia can also occur with other drugs such as some antibiotics (see below).

In one Canadian study, up to 30% of patients with dyspepsia were found to be taking an NSAID.

What helps: Try lowering your NSAID dose, but realize that some people cannot tolerate even a low dose. If this approach doesn't help, try switching to *acetaminophen* (Tylenol), which may be equally effective in treating pain but without stomach discomfort.

Note: Long-term use of an NSAID or acetaminophen can have side effects. Both types of pain relievers are for occasional use only.

- **Proton pump inhibitors (PPIs).** These stomach acid medications have been linked to higher rates of diarrhea caused by the dangerous *Clostridium difficile* bacterium.

Chronic PPI use (generally, more than six months) reduces the diversity of bacteria in your GI tract, possibly allowing unhealthy bugs to thrive.

Commonly used PPIs include *esomeprazole* (Nexium), *lansoprazole* (Prevacid) and *omeprazole* (Prilosec). If you experience persistent, watery diarrhea, stomach pain and fever, and are taking a PPI, talk to your doctor. He/she may test you for Clostridium difficile–associated diarrhea, which can be treated with antibiotics. If PPI use causes GI distress, ask your doctor about taking *ranitidine* (Zantac) on an as-needed basis—it's less likely to cause stomach problems than PPIs.

• **Antibiotics.** *Azithromycin* (Zithromax, Zithromax Z-Pak) and *erythromycin* (Eryc, Ery-Tab) are among the antibiotics most likely to cause diarrhea by speeding up food's transit time through the intestine. Typically, you just have to ride it out, being sure to stay hydrated.

Helpful: Water with a splash of orange juice and a pinch of salt is an effective, inexpensive substitute for store-bought, electrolyte-infused water.

Also: Ask your doctor whether your antibiotic can be taken with food—such as crackers—to help prevent GI symptoms. Some data suggest that taking probiotics may help counteract the GI effects of antibiotics. Get them via fermented foods such as kefir, sauerkraut, yogurt, kimchi and miso soup. Never stop an antibiotic without first consulting your doctor.

• **Selective serotonin reuptake inhibitors (SSRIs).** This class of antidepressants, including *fluoxetine* (Prozac), *sertraline* (Zoloft) and *paroxetine* (Paxil), can cause nausea and diarrhea in some patients. This usually subsides in a few weeks.

• **FODMAPs, or fermentable oligosaccharides disaccharides monosaccharides and polyols.** These are difficult-to-digest sugars such as lactose, found in dairy products...fructose, in fruit...fructan, in wheat and good-for-you veggies including asparagus, onions, garlic and artichokes...and galactans, in complex carbohydrates such as beans, including kidney beans, chickpeas and soybean products.

For unknown reasons, in some people, the carbohydrates in high-FODMAP foods don't get digested in the small intestine. The undigested carbohydrates advance to the large intestine, where bacteria feast on them, causing cramping and gas, and draw excess water into the colon, triggering diarrhea. If your GI discomfort flares up when eating one of the foods above, see a gastroenterologist to find out if FODMAPs are to blame.

Helpful: The American Gastroenterological Association offers a downloadable guide for following a low-FODMAP diet.

• **Stomach flu.** At least 20 million Americans are hit with acute gastroenteritis (commonly known as "stomach flu") every year. It's usually caused by the norovirus, which spreads rampantly through crowded areas such as hospitals, airplanes, cruise ships and nursing homes. The virus makes its way from an infected person's feces or vomit into your mouth, usually when you touch a contaminated surface (a toilet handle or an ATM machine, for example) or eat food prepared by a person who is infected.

Symptoms such as diarrhea, vomiting, stomach pain, fever, headache and body aches usually begin within 12 to 48 hours of exposure, and most individuals recover in one to three days. There is no effective treatment. Protect yourself with thorough handwashing using soap and water. An alcohol-based hand sanitizer should not be used as a substitute for soap and water. Good handwashing is essential to avoid transmission. If you become sick, avoid preparing food for others.

Note: Stomach flu is not the same as the flu, which is a respiratory illness caused by the influenza virus. For this reason, getting a flu shot won't protect you from stomach flu. Also, stomach flu is easily confused with food poisoning, which causes similar symptoms.

• **Too much fiber.** Following a high-fiber diet is a healthy move. But consuming too much fiber too quickly can cause cramping, bloating and gas.

Better: Gradually increase your consumption of produce (such as broccoli, carrots, avocado, apples, pears and figs) and beans by one to two servings a day—or a fiber supplement by one tablespoon a day. As long as you experience no adverse GI symptoms, continue increasing your intake slowly for a total of 30 g of fiber per day for men...and 21 g for women. If you are taking a laxative for constipation, synthetic fibers such as *methylcellulose* (Citrucel) may be less gas-forming than natural fibers such as *psyllium* (Metamucil).

- **Stress.** If you've ever been stuck on the toilet due to nerves, you know that the brain and belly are linked. Numerous studies have suggested that some GI problems may have a neurological component.

Why: More than 100 million neurons (cells that carry messages from the brain to other parts of the body) line the human GI tract—creating "the second brain." Not only can stress lead to upset stomach, new research suggests that the effect may also work in reverse, possibly explaining why many people with irritable bowel syndrome and other GI disorders develop depression and/or anxiety. Cognitive behavioral therapy or hypnotherapy tailored for GI issues may help. Ask your doctor for a referral.

What If It Is Food Poisoning?

Food poisoning is no fun! If you consume food that has been contaminated with bacteria, such as *E. coli* or *Staphylococcus aureus*, the telltale symptoms, including abdominal cramps, diarrhea and vomiting, often come on suddenly and typically last for 72 hours or so.

Due to the "transit time" it takes food to make its way through your body's digestive system, it's likely that something you ate a few hours before symptoms began—or even a few days earlier—is to blame.

Foods that most often cause food poisoning: Undercooked meat or poultry, ground meat, unpasteurized dairy, improperly washed fresh produce and food contaminated by a sick food handler.

Note: Many fast-food chains source their meat and eggs from multiple farms, increasing your risk for exposure to bacteria.

If you get food poisoning, be sure to stay hydrated (drink enough fluids so that your urine is light colored). Dizziness when standing can be caused by dehydration. Uncontrolled vomiting requires prompt medical attention.

Important: If you experience vomiting and diarrhea for more than 72 hours—or bloody diarrhea at any time—call your doctor. You may have a particularly virulent strain of E. coli that can cause kidney failure and may require IV fluids and perhaps even short-term dialysis.

6 Surprising Foods That Can Give You Food Poisoning

Robert B. Gravani, PhD, CFS, professor emeritus of food science at Cornell University, Ithaca, New York. He is past president of the Institute of Food Technologists.

Perfected by nature. That's the motto for Live Spring Water. It is "raw" water—unfiltered, untreated spring water—the latest trend in health-conscious circles.

Cost: $38 for a two-and-a-half-gallon jug...$16 for a refill.

Save your money...and you might be saving yourself something even more valuable—your health. According to the Centers for Disease Control and Prevention, the nation's top health protection agency, drinking "raw" water could increase the risk for serious food-borne illnesses including, potentially, cholera and typhoid. You also could swallow disease-causing parasites including *Giardia*, *Cryptosporidium* and *Cyclospora*. While no outbreaks have been reported from the bottled variety—and Live Spring, for one, says that it tests its water sources once a year for contamination—public health authorities believe that it's only a matter of time before someone gets sick from bottled raw water.

Unless you like to chase the latest trends, you probably don't have a cooler filled with raw water in your kitchen. *But chances are you do have one or more of the following five other surprising sources of food-borne illnesses…*

• **Melon and other fruits with thick skin.** You might assume that a fruit with a thick, inedible skin—such as cantaloupe, mango, papaya and even avocado—would be perfectly safe. After all, you're not eating the skin. But there have been several food-poisoning outbreaks associated with such fruits.

Risky moment: When you cut into the fruit, you can transfer bacteria from the skin to the flesh.

Protect yourself: Thoroughly wash fruits that have a thick skin before you cut through them, using water and a produce brush to get at nooks and crannies—soap isn't necessary.

• **Raw flour.** You're probably thinking, *Who eats raw flour?* But if you ever nibble raw cookie dough or lick cake batter off your finger—you do! Recently, dozens of people across the country got sick from eating raw dough made from flour contaminated with the *E. coli* bacterium. A whopping 10 million pounds of flour were recalled because of the outbreak.

Protect yourself: Don't eat raw cookie dough or anything that contains raw flour. And that's a doubly good idea because many recipes containing flour also include another food that is dangerous raw—eggs.

• **Homemade soups and stews.** If you have made a big pot of soup or stew and then left it on the stovetop for hours to cool, you are putting yourself at risk for a lesser known, yet pervasive, bacterium called *Clostridium perfringens*—estimated to cause a million cases of food-borne illness each year in the US. Even though the soup was boiled, the organism forms spores that can survive the cooking process—and then germinate as the food slowly cools.

Protect yourself: Cool soups and stews as quickly as possibly—only briefly on a countertop, then in the refrigerator.

Tip: Transfer hot liquids into large, shallow containers to let the liquid cool down quickly. As soon as it stops steaming, pop it in the fridge.

Alternative: Buy a nifty gadget called an ice paddle that you fill with water and then freeze—it cools hot liquids quickly with just a little stirring. Then put the now-cool soup or stew into the fridge. Eat within four days, and be sure to reheat to a simmer before serving.

• **Cooked meats—even ones that have been stored properly.** Everyone knows that raw meat can possibly harbor salmonella and other bacteria. But even foods that are cooked when you buy them, such as deli meats… smoked seafood…store-made deli salads… and precooked hot dogs can harbor *Listeria*. It's a bacterium that grows in moist, cool temperatures—such as a refrigerator or cooler.

Protect yourself: Eat meats that you buy cooked soon after purchasing them, and toss anything that remains five days after you opened the package. With unopened packages, use the "best by" date as a rule of thumb for when to toss. In this way, you won't be eating these foods after the bacterium has had a great deal of time to multiply.

Note: If you buy frozen hot dogs or freeze the hot dogs when you get them home, you're safer—Listeria won't multiply in the freezer.

If there are any spills from deli salads in your refrigerator, clean them up promptly. Once a week, wipe the walls and shelves of the fridge with warm, soapy water, then rinse…and keep the temperature at 40°F or lower.

Listeria is especially dangerous to pregnant women and people with compromised immune systems (from diabetes or cancer, for example). They should be especially cautious and heat not only hot dogs but also lunch meat and smoked seafood until they're steaming.

• **Raw pet food.** This one is a risk both for you and your cat or dog. Raw pet food (meat, bones, organs) is a popular "natural" trend. It's supposed to be closer to the kind of food that a feral dog or cat would eat in the wild. But it's very easy for these foods to get contaminated with salmonella, Listeria and other pathogens that can make pets and humans sick—the FDA has recalled several brands due to contamination.

As with humans, in pets these food-borne illnesses can lead to vomiting, diarrhea and sometimes fever. Even if your pet doesn't get sick, you can become ill if you contract these bacterial infections after handling pet food.

Protect yourself: It's best to avoid raw food entirely and serve your pet only food that has been cooked, either store-bought or homemade. If you do handle raw pet food, be sure to wash your hands in hot, soapy water for at least 20 seconds.

Staying Safe

Now that you know about these often-ignored dangers, you can protect yourself. But don't ignore the better-known food-safety risks, either. *These include...*

• **Rare or even medium-rare hamburgers.** Make sure burgers reach an internal temperature of 160°F.

• **Raw milk.** It's dangerous. Avoid it.

• **Bagged salad greens.** These have been the cause of many recalls. Better to buy bunches of spinach or heads of lettuce...rinse thoroughly in cold water (no need for soap)... dry thoroughly and refrigerate until use.

• **Sprouts.** Never eat any kind of sprout raw.

Signs of Food Poisoning

Think you've got food poisoning? Many cases are mild and go away on their own with a little home TLC including rest, staying close to the bathroom and restoring lost fluids.

But be certain to call your doctor if you have...

• **High fever** (over 101.5°F).

• **Blood in your stool.**

• **Frequent vomiting** that prevents you from keeping liquids down.

• **Signs of dehydration,** including decreased urination, a dry mouth and throat and/or feeling dizzy when you stand up.

• **Diarrhea that lasts more than three days.**

Update on Shingles: A New Vaccine and Better Self-Care

Lindsay C. Strowd, MD, assistant professor of dermatology at Wake Forest Baptist Health in Winston-Salem, North Carolina. Her research has appeared in *Journal of the American Academy of Dermatology, The American Journal of Dermatopathology* and other professional journals.

Shingles is one of those dreaded conditions that you may not think too much about—until it's your turn to endure the ravages of this painful viral infection.

Recent development: There's a new vaccine that provides better protection than the previous one. But despite all the attention it's getting, many people are still unaware of some key details.

Reality check: Because some people—vaccinated or not—still do develop shingles, you also need to know how to best treat the condition and use self-care measures to curb the suffering.

The Shingles Vaccine

The first vaccine for adult shingles, Zostavax, was FDA approved in 2006. It was found to prevent shingles in about half of people who received the single shot.

What you may not realize: Shingles is much more than a skin rash. It's a viral infection that starts with a rash but usually doesn't stop there. The rash can be intensely painful and can lead to severe nerve pain that's potentially permanent. And in some cases, shingles can increase stroke risk.

Shingrix, the shingles vaccine that was FDA approved in late 2017, is about 97% effective against shingles during the first year. Its effectiveness wanes over time, but experts predict that it will continue to reduce infections by about 85% over four years. Research has shown that it's particularly effective in older adults, who face the highest risk for shingles.

What you may not realize: The new vaccine is also recommended for those who were previously vaccinated with Zostavax. Even if you've already received the older vaccine, the CDC recommends getting the new one.

Also important: Just because you've already had shingles, it doesn't mean you're off the hook—you can get shingles more than once. *Other key facts to know about the new vaccine...*

• **It requires two doses instead of one.** While the original shingles vaccine was given in a single dose, Shingrix requires two doses—given about two to six months apart.

• **It's pricey.** Shingrix is about $280 for both shots total, roughly the same cost as the single-shot original vaccine. Most insurance, including Medicare, is expected to cover the new vaccine, but you'll want to check before getting the shots.

• **There's some discomfort from the shot,** which involves mainly arm swelling and localized pain—this is typical with most injections. But about half of patients age 70 and older report more bothersome side effects, including widespread muscle pain, fatigue and/or headaches. Most side effects are temporary and last about 24 to 48 hours.

• **The vaccine's duration is uncertain.** Most vaccines lose their protection over time. The older shingles vaccine seems to lose some of its protection after about five or six years. Shingrix has not been used long enough to determine exactly how many years of protection it will give. And patients may need revaccination at some point after the original vaccination series.

• **Shingrix uses killed viruses, while Zostavax uses live viruses.** Those with impaired immune systems cannot receive live vaccines. If you have been told in the past that you cannot get the shingles vaccine due to an impaired immune system, ask your doctor about Shingrix.

• **Shingrix can be given starting at age 50,** while Zostavax was given to those age 60 and older.

My advice: Everyone age 50 or older and any adult with an impaired immune system should ask a doctor about getting the new vaccine.

If You Do Get Shingles

If you get vaccinated but develop shingles anyway, the rash will typically be milder with less severe pain, and the illness will be shorter in duration. Plus, there will be less risk for serious complications such as permanent nerve damage.

Shingles typically starts with one to five days of shooting or burning pain, numbness, tingling, itching and/or skin sensitivity. Some people also have flulike symptoms—headache, chills and fever. The affected skin will then develop redness and small blisters filled with fluid. If you get these symptoms, see your doctor right away—early diagnosis and treatment can help shorten the course of the attack and improve symptoms. Antiviral medication may shorten the duration of the illness and help with pain relief. It also can reduce risk for nerve pain complications but must be given soon after the rash appears, ideally within 72 hours.

If the pain is severe: Ask your doctor about *gabapentin* (Neurontin), an antiseizure drug that also relieves nerve pain. Topical *lidocaine*, available over-the-counter, can help with pain as well.

Complications: The shingles rash sometimes occurs on the face or near the eyes. In these cases, the virus can enter the optic nerve and cause vision loss. And in very rare cases, the shingles virus can infect the brain and cause inflammation of the brain (encephalitis).

Important: Seek immediate medical care if the rash is near your eye or on your nose or it continues spreading to other parts of your body.

Best self-care options...

- **Try a cool-water compress...or oatmeal/baking soda baths,** which can reduce itching and discomfort. For a compress, soak and wring out a soft washcloth with cool water and apply it to the rash for five to 10 minutes, several times per day. For baths, add colloidal oatmeal/baking soda to cool bathwater. Soak for 10 minutes once a day.
- **Coat the rash with a thick ointment such as petroleum jelly,** Aquaphor or unscented A&D Ointment, then cover the area with a bandage. Ointments are soothing, and the bandage will protect the area from the friction caused by clothing.
- **Wear loose, natural-fiber clothes (such as cotton).** They're more comfortable than polyester or other synthetic fabrics.

The Shingles Trap

About 90% of adults had chicken pox (varicella-zoster virus) early in life. Once you've been exposed to this virus, it retreats to the nervous system and lies dormant. The virus can reactivate later in life, usually after age 50, and cause shingles.

Sometimes shingles will be reactivated during periods of extreme stress on the body—for example, during a bad illness. People with weakened immune systems—the elderly...those with chronic diseases...and/or patients taking immune-suppressing medications for conditions such as rheumatoid arthritis or lupus or using chemotherapy drugs—are at greater risk of developing shingles.

Is Shingles Contagious?

Albert M. Lefkovits, MD, associate clinical professor of dermatology, Icahn Mount Sinai School of Medicine, New York City.

Shingles itself is not contagious, but the virus that causes it is. *Here's what can happen...*

The *varicella zoster* virus that causes shingles also causes chicken pox. Shingles—characterized by flulike symptoms, itching, tingling and a painful rash with blisters—is actually a reactivation of this virus in a person who has had chicken pox. The virus can remain dormant in the central nervous system for years. People with weakened immune systems and the elderly are far more prone to a reactivation.

If you never had chicken pox (99% of Americans over age 40 have had it), you might become infected if you touch an open shingles blisters. However, you would develop chicken pox, not shingles. For those who do have shingles, the antiviral drug *valacyclovir* (Valtrex) is effective. Early treatment can help prevent a painful condition called postherpetic neuralgia. Any person who thinks he/she has shingles should see a doctor immediately.

Prevention: The Centers for Disease Control and Prevention recommends the shingles vaccine for most people over age 60.

Caution: Pregnant women, anyone with a weakened immune system or allergies to gelatin or neomycin antibiotics should not get the vaccine.

Contact Lenses and Bacteria

Lindsay Ciocco, OD, FAAO, instructor of ophthalmology, The Johns Hopkins Wilmer Eye Institute, Baltimore.

Bacteria can form biofilms (layers of microorganisms) that adhere to contact lenses, making them more resistant against antimicrobial solutions such as lens cleaners. *Biofilm formation is a major factor in eye infections related to contact lenses. To reduce chances of infection...*

- **Wash your hands with soap and water before inserting lenses.** Use the cleaning solution recommended by your doctor or labeled for your type of lenses. Follow the cleaning and storage instructions.

• **Avoid sleeping in contact lenses,** even if you have the "continuous wear" type, since overnight wear is a big risk factor for infection. If you are not careful about cleaning, consider a daily disposable lens. Smokers and those who have diabetes or a weakened immune system are at a greater risk for infection.

Water Purification Concern

Jessica Fairley, MD, MPH, assistant professor of medicine and global health, Emory University, Atlanta.

If you like to "rough it" when you travel, you might be concerned about the drinking water. Do water-purification devices really work?

Devices, tablets and liquids that filter and/or purify water are effective, though some are better than others for specific needs. For example, filtration devices (pump or gravity-drip devices) can remove bacteria and parasites such as *Giardia*, but only those devices that also use chlorine, iodine or a microfiltration process can remove viruses such as *enterovirus*. These cost $20 and up. Devices using ultraviolet light cost under $100 and can disinfect small amounts of water (about 25 ounces) quickly, though you may need to filter the water first. Some pocket-size, battery-powered units use a technique called salt electrolysis in which briny water is electrically charged to kill pathogens. And boiling water for 60 seconds is a tried-and-true way to purify water, although it may still look discolored.

Visit CDC.gov/travel and click on "Destinations" to find precautions for each country before selecting a device to buy. Or opt for sealed bottled water.

Caution: Use iodine in the filtration devices mentioned earlier for no more than a few weeks, and avoid it if you are pregnant or have a thyroid condition.

Chapter 9

KIDNEY, LIVER AND BLADDER HEALTH

Medications That Don't Mix with Alcohol

Many of us have become so accustomed to seeing the "avoid alcohol" warning on every new prescription we get that we've begun to tune out this advice...and few of us even consider that alcohol might react with over-the-counter (OTC) medications.

That's a huge mistake! Alcohol is a powerful drug that has widespread and sometimes unpredictable effects in the body. It makes some medications less effective...amplifies the effects of others...and can cause a toxic—or even fatal—reaction with some medications.

Below, some medications that are adversely affected by alcohol...*

Acetaminophen

Acetaminophen (Tylenol) by itself can be harmful to the liver—in fact, acetaminophen overdose is the number-one cause of acute liver failure. But the likelihood of liver failure is much greater if you also drink alcohol.

Why acetaminophen and alcohol don't mix: Alcohol is a toxin, but there's a reaction in the body that breaks apart alcohol molecules so they are less dangerous. This reaction requires a coenzyme called NAD (*nicotinamide adenine dinucleotide*) that's found in all living cells. However, we also need NAD to deal with the toxic effects of acetaminophen. The breakdown of acetaminophen in the liver creates a highly toxic by-product.

Main danger: If stores of NAD are depleted by drinking alcohol and taking acetaminophen, liver problems or even permanent liver damage can result. Acetaminophen is particularly dangerous when taken during or within a couple hours of alcohol consumption.

Ibuprofen

Ibuprofen (Advil, Motrin) blocks the production of prostaglandins. These hormones, which the body releases in response to illness and injury, can cause pain, swelling and

*It's best to abstain from alcohol when taking any of these medications. However, if you do drink alcohol while taking these meds, be sure to accurately report the amount to your doctor so that you can be appropriately monitored.

Kevin T. Strang, PhD, distinguished faculty associate in neuroscience and physiology in the department of neuroscience at University of Wisconsin-Madison School of Medicine and Public Health. He is also coauthor of *Vander's Human Physiology.*

fever. But prostaglandins also play a critical role in blood clotting and blood vessel control, which impacts kidney function.

When blood flow to the kidneys is reduced for any reason—for example, during exercise or dehydration—prostaglandins are released to prompt blood vessels in the kidneys to dilate, which helps protect them from oxygen deprivation.

Why ibuprofen and alcohol don't mix: Drinking alcohol causes excess urination that can lead to dehydration. Alcohol also inhibits prostaglandins. If you take ibuprofen to help relieve a hangover or use it on an ongoing basis while drinking excess alcohol, it could block the prostaglandins that are released to protect the kidneys.

Main danger: Every episode of alcohol plus ibuprofen potentially kills a few more kidney cells, which makes kidney failure more likely over time. But acute renal failure can occur with just one episode of excess alcohol and ibuprofen.

Note: Ibuprofen combined with dehydration from diarrhea, vomiting or exercise, for example, can adversely affect the kidneys as well.

Blood Thinners

Aspirin and other blood thinners, such as *warfarin* (Coumadin) and *clopidogrel* (Plavix), are often used by people who have heart disease. They work by inhibiting prostaglandins, which, as mentioned above, are involved in blood clotting.

Why blood thinners and alcohol don't mix: Because alcohol also inhibits prostaglandins, this combination results in an exaggerated anticlotting effect.

Main dangers: A higher, unpredictable anticoagulant effect in the system, which could cause dangerous bleeding anywhere in the body, such as a stroke or bleeding ulcer. Additionally, both aspirin and alcohol are known stomach irritants. Over time, the combination can increase the risk for stomach problems including gastritis and ulcers.

Anxiety Meds or Narcotics

Benzodiazepines (such as Valium and Xanax) and the narcotic pain relievers *oxycodone* (OxyContin) or *hydrocodone* (Vicodin) target specific neurotransmitter receptors in the brain. When triggered, these receptors depress brain activity, which helps ease anxiety and pain.

Why anxiety medications OR Narcotics and alcohol don't mix: Alcohol is also a central nervous system depressant. If it's consumed when either drug is still in a person's system, the drug effect is amplified.

Main danger: The circuit in the brain that's responsible for regulating breathing contains *gamma-aminobutyric acid* (GABA) neurons. When there's excessive activation of GABA—which can happen when mixing these drugs and alcohol—the breathing circuits can shut down.

If you are unconscious—passed out or sleeping—you could stop breathing if you've had anxiety or pain medications and alcohol. These combinations are a major cause of alcohol-related deaths.

Blood Pressure Drugs

There are two main types of drugs prescribed for high blood pressure—diuretics, such as *chlorothiazide* (Diuril), and *vasodilators*, such as nitroglycerin. Diuretics work by reducing blood volume, namely by ridding the body of excess water via urination. Vasodilators work by widening the blood vessels to lower blood pressure.

Why blood pressure drugs and alcohol don't mix: Since alcohol is a diuretic and a potential vasodilator, it intensifies the actions of blood pressure medications. In other words, combining alcohol and any of these drugs is like taking multiple doses of the medications.

Main danger: You can have a dangerous drop in blood pressure that may cause dizziness, fainting, seizures or cardiac arrhythmias.

Alcohol and Other Meds

The effects of alcohol aren't limited to the drugs listed above. The cytochrome P450 system in the liver helps the body to eliminate all foreign substances—alcohol, prescription and OTC drugs and pesticides. The more foreign substances you're exposed to, the more robust this system becomes. Heavy drinkers have a very hearty cytochrome P450 system—this helps them detoxify large amounts of alcohol but also clears desirable drugs. This means a heavy drinker may not get the full benefit of any medication!

Kidney Stones on the Rise Among Women

Andrew Rule, MD, consultant, division of nephrology and hypertension, Mayo Clinic, Rochester, Minnesota.
Mayo Clinic, news release.

Kidney stones are becoming more common, especially in women, new research has found.

The Study

Lead researcher Andrew Rule, MD, and his colleagues analyzed the records of more than 7,200 residents of Olmsted County, Minnesota, who were diagnosed with kidney stones for the first time between 1984 and 2012.

The investigators found that women—especially those 18 to 39 years old—developed stones more often than men. They were most likely to have so-called infection stones, blamed on chronic urinary tract infections.

Bladder stones were less common. However, they were found more often in men, because of blockages involving the prostate gland.

The findings are published in *Mayo Clinic Proceedings*.

Possible Explanation

Better diagnostic tools could be part of the reason for the steady rise in diagnoses, according to researchers.

By using CT scans, "we are now diagnosing symptomatic kidney stones that previously would have gone undiagnosed because they would not have been detected," said Dr. Rule.

Whether something besides better imaging techniques is responsible for kidney stones being found more often in women will require further study, the researchers said.

The researchers noted that their findings may not apply to everyone because study participants were mainly white. White people have a higher risk for kidney stones than other racial groups, they said.

How to Prevent Kidney Stones

People prone to kidney stones should make some changes to their diet to help prevent recurrences, the researchers advised. This may include drinking more water, reducing salt intake and eating less meat.

The American Urological Association has information on kidney stones at UrologyHealth.org. Search "kidney stones."

One More Heartburn Drug Danger

Long-term use (over two weeks) of proton pump inhibitors (PPIs), such as *omeprazole* (Prilosec) and *esomeprazole* (Nexium), is known to increase risk for acute kidney problems, such as fluid retention and fatigue.

New research: PPIs can cause serious long-term kidney problems (even renal failure) without initially causing symptoms.

If you use a PPI: Follow label directions unless your doctor advises otherwise. If you're using PPIs for longer than 14 days, make sure your doctor is monitoring your kidney function.

Ziyad Al-Aly, MD, assistant professor of medicine, Washington University School of Medicine, St. Louis.

Vegetarian Diet May Stave Off Dialysis

According to recent research, people with chronic kidney disease avoided rapid reduction in kidney function (possibly postponing dialysis) by following a low-protein vegetarian diet and taking ketoanalogues, a mixture of modified essential amino acids.

Possible reason: This combination appears to aid the body in processing protein, which helps protect the kidneys.

Liliana Garneata, MD, PhD, assistant professor of nephrology, Dr. Carol Davila Teaching Hospital of Nephrology, Bucharest, Romania.

Kidney Disease Linked to Diabetes

Kidney disease boosts diabetes risk. It's well known that diabetes increases risk for kidney disease. Now it appears that the reverse is also true.

Recent study: Among 1.3 million nondiabetic adults, those with higher levels of blood urea nitrogen (a sign of reduced kidney function) were 23% more likely to develop diabetes over the five-year study period than those with normal urea levels.

Why: Blood urea nitrogen results in increased insulin resistance and impaired insulin secretion—both hallmarks of diabetes.

Ziyad Al-Aly, MD, assistant professor of medicine, Washington University School of Medicine, St. Louis.

Hidden Infection Risk

As kidney function declined, the risk for infections, such as urinary tract infections and sepsis, grew almost sixfold, a study of 1.1 million people found. Because kidney disease often goes undiagnosed, many people are at high risk for such infections without knowing it.

What to do: Be sure your doctor monitors your kidney function with a serum creatinine blood test or an albuminuria urine test—especially if you've had more infections than usual.

Juan-Jesus Carrero, PharmD, associate professor of renal epidemiology, Karolinska Institutet, Stockholm, Sweden.

Healthy Liver, Healthy Hormones...Better Menopause (and Beyond!)

Holly Lucille, ND, RN, a naturopathic doctor whose private practice, Healing from Within Healthcare, in West Hollywood, California, focuses on comprehensive naturopathic medicine and individualized care. She is author of *Creating and Maintaining Balance: A Woman's Guide to Safe, Natural Hormone Health.* DrHollyLucille.com

Not to slight any other organ or process our beautiful bodies have, but the liver, when it comes to hormones, has got to take center stage. What the heck does the liver have to do with hormones anyway, you might say? Well, I am going to tell you!

Let's start with the basics. The liver is our largest internal organ and our primary detoxification organ. It is about the size of a football, and is located mostly in the upper right quadrant of your abdomen, beneath the diaphragm and above the stomach. It bears the responsibility for more than 500 different functions including breaking down alcohol, medications, chemicals and other toxins, thyroid hormone conversion, helping your blood clot and making glucose so you can have a quick burst of energy. The liver is also involved in fat, carbohydrate and protein metabolism as well as vitamin and mineral storage. Fascinatingly enough, your liver is the only organ that can regenerate (re-grow) itself.

Hormones and Your Liver

Let's consider the liver and hormones. The liver uses a pathway called the *enterohepatic circulation*. The health of your liver and how well this particular pathway is functioning determines whether our estrogens and other hormone levels stay balanced. First, hormones, such as estrogens, are broken down in the liver and bound, or "coupled." with another substance and excreted into the bile. Then the liver secretes bile into the small intestines where most of it, along with its load of substances, is eliminated through your bowel movements.

Any disruption in this process contributes to increased levels of both hormones and chemicals in the body. If the liver is overloaded by the myriad environmental toxins and estrogen mimickers you are exposed to on a daily basis or if the bowel is toxic with, perhaps, a microflora imbalance due to poor dietary choices and antibiotic use, you can have a liver that is underfunctioning and, subsequently, a decreased excretion of estrogens. This can be a big problem, leading to signs of estrogen dominance and symptoms of hormonal imbalances like hot flashes, weight gain and irritability.

The liver also requires nutrients such as niacin, vitamin B-6, magnesium and amino acids to couple, or conjugate, hormones. Nutritional deficiencies can alter this process as well, leading to estrogens being reabsorbed into the blood stream, biologically active and having to be processed all over again...leading to more work for you liver.

Lovin' Your Liver!

Even though the liver takes a beating in our modern day, there are things you can do to love, support and protect it. *Here are my favorites...*

- **Reduce exposure to environmental toxins.** One of the best resources to help you do this on a daily basis are the shopping guides from the Environmental Working Group.
- **Eat liver-cleansing foods.** Nutritious foods like beets, cruciferous vegetables (broccoli, Brussels sprouts, cabbage, etc.), artichokes and dandelion greens are wonderful for liver health.
- **Take a liver-supporting supplement.** One of my favorites is milk thistle (*Silybum marianum*). It contains some of the most powerful liver protective substances known, silymarin. It has the ability to inhibit the action of harmful free radicals that damage liver cells. It also stimulates protein synthesis, which can help in the production of healthy new liver cells to replace the damaged ones. I recommend a dose of 175 mg daily of standardized Milk Thistle Extract (seed) containing 80% silymarin (140 mg).
- **Use castor oil packs.** Although they can be a bit laborious, they are very effective as a remedy to help decrease liver congestion.
- **Start your day out bright.** Fresh lemon juice—I use the juice of an entire lemon—in water is a superb way to flush the liver and get it ready for the assaults of the day ahead.

Although the connection isn't obvious, having a healthy liver can help you have a healthy hormonal balance through menopause and beyond. Just a few steps each day can pave the way.

Learn from Your Urine: What Your Pee Says About Your Health

Jonathan M. Vapnek, MD, a urologist and clinical associate professor of urology at Mount Sinai School of Medicine in New York City. A member of the American Urological Association, he's been named by *New York Magazine* as one of New York City's best urologists.

You would be surprised by how much information can be gleaned from the urine that you produce each day (one to two quarts, on average). For example, the simple "dipstick" urine test that doctors often use to check for a urinary tract infection also can help them diagnose kidney disease, diabetes, cancer and other conditions. But there is more.

What you may not realize: If you know what to look for, you can tell a lot about your health just by being aware of the physical characteristics of your urine—such as color, smell and frequency. *What to watch out for...*

Color

When you're healthy and drinking enough water, your urine should be mainly clear or straw-colored with just a hint of yellow. The yellow color comes from *urochrome*, a pigment produced by the breakdown of a protein in red blood cells.

Urine is naturally darker in the morning because you don't drink water while you sleep. If a color change persists, however, it could be a problem. *For example...*

- **Brown or dark brown. Pay attention if your urine is dark for more than a week.**

What this usually means: Liver disease. The liver normally breaks down and excretes *bilirubin*, a pigment that's produced by the turnover of red blood cells. Patients with liver disease accumulate bilirubin. This initially will cause jaundice, a yellowing of the skin or the whites of the eyes. As more bilirubin accumulates, it can cause the urine to become brown. A combination of dark-colored urine and jaundice means that liver disease might be getting worse. See your doctor right away.

Dark-colored urine also can be a side effect of some antibiotics, laxatives and muscle relaxants. Eating large amounts of fava beans, rhubarb or aloe can cause brown urine as well. In some cases, dark-colored urine can signal kidney failure.

- **Red or pink.** Urine that's tinged with red or pink could simply mean that you have been eating beets. (The medical term for beet-induced urine changes is *beeturia*). Or it could mean that you're urinating blood.

The amount of blood will affect the color. If the urine resembles cabernet wine, you're bleeding a lot...urine that's pinkish or just slightly red contains only traces of blood. A microscopic amount of blood won't be visible—it can be detected only with a laboratory test.

What this usually means: Blood in the urine is always a problem. Make an appointment to see your doctor. If you see blood and it also hurts when you urinate, you could have an infection—in the urethra, bladder or kidney or even a malignancy in the bladder, for example. Bleeding without pain also can indicate these conditions.

- **Green.** Though rare, a person's urine can turn a greenish color.

What this usually means: Green urine can appear when you've consumed a chemical dye—from food coloring, for example, or from taking medications such as *amitriptyline* (Elavil), an antidepressant, or *indomethacin* (Indocin), a nonsteroidal anti-inflammatory drug. In some cases, urine with a greenish tint can signal a urinary tract infection with certain bacteria (such as pseudomonas) that affect the color.

If your urine is greenish, increase fluid intake to see if it clears. If it doesn't in two days, see your doctor or a urologist.

Odor

If you're healthy, your urine should be highly diluted, consisting of about 95% water, with only small amounts of dissolved chemical compounds and metabolic by-products. It typically has no—or only a faint—odor.

Of course everyone is familiar with the effect that asparagus and some other foods, such as onions or fish, have on the smell of one's urine. This strong "rotten" smell is due to the chemical compounds in certain foods, particularly molecules that are not completely broken down by the body. The smell usually disappears within a day or so.

Some other less common urine smells include...

- **Ammonia-like.** If your urine is concentrated, with a larger-than-normal amount of *urea* (a chemical compound in urine), you might smell an aroma that resembles ammonia. Or you might just notice that it has a stronger smell than usual.

What this usually means: Dehydration. The less water you drink, the higher the concentration of urea and other substances—and the stronger the smell. You can diagnose this yourself by drinking, say, one extra glass of water an hour for several hours to add water to your urine. The strong urine smell will probably disappear within a few hours. If it does not, see your doctor.

• **Foul-smelling.** If your urine smells foul or unusual in any way for more than a few days, pay attention to the odor.

What this usually means: If it's not caused by a food that you've eaten, it could signal an infection in the bladder or kidneys. Less often, it's due to a metabolic disorder that reduces the body's ability to fully break down foods during digestion.

Uncontrolled diabetes can cause an abnormally sweet odor, and penicillin can cause a distinctive medicinal odor.

Even if you have no other symptoms, such as pain while urinating, but your urine continues to have an unusually strong smell for more than a couple of days, talk to your doctor.

Foamy or Bubbly

It's natural to see foam in the toilet when you really have to go and have a heavy stream. But urine that's consistently foamy or bubbly could mean that you're losing protein.

What this usually means: Kidney disease. Large amounts of protein in the urine is one of the main signs of chronic kidney disease. See your doctor right away.

Mucus or Cloudy

Mucus in urine could indicate inflammation in the urinary tract.

What this usually means: Urinary tract infection. See your doctor.

Cloudy urine also can be related to infection but often is just an indication that your urine is alkaline, which is harmless at low levels.

Volume and Frequency

The average adult typically urinates four to eight times in 24 hours. A change in the frequency of your urinary habits, including getting up more than twice a night to urinate, or an increase or decrease in the amount that you urinate, warrants attention.

What this usually means: An increase in the frequency of urination, along with an increase in volume, is one of the telltale signs of diabetes.

If the amount of urine seems the same but you're urinating more often, you could have a urinary tract infection. If this is the case, you'll probably have very strong urges to urinate even when just a small amount comes out.

Frequency of urination and/or urinary urgency in the absence of a urinary tract infection can indicate an overactive bladder.

Don't worry if there's been a decrease in the amount or frequency of urination. You probably just need to drink more water. If this doesn't help, see your doctor.

Daily Aspirin for Hepatitis B

Daily aspirin is linked to reduced risk for liver cancer in people with hepatitis B. Hepatitis B attacks the liver and can cause cirrhosis and cancer. Antiviral medicines reduce the cancer risk but do not eliminate it—and cannot be used by all patients. In patients with chronic hepatitis B, those who took aspirin daily were 37% less likely to develop liver cancer within five years.

Teng-Yu Lee, MD, PhD, a researcher in the division of gastroenterology and hepatology, department of internal medicine at Taichung Veterans General Hospital, Taichung, Taiwan.

This Cancer Has the Fastest-Rising Death Rate, But It's Very Preventable

Pankaj Vashi, MD, AGAF, FASPEN, chair of the department of medicine and chief of the department of gastroenterology/nutrition at Cancer Treatment Centers of America at Midwestern Regional Medical Center, Zion, Illinois.

In June 2017, a team of scientific experts from the American Cancer Society issued a special report about liver cancer.

Sobering statistics: Death rates from liver cancer (*hepatocellular carcinoma*) are rising faster than those of any other cancer—with rates doubling since the mid-1980s, said the report, published in *CA: A Cancer Journal for Clinicians*. This year, about 41,000 Americans will be diagnosed with the disease. The report also grimly notes that only one in five people with liver cancer is alive five years after diagnosis.

That is the bad news. *Here's the good...*

"A substantial proportion of liver cancer deaths could be averted" by prevention and early detection and treatment of the leading causes of liver cancer, the experts wrote.

More good news: The main risk factors behind the rise in deadly liver cancer have been identified, and medical care and lifestyle changes usually can keep them under control.

Here's how to protect yourself from this deadly disease...

Critical Risk Factors

The three-pound liver is the largest internal organ and for good reason—it performs a wide array of indispensable functions.

It filters and detoxifies your blood and makes proteins that help the blood clot. Food would be unusable without the liver—it's a must for the digestion of carbohydrates, protein and fat. The liver also stores glycogen, a type of carbohydrate called a *polysaccharide* that is used for fuel when blood sugar (glucose) is low. And the liver helps produce several crucial hormones such as *angiotensin*, which regulates blood pressure.

Because the liver is involved in such a broad range of metabolic activities, it is exposed to many factors that can weaken and damage it, increasing the likelihood of liver cancer. The two main factors are blood-borne viruses such as hepatitis C...and excess dietary fat.

• **Hepatitis C virus.** Half of all cases of liver cancer are caused by hepatitis C, which infects liver cells. Over the decades, a chronic case of hepatitis C can first cause liver inflammation and damage and then lead to cirrhosis (liver scarring, or fibrosis) and liver cancer.

About 3.5 million Americans are infected with hepatitis C, and 81% of them are baby boomers, people born from 1945 to 1965. Not surprisingly, baby boomers have the highest death rates from liver cancer, but older and younger people get it, too.

In the case of baby boomers, most with hepatitis C were probably infected in the 1960s, '70s and '80s by blood transfusions and organ transplants...contaminated medical equipment or procedures that exposed them to other people's blood...sharing needles in recreational drug use...or having sex with someone who was infected. This virus was discovered in 1989 and eliminated from America's medical blood supply in 1992.

Hidden time bomb: Most people (of any age) who have chronic hepatitis C infection don't know that they're infected—because the infection rarely creates symptoms until the disease has reached an advanced state.

What to do: If you're a baby boomer, you must be tested for hepatitis C—it's that simple. (It also is the recommendation of the Centers for Disease Control and Prevention.)

If you're not a baby boomer, you still should be tested for the hepatitis C virus if you had a blood transfusion before 1989 or if you have a history of intravenous drug use.

The test detects antibodies to the virus. Some people infected with hepatitis C "clear" the virus and are no longer infected—but they still will test positive for antibodies that were formed at the time of the infection. That's why positive antibody tests are followed up with liver scans that can detect cirrhosis, and if you have cirrhosis, you definitely have an active infection. A liver biopsy is the medical "gold standard" for confirming hepatitis C.

If you find out that you're infected, be happy you found out—and don't despair. A few years ago, it was next to impossible to stop chronic hepatitis C from damaging the liver. But in the past few years, the FDA has approved daily drug regimens that can cure hepatitis C, eradicating the virus from the body in more than 90% of cases. The risk of developing liver cancer depends on the damage already done by the virus. But after successful treatment of hepatitis C, the risk decreases with time. If you're diagnosed with hepatitis C, talk to your doctor about the drug regimen that is best for you.

- **Hepatitis B virus.** Infection with hepatitis B is the main cause of liver cancer worldwide, but it is less common in the US, where it causes about 15% of cases.

What to do: As with hepatitis C, most people who are infected with hepatitis B don't know it. You should be tested for hepatitis B if you were born in Asia or Africa, where it is more common...you were never vaccinated for hepatitis B (a standard vaccination in the US)...you had sex with a person known to be infected with hepatitis B...you have an HIV infection...you're on hemodialysis for kidney failure...you are on chemotherapy or another immunosuppressive treatment...or you have ever used recreational drugs intravenously.

If you are infected with hepatitis B, treatment will depend on whether the infection is acute or chronic and the degree of liver damage. Talk to your doctor about the liver-protecting regimen that's right for you.

- **Obesity and diabetes.** The twin US epidemics of obesity and diabetes have led to a third epidemic—nonalcoholic fatty liver disease (NAFLD)—and NAFLD can lead to liver cancer. Obesity, of course, includes excess fat...and in diabetes, excess blood sugar eventually gets stored as excess fat. Fatty liver afflicts an estimated 20% to 30% of American adults, including more than 60% of those who are obese.

What happens: Between 10% and 20% of people with NAFLD develop an even more serious form of fatty liver disease called *nonalcoholic steatohepatitis* (NASH). In NASH, liver cells are inflamed and swollen, and there often is cirrhosis.

Warning: NASH puts you at the same risk for liver cancer as someone with hepatitis C.

What to do: There are no long-term medical therapies that successfully control NASH. But lifestyle changes have proved to both prevent and reverse the condition.

Healthy Liver Lifestyle

If you're obese or have diabetes, you probably have NAFLD, and it's possible that you have NASH. Either way, your risk for liver cancer is elevated. Make the following lifestyle changes—starting today.

Note: The same lifestyle changes also are effective for strengthening the liver in people diagnosed with hepatitis C or hepatitis B.

- **Eat a Mediterranean diet.** It's the best dietary approach for managing NAFLD and NASH.

Latest development: A scientific paper in the July 2017 issue of the medical journal *Liver International* declared the Mediterranean diet "the diet of choice" for NAFLD. The paper's authors point out that the diet can reduce fat in the liver even without weight loss...reduces liver inflammation and liver scarring (cirrhosis)...can prevent or treat diabetes...and is better than a low-fat diet for weight loss. (Losing as little as 7% to 10% of your total body weight can reverse NASH.)

Bottom line: Eat more fruits, vegetables, beans, whole grains, olive oil, nuts and seeds, and fish. Eat less saturated fat from red meat and dairy products, less sugar and less processed food, and drink fewer or no sodas, including diet sodas (which, research shows, increases the craving for sugar).

• **Don't fail to exercise.** The more physically active you are, the less likely it is that you will develop NAFLD.

My recommendation: Go for a brisk walk of 30 minutes at least five days a week—a study shows that this regimen reduces liver fat by up to 43%.

• **If you're drinking coffee, don't stop.** Many studies link coffee intake to a healthier liver.

Standout scientific research: Coffee drinkers have a 40% lower risk for liver cancer than people who don't drink coffee, according to a study published in *Clinical Gastroenterology and Hepatology*. Those who drank the most coffee—three or more cups a day—had a 56% lower risk. The beverage is proved to reduce liver enzymes (a sign of inflammation) and to slow the progression of fibrosis.

• **Consider taking liver-supporting nutritional and herbal supplements.** Scientific studies show that certain nutritional and herbal supplements can decrease liver fat and fibrosis and improve liver function. *Check with your doctor about taking these top three supplements...*

• Omega-3 fatty acids. *Typical dose:* 500 milligrams (mg) to 2,000 mg daily.

• Vitamin E. *Typical dose:* 400 IU, twice daily.

• Silymarin (active ingredient in milk thistle). *Typical dose*: 250 mg, three times daily.

Pancreatitis Risk

Triglycerides are blood fats known to raise the risk for heart attack—and new research shows that they also are linked to acute pancreatitis, a sudden, potentially fatal inflammation of the pancreas. Triglyceride levels below 150 milligrams per deciliter (mg/dL) are considered normal. People with levels of 177 mg/dL to 265 mg/dL had a 130% increased pancreatitis risk...for those with levels above 443 mg/dL, the risk increased by 770%. Absolute risk for acute pancreatitis remains small—but the findings are another reason to ask your doctor how to keep your triglyceride level at 150 mg/dL or less.

Study of 116,550 men and women led by researchers at University of Copenhagen, Denmark, published in *JAMA Internal Medicine.*

When Tears Roll Down Your Leg...Urinary Stress Incontinence

Holly Lucille, ND, RN, naturopathic doctor whose private practice, Healing from Within Healthcare, in West Hollywood, California, focuses on comprehensive naturopathic medicine and individualized care. She is author of *Creating and Maintaining Balance: A Woman's Guide to Safe, Natural Hormone Health.* DrHollyLucille.com

"I laughed so hard tears ran down my legs." When you can't hold back the tears...OK, what I really mean is urine...while coughing, exercising, sneezing, laughing, or lifting something heavy, it is called "urinary stress incontinence" and it's a common occurrence in postmenopausal women. The result is either a small little tinkle of urine or a complete flood and loss of control.

First, we need to identify and treat the cause. The calamitous release of pee at the wrong times happens for a variety of reasons—and simply being aware of them can help you manage and "keep it inside."

It's Probably Menopause...Again!

As you near menopause, your estrogen levels begin to drop, and this can contribute to not only your pelvic muscles weakening but the urethral tissue becoming thinner, less resilient and less elastic...leading to reduced control over urination.

Other contributing factors to be aware of are certain medications such as diuretics or steroids, which can have urinary incontinence as a side effect. With my patients, I always go through the side effects listed of any medications that they are on. You would be surprised how many clinical complaints are actually due to them.

Chronic constipation can also weaken the pelvic floor muscles, making it harder to hold urine. Being overweight can put extra pressure on your bladder as well, worsening the situation.

Believe it or not, food sensitivities can also exacerbate the issue, causing irritation and inflammation to the bladder.

Your Bladder Is Not Your Boss

Although associated with menopause, urinary stress incontinence is not a given! By taking charge and correcting the specific contributing factors, this—like so many other "menopausal symptoms"—can be an "optional" issue.

Here are some tips and tricks...

- **Review and increase awareness of the side effects of any medications you are taking.**
- **Rule out food sensitivities.** I often recommend the "Eat Right for Your Type" blood-type diet for a period of four weeks to effectively help rule out foods that might have become irritants. It is an inexpensive and effective modality.
- **Reach and maintain an ideal weight to reduce pressure on the bladder wall.**
- **Correct constipation.** Increase fiber and by all means stay hydrated...drinking at least half your body weight in ounces a day...and reduce caffeine and alcohol.
- **Strengthen your pelvic floor muscles by using Kegel exercises.** Regular exercise can strengthen and build endurance to the group of muscles that control the opening and closing of your urethral sphincter (where the pee comes out). Kegel exercises are the standard and most effective treatment for incontinence caused by poor muscle tone, but you have to do them! The first step is to properly identify the correct muscle group. As you begin urinating, try to stop the flow of urine without tensing the muscles of your legs. It is very important not to use these other muscles, because only the pelvic floor muscles help with bladder control. When you are able to stop the stream of urine you have located the correct muscles. Feel the sensation of the muscles pulling inward and upward. It feels like squeezing your buttocks so as to not pass gas. Consistency is the key when doing these exercises, so plan on 10 minutes, two times each day. Morning and evening are good times for most people, but the important thing is to choose times that are convenient for you so you can develop a routine. No one will know what you are doing, so you can do these anywhere! Begin with tightening and relaxing the sphincter muscle as rapidly as you can for one minute. Take about a minute rest and then contract the sphincter more slowly holding for a count of three, gradually working to increase the count to 10. Then go back to the rapid contractions for a minute. Make sure to relax completely between contractions. If you stay consistent, you will start to see marked improvement within three to six weeks.

Vaginal estrogen therapy might also be helpful, so see a qualified menopause practitioner, such as a licensed naturopathic doctor to assist in treatment options.

These simple and noninvasive interventions can not only lead you once more to crying tears of joy, but can contribute to your overall well-being!

When All Else Fails for Overactive Bladder... Botox or a "Pacemaker"

Cheryl Iglesia, MD, director, section of female pelvic medicine and reconstructive surgery (FPMRS), MedStar Washington Hospital Center, Washington, DC.

If you suffer from an overactive bladder (OAB), you're no stranger to those alarming gotta-go-now moments that can strike day or night.

Lifestyle approaches are often effective and should always be your first line of defense. If these fail, there are medications—but they have lots of drawbacks, including dry mouth, constipation and dizziness. So what if lifestyle approaches don't work for you and medications either don't provide relief or you can't stand the side effects?

Then it's time for what doctors call "third-line" treatments. One is Botox, which was approved for this condition in 2013. Another is a kind of bladder "pacemaker" called sacral neuromodulation (SNM). It has been available since the 1990s, but the technology has improved and it's gaining adherents among patients and doctors.

Is either approach right for you? And if so, which one? The good news for women struggling with this serious problem is that there is now a head-to-head clinical comparison of Botox and SNM. To learn more, we spoke with Cheryl Iglesia, MD, director of the female pelvic medicine and reconstructive surgery division at MedStar Washington Hospital Center in Washington, DC.

OAB—When Your Bladder Sends the Wrong Signals

Before looking at the pros and cons of SNM and Botox, it's important to understand OAB. Bladders are considered overactive when the muscles contract to squeeze out pee when you're trying to hold it in. Sometimes nerves mix up the signals the bladder sends to the brain, so your bladder contracts when it should be relaxed and filling up with urine.

For people with OAB—slightly more women than men are affected—social gatherings, traveling and sitting through a meeting or movie can become an ordeal even when you know where to find the nearest bathroom. OAB goes hand-in-hand with incontinence—involuntary leakage—which just compounds the embarrassment. For women, menopause makes both conditions more likely.

Easy UTI Fix

Cut your risk for urinary tract infections (UTIs) in half by drinking an extra six cups of water a day. Young women who had frequent UTIs and drank six more cups of water daily were 48% less likely to have another UTI (the women had been drinking about four cups of fluid a day before the study). And the water drinkers were able to reduce their use of antibiotics by 47%. Fluid intake may reduce UTI risk by preventing bacteria from adhering to the bladder and reducing overall bacterial concentration.

Thomas Hooton, MD, clinical director, division of infectious diseases, University of Miami School of Medicine, and coauthor of a study of 140 healthy premenopausal women who had at least three UTIs in the previous year, presented at the recent IDWeek 2017 conference in San Diego.

Third-Line Treatments: When All Else Fails

The best first approach is to try lifestyle changes, including Kegel exercises to strengthen the pelvic floor and help stop leaks. Diet changes (such as cutting out caffeine) and mind-body approaches such as visualization may also help. While lifestyle changes work for many patients, those who can't find relief from their symptoms with medication—or who can't tolerate the side effects—have two other options, both of which are covered by insurance...

- **Botulinum toxin (often sold under the brand name Botox).** Given as a series of injections directly to the bladder, Botox temporarily paralyzes your muscles so that they no longer contract involuntarily. For many patients, Botox works at reducing OAB symptoms. But success comes at a price. There's an increased risk for urinary infections. And for about one in six patients the bladder becomes so relaxed that they have problems emptying it completely. They require catheters to drain their urine—at least for a few weeks. You'll also need to get another shot every six to nine months, on average.

• **Sacral neuromodulation (SNM) works like a bladder pacemaker.** Doctors implant a device at the base of your spine that sends a mild electric current to nerves that control the bladder. The current restores the normal signals between the brain and the bladder so you'll only feel the need to go to the bathroom when your bladder is actually full. While SNM has been around for 20 years, the two-step treatment has become easier and less invasive than it used to be.

The first step is a "testing phase." During an outpatient procedure, a temporary electrode is placed under the skin near the tailbone. The electrode is attached to a wire that leaves the body through the skin over your tailbone and hooks up to a stimulator the size of a battery pack that you carry around. During this two-week phase, you'll be asked to keep a diary describing how often and how urgently you have to urinate. You'll also have to stay hooked up most of the time, except for when you bathe.

If the trial is a success—you're making much fewer runs to the bathroom—a surgeon will replace the temporary electrode and stimulator and implant permanent ones. This part of the process takes less than one hour and is generally performed under local anesthesia with sedation. Once the surgery is over, you or your doctor can adjust the device with a hand-held controller to maximize its effectiveness and comfort level. Then you'll need to check in with your doctor every six to 12 months to make sure that the device is working well. Depending on the settings, the device will need to be replaced about every five years.

For many women and men, SNM can be a game-changer. One long-term study found that significant improvement in OAB symptoms was sustained over two-and-a-half years—of the 96 women followed, 85 chose to keep the devices implanted. The results are comparable to medications but without the side effects of the drugs.

How SNM Stacks Up to Botox

When researchers compared the two treatments in a recent clinical trial, they found that both worked equally well in reducing symptoms and the Botox injections were slightly better at reducing daily leaking. But unlike Botox, if SNM isn't treating your OAB, you can simply have the device removed without any lingering side effects.

That doesn't mean SNM is risk-free. Medtronic, maker of the InterStim System used for SNM, did its own clinical study.

Results: Out of the 219 men and women in the study, 52% experienced adverse effects ranging from temporary pain at the site of implantation (the most common) to occasional electric shocks (reprogramming the device usually fixes this problem).

What's best for you? The choice is yours, of course, but it's worth noting that in one study of 272 patients using SNM for one year, only seven chose to have the devices removed. If your battle with OAB has made you desperate and nothing else seems to help, SNM may be a way to get your life back.

Shocking Help for Incontinence

When 500 women received 18 real or sham electroacupuncture treatments (acupuncture with electrical stimulation) with the needles placed on the lower back over a six-week period, two-thirds of those receiving the actual treatments had a decrease of 50% or more in the amount of leakage. For longer-lasting effects, an additional round of electroacupuncture is recommended.

Theory: Acupuncture may strengthen the muscles in the pelvic floor that help control the bladder.

To find an acupuncturist: Consult the National Certification Commission for Acupuncture and Oriental Medicine, NCCAOM.org.

Baoyan Liu, MD, researcher, China Academy of Chinese Medical Sciences, Beijing.

New UTI Medication

The FDA recently approved *meropenem* and *vaborbactam* (Vabomere) for the treatment of "complicated" urinary tract infections (UTIs), including pyelonephritis (kidney infection). The bacteria-fighting drug is administered intravenously for up to 14 days. In trials, 98% of UTI patients were either cured or had improvement when treated with Vabomere, compared with 94% using another intravenous antibiotic drug therapy.

Jonathan Vapnek, MD, associate clinical professor of urology, Icahn School of Medicine at Mount Sinai, New York City.

Belly Fat Tied to Lower Kidney Cancer Survival Odds in Women

Joseph Ippolito, MD, PhD, instructor in radiology, Washington University School of Medicine, St. Louis.

Washington University School of Medicine in St. Louis, news release.

Belly fat reduces a woman's chances for surviving kidney cancer, but not a man's, a new study suggests.

Recent Study

The study included 77 women and 145 men with kidney cancer. Half of the women with high amounts of belly fat died within 3.5 years of diagnosis. Meanwhile, more than half of women with low amounts of belly fat were still alive after 10 years.

Researchers at Washington University School of Medicine in St. Louis found no link between belly fat and men's kidney cancer survival.

The report was published in the journal *Radiology*.

Implications

The findings suggest kidney cancer develops and progresses differently in men and women, the study authors said.

"We're just beginning to study sex as an important variable in cancer," said study senior author Joseph Ippolito, MD, PhD. Dr. Ippolito is an instructor in radiology.

"Men and women have very different metabolisms. A tumor growing in a man's body is in a different environment than one growing inside a woman, so it's not surprising that the cancers behave differently between the sexes," he explained.

Excess weight is a major risk factor for kidney cancer, but does not necessarily affect a patient's chance of survival. This study suggests, however, that the distribution of body fat affects women's survival odds. But it does not prove a cause-and-effect relationship.

"We know there are differences in healthy male versus healthy female metabolism," Dr. Ippolito said.

"Not only in regard to how the fat is carried, but how their cells use glucose, fatty acids and other nutrients. So the fact that visceral [belly] fat matters for women but not men suggests that something else is going on besides just excess weight."

This line of research could lead to better ways to treat women with kidney cancer, Dr. Ippolito added.

The National Cancer Institute has more information on kidney cancer at Cancer.gov. Search "Kidney cancer."

Chapter 10

PAIN AND AUTOIMMUNE DISEASE

Menopause Is a Pain in the Back!

That pain in your lower back may not be caused by sprains or strains, sleeping on a saggy mattress or just the wear and tear of life. If you're a woman in midlife or older, your aching back may be set off by menopause.

Background: Women don't have exclusive rights to lower back pain. It's quite common in men, too. The cause is often degeneration of the rubbery, cushioning discs in the lumbar region of the lower back—and it tends to get worse as we get older. But some studies have also found that estrogen helps keep these discs in good shape and that the loss of estrogen that comes with menopause can weaken discs. So researchers set out to learn more about how menopause affects this common cause of back pain in women.

Study: Researchers from China used MRI images, rather than simple x-rays, to evaluate disc degeneration in 1,566 women and 1,382 men of similar ages with low back pain. None of the women were taking hormone therapy. The women ranged in age from 30 to 93—some were premenopausal, others perimenopausal and many postmenopausal. Average age at menopause—defined as one year after the last menstrual period—was 51, and the average age of women in the study was 68. The researchers used an eight-point grading system to identify the level of lumbar disc degeneration.

Results: Postmenopausal women had significantly more severe disc degeneration than age-matched men. A serious level of degeneration (grade five or above) was found in 61% of postmenopausal women but only 42% of men the same age.

Surprising finding: Before menopause, women had *less* disc degeneration than men of the same age. Researchers believe one reason is that women tend to experience less mechanical stress and physical injury in their jobs. But around the ages of 50 to 60, the discs of women began to degenerate much more quickly than those of men. It didn't happen all at once—the discs of postmenopausal women degenerated progressively throughout the first 15 years after menopause. After 15 years, disc degeneration in women slowed down and kept pace with degeneration in men.

Study titled "Association between menopause and lumbar disc degeneration: an MRI study of 1,566 women and 1,382 men" by researchers at Wenzhou Medical University in Zhejiang, China, published in *Menopause*.

Bottom line: You are now free to blame menopause for your aching back. But you're not helpless. Now is the time to strengthen the muscles that support your spine—that can take pressure off your lumbar discs. Consider a yoga program, which helps with strength and balance—and also strengthens bone and helps prevent and even treat osteoporosis.

Is Your Back Pain an Imposter?

Stuart M. Goldman, DPM, a podiatrist in private practice in Baltimore who specializes in nonsurgical treatment of pain. Board-certified by the American Board of Foot and Ankle Surgery and a Fellow of the American College of Foot and Ankle Surgeons, he is author of *Walking Well Again: Neutralize the Hidden Causes of Pain.*

"Baby boomer back" is the nickname doctors have for lumbar spinal stenosis. That's because the condition mainly strikes adults over age 50. But even people in their 70s and up—or those only in their 20s—can be afflicted by spinal stenosis, a condition in which the spinal canal narrows and may compress the spinal cord or spinal nerves.

The symptoms are unpleasant, to say the least—low back, leg or foot pain that worsens when walking or standing, along with weakness, burning and/or tingling in the affected areas.

The first line of defense is usually pain medication—a nonsteroidal anti-inflammatory drug (NSAID), such as *ibuprofen* (Motrin), or nerve pain medication such as *gabapentin* (Neurontin). If that doesn't ratchet down the pain, the next step may be physical therapy, cortisone injections and/or back surgery to alleviate pressure on the spinal nerve roots.

The problem is, these treatments don't always work, and when they do, the relief may last only months, weeks or, in some cases, just days. Surgery can fail and, of course, it carries the risk for infection, blood clots and damage to structures, including nerves.

Surprising discovery: In many patients diagnosed with spinal stenosis, the symptoms are actually caused by pseudostenosis. This condition, in which the lower body structures (from feet to hip bones) are not functioning perfectly, can cause positional changes of the spine that exert pressure on bone structures or nerves, causing symptoms identical to those of spinal stenosis.

The tricky part is that an MRI may, in fact, reveal spinal stenosis—the two conditions often occur simultaneously. In my practice, I've found that pseudostenosis contributes to more than half of spinal stenosis cases.

Pseudostenosis is not a well-known concept—as a result, it is not considered by most doctors. Although the pain is coming through the spine, the actual cause is the poor function of the lower extremities. This is why standard treatments for spinal stenosis may be doomed to fail in these cases, even if they are done extremely well.

Note: Pseudostenosis can also occur on its own, even if spinal imaging (such as an MRI or a CT scan) is negative.

Good news: Based on my clinical experience, 70% of patients with pseudostenosis experience near-complete relief of symptoms often within a day or two by making a few simple positional changes. If someone does not improve within two days, it means that the treatment did not properly address the true cause of pain.

Discovering the Real Cause

Pseudostenosis has several causes. The most common are limb length discrepancy (one leg is shorter than the other) and flexible flat feet (the arch flattens when you step down). Other culprits may be any pain-inducing condition that affects the way a person walks. This may include arthritis of the feet, ankles, knees or hips…imperfect walking because of a nerve problem due to stroke or multiple sclerosis…tightness of the Achilles tendons…or a rigid flat foot.

Each of these conditions can affect your body in a way that mimics the effects of spinal stenosis, and more than one may be present at the same time, even if the patient is not aware of it. *Here's what you can do about the most common causes of pseudostenosis...*

• **Limb length discrepancy (LLD).** Either limb may be structurally shorter than the other, or one limb may function as if it is shorter, often because of an injury. Most people are unaware of the difference.

Red flags: With LLD, standing may cause more back and/or leg pain and leg tiredness than walking. To alleviate symptoms, people with LLD often feel the need to periodically "shake a leg" or shift their weight from side to side when standing. Even a mild LLD of 2 mm to 3 mm can cause symptoms.

Another sign of LLD: You have asymmetric wear-and-tear of your shoes. Often the wear is worse on the outer heel of your shoe worn on the shorter leg.

Quick test that may suggest LLD: Stand in front of a tall mirror, and look to see if your head tilts to one side and/or if your shoulders and hips are not horizontal. This asymmetry may be seen with either an LLD or scoliosis, which often occur together. (Wearing horizontal stripes and a belt makes the assessment easier.)

Next, put on a pair of shorts and stand in front of a long mirror to look at your legs. An LLD will often cause the foot of the longer leg to turn out more than the other. Then check your feet. Each leg may have different foot deformities, such as bunions, hammertoes, calluses or a flat foot.

How to treat LLD: A lift in the shoe of the shorter leg may quickly improve pseudostenosis symptoms. Don't go for the one-size-fits-all, shock-absorbing pharmacy inserts. A customized heel lift is critical in treating LLD. And no one will even notice that you're using it.

Websites such as GWHeelLift.com...and my site, WalkingWellAgain.com, offer solid heel lifts made of 1-mm to 12-mm durable plastic that can be stacked to achieve the perfect height.

Helpful: You can slip the heel lift under your shoe's insert to keep it in place.

• **Flexible flat feet.** Flexible flat feet are another common cause of pseudostenosis. This condition is usually easier to treat than rigid flat feet. If your foot has an arch when you're sitting but flattens out when standing, you have a flexible flat foot.

To test yourself for flexible flat feet: Take off your shoes and socks. If you have an arch when sitting, wet your foot and step on a brown grocery store bag. If the entire sole makes a print, that means that the arch has flattened, and you have a flexible flat foot.

How to treat flexible flat feet: Both orthotics and braces are available. Orthotics are custom-designed inserts that fit entirely inside a shoe. Ankle braces include a custom foot insert as well as an extension that goes above the ankle to increase stability.

To determine if orthotic control can help, a podiatrist may apply a tape strapping to your feet to control the foot function. If done well, it may simulate the effects of custom orthotics. The Unna Boot, a type of compression bandage that is embedded with zinc oxide paste to make it more supportive, can test for more aggressive control, such as a custom brace. Patients wanting to try self-taping may use Quick Tape, available at SupportTheFoot.com.

If symptoms improve with the tape strapping, podiatrist-fitted orthotics are the go-to treatment. Custom orthotics usually cost hundreds of dollars and are often not covered by insurance. If cost is a factor, excellent over-the-counter (OTC) orthotics are available from Vasyli Medical, at Amazon.com or from a distributor at VasyliMedical.com. Even though OTC orthotics are not necessarily as effective as custom devices, they sometimes do help and cost less than $100. Ankle braces are usually covered by health insurance.

With either heel lifts for LLD or supportive orthotics or braces for flexible flat feet, long-term treatment is often needed.

Takeaway: If you've been diagnosed with spinal stenosis, and your symptoms did not improve or returned after treatment, consider consulting a podiatrist to see whether pseudostenosis may be the real problem. To find a podiatrist near you, get a referral from your physician or check the website of the American Podiatric Medical Association, APMA.org.

Yoga Works as Well as Physical Therapy for Back Pain

When patients took yoga classes every week for three months, then attended more yoga sessions or practiced at home for nine months, they reported the same improvement in pain and activity limitation after one year as patients who had 15 visits with a physical therapist during the three-month period, then for the nine months had further sessions every two months or did prescribed home exercises.

Robert B. Saper, MD, MPH, director of the program for integrative medicine and health disparities, Boston Medical Center.

The Right Moves to Fight Your Pain

Vicky Saliba Johnson, PT, FFFMT, FAAOMPT, cofounder of The Institute of Physical Art, an international post-professional continuing-education organization in Steamboat Springs, Colorado.

If you have nagging joint pain in your hip or shoulder or suffer from mobility problems due to a neurological condition, such as Parkinson's disease or complications from a stroke, there is an approach used by physical therapists that you should know about... but probably don't.

Its official name, proprioceptive neuromuscular facilitation, is a bit of a mouthful, so it's known simply as PNF.

How PNF works: PNF-trained physical therapists use the brain and nervous system's complex feedback system to facilitate optimum patterns of movement and posture. The key to PNF is using the input from the skin, muscles and other sensory organs to influence the brain's ability to activate the right muscles and movement patterns, especially the proprioceptors, which tell the brain where your body is in space.

With PNF, practitioners observe and assess how problems in a patient's posture (such as a forward head position due to computer use) and/or movement such as walking without properly engaging the pelvis and trunk, may be causing or worsening an underlying condition. Performed repeatedly, such postures and movements not only place undue stress on our fascia (connective tissue) muscles and joints but also become ingrained in our "muscle memory." Eventually, these ingrained patterns can lead to pain and injury.

Once the problem is identified by the PNF-trained physical therapist, he/she designs a plan to retrain the patient's brain and body to move in safer, more effective ways.

This plan combines specific positioning with manual resistance and active stretching to remind the brain of the healthy alignment it used to know—before it was compromised by injury, disease or repetitive poor movements.

How PNF has evolved: The technique was originally developed in the 1940s by neurophysiologist and medical neurologist Dr. Herman Kabat and physical therapist Maggie Knott to address postural control and movement deficiencies in patients with neurological disorders. The practice later expanded to include head injuries, Parkinson's disease and more.

Over time, PNF has become an approach used for all patients, including orthopedic patients with knee, hip, neck, shoulder and ankle pain. More physical therapists are seeking this specialized training.

Scientific evidence: An important study published in the *Journal of Human Kinetics* found that PNF improves range of motion and increases muscle strength—both of which play a significant role in curbing pain and improving mobility.

How PNF may help you…

Hands That Heal

At the root of PNF theory is a principle called "overflow." When an area of the body has physical pressure applied to it with appropriate resistance and with proper manual contact, the brain responds by sending neurological impulses to the muscles of that area.

If the therapist continues to apply the appropriate amount of pressure over time, these impulses begin to overflow into the nerves that stimulate other muscles. PNF allows the therapist to direct this overflow to the weaker or inhibited muscles.

For example, a patient who has suffered a stroke or spinal cord injury may find it difficult to simply turn over in bed. In this case, the physical therapist might resist the hip flexors or shoulder extensors, which tend to be stronger, and direct the overflow toward the person's core muscles, which are probably weak as a result of the neurological event. Eventually, the brain will remember what it used to do to direct the body to roll over.

The length of treatment and the patient's ability to participate are dependent upon the injury and the patient's mental capacity. Most patients are given a home program for repetition to promote motor learning. An orthopedic patient with no neurological damage may need only a few treatment sessions. Patients who have neurological issues will require more sessions. Some insurance plans cover the cost of treatment.

Is PNF for You?

There are easy tests you can do on your own to help you determine whether you're a candidate for PNF. *For example, you can try the following if you are affected by…*

- **Low-back pain.** Try standing on one leg at a time. If you feel that you do not have good balance or your back arches while trying to stand on one leg, you are probably not using your pelvis to effectively connect your core to your legs. The low-back pain you are feeling is being aggravated with every step you take when your core is disconnected from your legs.
- **Shoulder pain.** Stand with your back against a wall. Press your lower back against the wall, then your middle and upper back. Now pull your shoulder blades together and rotate your palms forward. You should be able to keep your back flat against the wall.

If your back begins to arch as you do this, it indicates one of two things: Poor range of motion is compromising your ability to move the shoulder blade on the rib cage…or the brain cannot properly connect with the muscles needed to move the shoulder blade on the rib cage. In either case, a PNF-trained physical therapist will restore the brain's ability to connect with the muscles and create appropriate positioning of the shoulder blade.

- **Stroke.** If you have been discharged from medical care but everyday activities, such as getting out of bed or walking short distances, still feel challenging, PNF could help.

PNF is always done in conjunction with other physical therapy techniques. Depending on the problem, acupuncture and acupressure might also be appropriate.

To find a PNF clinician near you: Consult The Institute of Physical Art (InstituteofPhysicalArt.com), which provides certification that ensures each certified therapist (CFMT) uses PNF in the most effective manner.

Dr. Levin's Anti-Migraine Plan

Morris Levin, MD, chief of the Division of Headache Medicine and director of the Headache Center at UCSF Medical Center in San Francisco. He is coauthor of *Understanding Your Migraines: A Guide for Patients and Families*. Dr. Levin is board-certified in neurology, pain medicine and headache medicine.

Medications can help prevent and treat migraine, but fortunately there are many lifestyle and other treatment options that can help dramatically—without drugs.

The advice I give the migraineurs I treat...

Know Your Triggers

Identifying your migraine triggers and avoiding them is key to preventing an attack. Triggers are highly individual, including particular smells, sounds, lighting, 3-D movies—even weather changes. *Common food triggers include...*

- **Alcohol**—especially red wine, perhaps because of its high levels of histamine.
- **Nitrites.** Found in hot dogs, bacon, sausage and processed meats.
- **Monosodium glutamate (MSG).** A flavor enhancer that goes by many names, it is a powerful trigger for many people.

Taking the right steps at the first sign of a migraine coming on can lessen an attack—or avert it. *These natural remedies can help...*

- **Apply a cold pack to the site of the pain.** Cold may reduce blood vessel inflammation. A bag of frozen peas makes a good cold compress. It conforms to the shape of your head, and you can refreeze the bag for reuse. (*Note*: Don't eat thawed and refrozen peas—they can harbor unhealthy bacteria.)
- **Aromatherapy,** a popular migraine treatment in Europe, is not backed by strong scientific evidence, but some patients find it helps them relax and eases their headache pain. Tiger Balm—a mixture of camphor, menthol, cajuput oil and other herbals—is particularly effective and is available in supermarkets and pharmacies. Rub a small amount into your temples at the first sign of migraine.

Other essential oils to try: Eucalyptus, lavender and peppermint.

- **Drink a caffeinated beverage**—but not more than 100 mg of caffeine (one cup of medium-roast coffee).

Other options: Strong black tea (50 mg/cup)...green tea (25 mg/cup).

Warning: Caffeine triggers migraines for some people.

Regular tea and coffee drinkers: To avoid a caffeine-withdrawal headache—another migraine trigger—drink the caffeinated beverage at the same time each day.

Vitamins and Herbs That Help

Certain supplements can reduce the frequency and/or intensity of migraines. *Try these one at a time for two or three months...*

- **Vitamin B-2 (riboflavin) may reduce migraine frequency.**

Try: 400 mg/day. Vitamin B-2 usually doesn't have adverse side effects.

- **Magnesium gluconate and magnesium taurate may both prevent migraine.**

Try: 500 mg to 600 mg/day of either one. Lower the dose if you have loose stools.

Option: 100 mg of either at the start of a migraine can reduce its intensity.

- **Feverfew has been used for centuries to prevent and relieve migraine.** Studies show that it can reduce migraine frequency and severity.

Try: A total of 50 mg to 125 mg/day (tablet or capsule) divided into three doses. Feverfew thins blood—don't take it if you are on aspirin therapy or take a blood thinner such as *warfarin* (Coumadin). Also avoid it if you are allergic to ragweed. Other side effects include joint aches and gastrointestinal disturbances.

Nerve Stimulation

The FDA recently approved Cefaly, a noninvasive nerve stimulator that looks like a headband and is worn across the forehead. It delivers tiny, painless electrical pulses to the upper branch of the trigeminal nerve—the nerve responsible for sensations in your face and head. When inflamed, the trigeminal nerve overresponds to stimuli, possibly causing migraine pain.

Theory: Repeated pinging with electrical pulses might make the trigeminal nerve less sensitive to stimulation. In a recent Italian study, using Cefaly 20 minutes daily for four months reduced migraine frequency by more than 50%.

The device costs $349, plus $25 for three sets of electrodes (each set lasts about one month), and can be ordered online at Cefaly.us. It requires a prescription from your doctor and may not be covered by insurance. (Cefaly should not be used if you have a cardiac pacemaker, an implanted or wearable defibrillator, an implanted metallic or electronic device in your head or have pain of unknown origin.)

New Hope for a Cure

New research shows that calcitonin gene-related peptide (CGRP), a strong vasodilator produced in neurons involved in the transmission of pain, could trigger and maintain migraines. During a migraine headache, CGRP binds to receptors in the trigeminal nerve. In recent clinical trials, an antibody treatment that blocks the activity of CGRP modestly reduced the number of days per month that patients were disabled by migraine and even eliminated migraines for up to 15% of patients. The treatment could become available as an injection later this year.

What Is a Migraine?

A migraine headache is a cascade of electrical, chemical and inflammation-related blood vessel changes that occur in the brain, typically in distinct stages, but they can overlap...

- **Prodrome.** The warning stage. You may feel "off," irritable or moody...have amplified senses, such as a heightened sense of smell... and crave certain foods, such as sweets.
- **Aura.** Usually occurring five to 60 minutes before an attack, it involves visual disturbances such as flashing lights, zigzag lines or blind spots.
- **Headache.** Pain, mild to severe, often described as intense pounding or pressure, usually on one side of the head.
- **Postdrome.** The recovery period. You may feel fatigued over the next few hours or days.

The Posture Cure for Migraines and Other Chronic Headaches

Dr. Mitchell Yass, DPT, creator of The Yass Method, which uniquely diagnoses and treats the cause of chronic pain through the interpretation of the body's presentation of symptoms. Dr. Yass is the author of two books, *Overpower Pain: The Strength Training Program That Stops Pain Without Drugs or Surgery*, and *The Pain Cure Rx: The Yass Method for Resolving The Cause of Chronic Pain.*

There are certain possible causes of headaches—like a cerebral bleed, meningitis, a tumor in the brain—that are very dangerous and can be life threatening. Most of these can be identified by the use of diagnostic tests like MRIs and CAT scans. And there is no question that these types of tests should be run in the case of severe headaches.

But what happens when all the tests come back negative? With no "cause" established, the goal simply becomes finding ways to reduce the intensity of the headaches. This leaves medical practitioners with little alternative but to prescribe pain medications or Botox injections. The problem here is that the side effects of most of these medications can be worse than the headaches they are intended to address...and Botox is only temporary. The headaches could continue indefinitely!

I have been able to resolve the headaches of many people—including those suffering with migraine headaches and cluster headaches—by addressing a postural deviation called "forward head and shoulder posture," where the head is forward and the shoulders rounded.

It All Starts with Posture

When standing with proper posture, your ears and shoulders should be directly aligned over the hips.

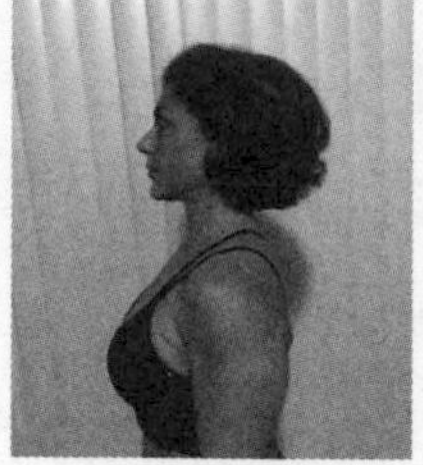

Proper

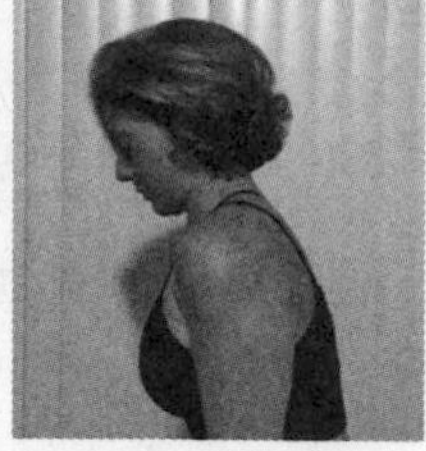

Forward head and shoulder

Forward head and shoulder posture is where these landmarks are in front of the hip when looking at a person from the side. The posture creates a hunching at the upper back.

This hunched posture is caused by a muscle imbalance between the chest muscles, front (anterior) shoulder and biceps versus the muscles between the shoulder blades, rear (posterior) shoulder and triceps. And it's this imbalance that could be the root of migraines and other chronic headaches.

The Slow Train to Head Pain

If you just want to trust me and don't want all of the details, skip to the exercises that can relieve your headache pain (located on the next page)...but my patients do better when they understand the mechanism they are working to correct. *Here's what happens, step-by-step, when headaches are caused by poor posture...*

- **The front set of muscles** (chest, front shoulder and biceps) tend to be excessively used because everything we do with our hands is done in front of us.
- **When this imbalance grows, the chest muscles can especially shorten.** Shortened chest muscles pull the shoulders forward, creating rounding of the upper back.
- **At the same time, the shoulder blades will be moving laterally farther away from the spine.** The muscles that support the head (called the levator scapulae and upper trapezius) attach from the shoulder blades to the upper cervical spine and skull. When the length of these muscles is increased, they can lose their ability to support the head.
- **These head-supporting muscles will strain,** which can create pain at the upper neck region and cause the head to move more forward.
- **As the head moves more forward, it increases the load on those supporting muscles** because the weight of the head is moving farther away from being properly supported over the cervical spine.
- **Since the upper trap muscles attach to the skull at its base,** the forward tilt of the

MUSCLES OF THE UPPER BACK AND NECK

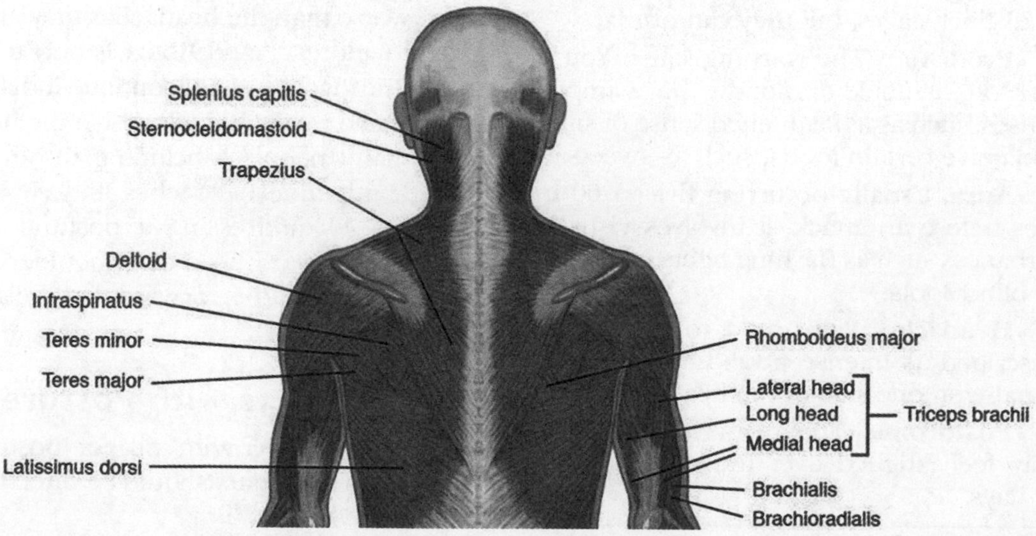

head will begin to create an excessive pulling. Muscles don't actually attach to bones; they attach to the periosteum, connective tissue that surrounds bone. Connective tissue has a very high density of pain receptors in them. By pulling excessively on the periosteum, there is a good opportunity for the pain receptors to be ignited anywhere around the skull—causing headaches—because periosteum also surrounds the skull.

The 4 Exercises for Headache Relief

To resolve headaches generated by poor posture and the resulting muscle imbalance, you simply need to strengthen the weaker muscles. As these muscles are strengthened, you'll see improving posture and a reduction in headaches. Then you can say farewell to painkillers and bye-bye to Botox. Here are the four exercises—all you need is a resistance band, a door and a chair!

For each exercise, perform three sets of 10 repetitions with a minute rest in between each set. The series of exercises are performed three times a week with a day rest between. Resistance should be progressed to eventually get the muscles strong enough to perform all functional tasks without straining and eliciting symptoms.

1. Lat Pulldown (interscapular muscles: midtraps and rhomboids)

Tie a knot in the center of a resistance band and secure it in place at the top of a closed door. Sit in a sturdy chair and lean

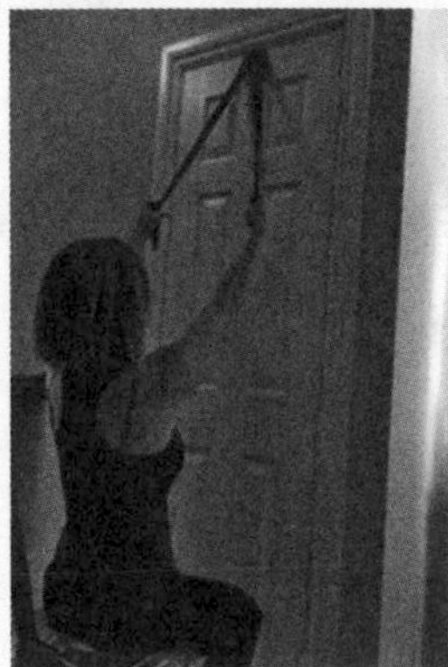

START

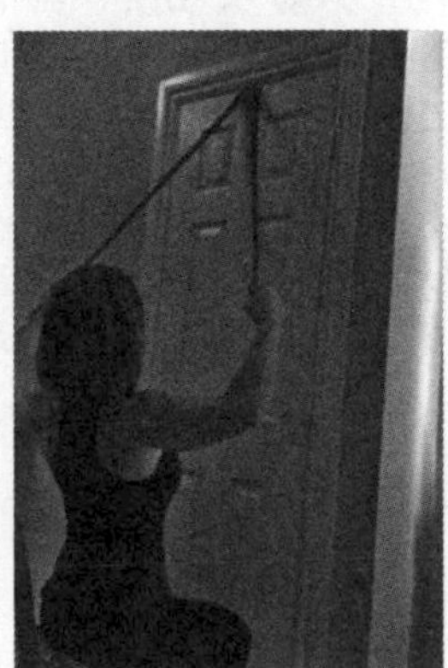

FINISH

back with an angle at the hip of about 30 degrees. Reach up for the ends of the band so that the start position begins with the arms nearly straight and the elbows just unlocked. Pull the band down keeping your arms wide and bringing the elbows just below shoulder height and slightly behind the line of the shoulders. At this point, you should feel the shoulder blades squeeze together (the elbows will barely reach behind the line of the shoulders if performing this exercise correctly). Then return to the start position. *Important*: If the elbows start to drop so they are lower than the shoulders, you are using the incorrect muscles to perform the exercise.

2. Lower Trap Exercise (lower trapezius muscle)

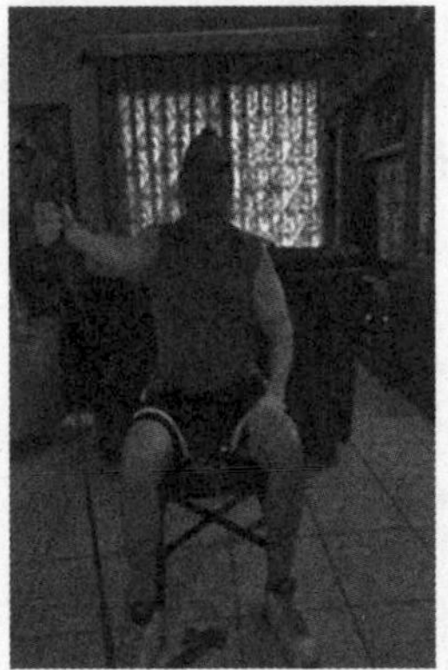

START

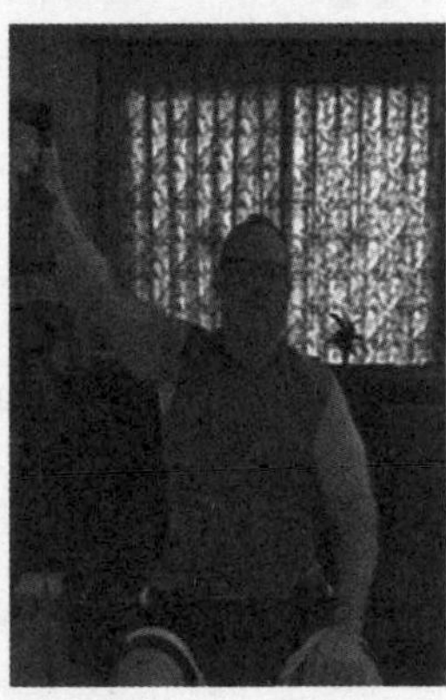

FINISH

Sit in a sturdy chair with a back and lean back slightly—about 10 degrees. This posture will prevent the resistance from pulling you forward. Step on one end of the resistance band to secure it and hold the other end in your working hand. Start with your arm halfway between pointing straight forward and pointing straight to the side, with your hand at shoulder height and your elbow just unlocked. Begin to raise the resistance until the arm reaches about 130 to 140 degrees (about the height of the ear). Then return to the start position at shoulder height.

3. Posterior Deltoids (posterior deltoids)

Stand with your feet more than shoulder width apart, knees slightly bent and your butt pushed behind you. Your weight should

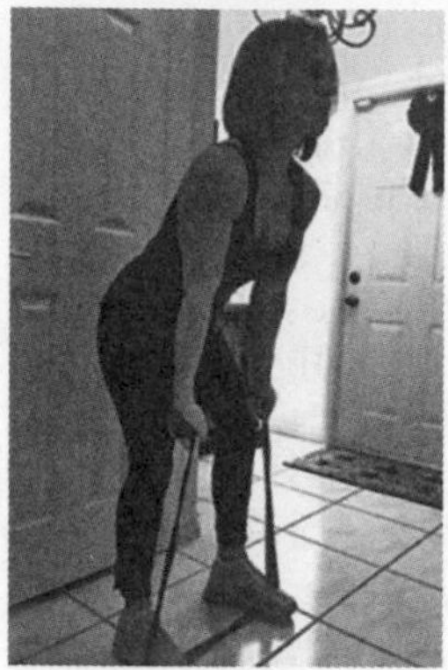

START

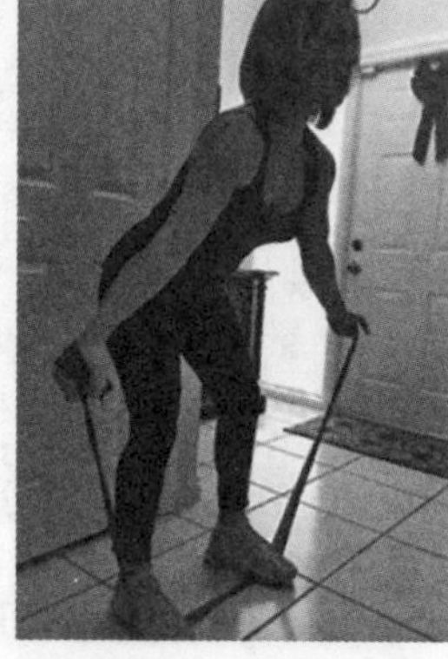

FINISH

be mostly on your heels. Step evenly on the band and hold the ends in front of your thighs with your palms facing in and your elbows unlocked. Begin to move the resistance out to your side from the shoulders like a pendulum. Go out until you feel the shoulder blades start to move inward (about 60 degrees), and then return to the beginning position.

4. Skull Crushers (triceps, single and both arms)

There are a multitude of exercises that strengthen the triceps. This particular one is the most effective because it puts the long head of the triceps in the optimal position. The long head of the triceps is the only part of the triceps muscle that passes the shoulder joint. Therefore, it is the only part of the muscle that can affect the position of the arm bone in the shoulder joint. The exercise can be performed with one arm or both, depending on whether your pain is associated

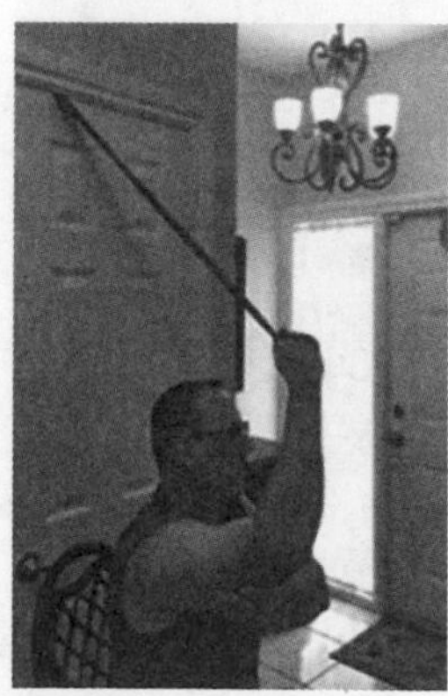

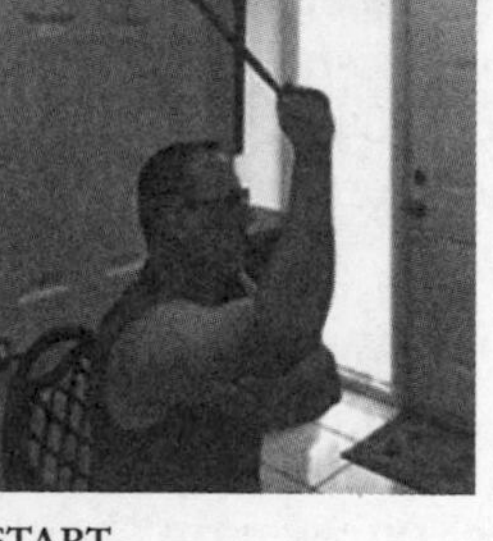

START FINISH

with one side or requires both arms to be strengthened to resolve it.

To perform the exercise, tie a knot in one end of a resistance band to secure it behind a closed door. Sit upright in a chair, back supported facing away from the door, with your legs comfortably open and feet firmly on floor. Start with your arm in front of you, upper arm just above parallel to the floor and elbow bent at 90 degrees. Keeping the upper arm in place (you can support with your other hand), begin to straighten the elbow, lowering the forearm until the elbow is just short of locked. Slowly return to the starting position.

Headache When Bending Down

Alan Rapoport, MD, clinical professor of neurology, The David Geffen School of Medicine, UCLA, California.

Anytime someone has a headache or increased pressure in the head from bending, coughing or straining in some way, that person should be evaluated by a physician, who may recommend a neurological consultation and/or an MRI.

Although it is unlikely that there is any serious problem going on, especially if you have no other symptoms such as nausea, visual problems or severe pain, a doctor can assess whether there is some change in pressure in the brain upon changing head position.

Irregularities in cerebral spinal fluid pressure, lack of cerebral spinal fluid flow or structural abnormalities in the back of the brain all can be possible problems.

The good news is that most of the time nothing serious is found after a thorough evaluation from a doctor.

Pain, pressure or light-headedness when bending down may be due to a sinus problem. Or headache-like symptoms might be a sign of high or low blood pressure, which can be easily treated with medication and lifestyle changes.

Again, if headaches persist, make an appointment to see your doctor so that you can find out what's going on.

Acupuncture: The Go-to Pain-Fighter

Roger Batchelor, DAOM, LAc, doctor of acupuncture and Oriental medicine and associate professor of acupuncture at the National University of Natural Medicine in Portland, Oregon. He was the primary acupuncturist at the Hooper Detoxification Stabilization Center, a 54-bed public-health facility and regional detox center, also in Portland.

Got a backache? If you're like most people, you probably reach for a bottle of *ibuprofen* (Motrin). If the pain is more severe—say, a broken bone or a piercing ache after surgery—you, like millions of Americans, may be prescribed a highly addictive opioid, such as *oxycodone* (OxyContin) or *hydrocodone* (Vicodin).

Now: Acupuncture, an ancient form of healing that has been practiced and refined for centuries, is increasingly being used in the US as the go-to treatment for pain relief. About three million American adults receive acupuncture each year, with chronic pain being the number-one reason—whether it's back, neck or shoulder pain, chronic headache or osteoarthritis.

How Acupuncture Eases Pain

If the thought of being stuck with needles sounds more pain-inducing than pain-relieving, there are a few details you need to know. It's true that acupuncture involves "needling"—or the insertion of needles through your skin. But it's worth noting that the typical acupuncture needle is sterile and no wider than a strand of hair.

When these needles are inserted by a skilled acupuncturist, it doesn't hurt. The most that some people feel is a mild tingling or pinprick sensation at the outset. During a typical session for a pain-related condition, the acupuncturist might use 10 to 20 needles, often placed in such areas as the limbs, back and scalp.

The needles are inserted into specific "acupoints" throughout the body, based on the ancient Chinese philosophy that our health is governed by the uninterrupted flow of qi (pronounced "chee"), or bioenergy, through the body. According to the principles of traditional Chinese medicine, when one's bioenergy becomes blocked, it builds up like water behind a dam, leading to pain and/or dysfunction. Needling a combination of acupoints—there are thousands of them—can relieve qi blockages and elicit the body's natural healing response.

Needling also signals the brain and spinal cord to produce chemicals and hormones, such as endorphins, that function as the body's own pain relievers, as well as natural anti-inflammatory compounds.

The result: Less need for pain medication. Many patients also feel less stress and sleep better following acupuncture—benefits that also help them cope with pain.

So what happens when you go for acupuncture? You'll be asked to lie on an exam table for the treatment. You can usually remain clothed, though you may need to remove a shirt or your socks, for example, if they are covering an area that will be needled. In some cases, you may prefer to change into a gown provided by the practitioner. You can expect to see your acupuncturist once or twice weekly for five to 10 sessions that last about one hour each. Not all insurance (including Medicare) covers acupuncture. Check with your insurer.

Acupuncture for Opioid Withdrawal

On the heels of a shocking report that more than 64,000 Americans died from drug overdoses in 2016, the US Department of Health & Human Services recently declared the abuse of pain-relieving opioids a public health emergency.

Not only does acupuncture lessen the need for opioids, it can help opioid-addicted individuals through the painful withdrawal process. When a person addicted to opioids first quits, he/she will experience unpleasant withdrawal symptoms, including insomnia, pain, leg cramps, irritability, nausea and constipation.

Medications such as *methadone* (Dolophine or Methadose) and *buprenorphine* (Subutex) are prescribed to ease withdrawal but tend to backfire. Methadone must be taken daily, with each dose providing pain relief for about four to eight hours. However, methadone is highly addictive, and misuse of this drug can be fatal. Buprenorphine can cause side effects such as muscle aches, nausea, constipation, sleep problems, irritability and more.

Acupuncture, on the other hand, has no side effects...may help prevent relapse... quells cravings...and does not require the patient to take yet another drug.

It's all about the ears: When treating people addicted to opioids, many acupuncturists follow an *auricular*, or ear-focused, acupuncture protocol endorsed by the US National Acupuncture Detoxification Association (NADA). Auricular acupuncture is based on the belief that points on the ears correspond to different areas of the brain and body. The NADA-approved protocol, also called acudetox or 5-Needle or 5NP ear acupuncture protocol, involves inserting three to five needles into each ear at specific points.

For opioids such as OxyContin, one to three months of daily acupuncture are needed to get through the worst of the detox process.

To get more information on the NADA-approved protocol, visit Acudetox.com. For general pain relief, you can find an acupuncturist with multiple years of training and certification at NCCAOM.org.

A Newer Approach

With electroacupuncture (EA), a newer form of acupuncture that was developed in the 1950s, the needles may be connected to a small unit that provides painless mild electrical stimulation. The electricity mimics the act of a practitioner physically maneuvering the needle, sending a stronger signal to the body. Even though you may feel a mild electric tingle with electroacupuncture, it is not uncomfortable and should feel relaxing.

Numerous studies show that different types of naturally occurring pain-relieving hormones are released at different EA frequencies. Needles are typically left in for 20 to 40 minutes.

Important finding: In a study in the journal *Pain*, women who received EA prior to abdominal surgery needed 60% less morphine in the 24 hours following the operation. Besides reducing the need for addictive pain medications, acupuncture also counters the most common side effects of opioids—including nausea, dizziness, urinary retention, constipation and lethargy.

Note: People with pacemakers should avoid EA to prevent unnecessary interference with the device.

What About Acupressure

For certain conditions, acupressure—applying pressure or massaging acupoints—can be as effective as acupuncture.

How it works: Massaging one point on the body can relieve symptoms in other parts of the body via pathways called meridians.

You can try acupressure for 30 to 60 seconds once or more daily on yourself or another person for...

Frontal headache:. Massage the fleshy spot between the thumb and pointer finger with firm pressure. This point is known as Large Intestine 4.

Nausea: Massage the spot on the palm side of the forearm, three finger widths from the base of the palm, between the two tendons in the middle of the forearm. This point is known as Pericardium 6.

Note: During opioid withdrawal or after surgery, traditional acupuncture is more appropriate than acupressure.

Menopause May Worsen Rheumatoid Arthritis Symptoms

Elizabeth Mollard, PhD, APRN-NP, assistant professor of nursing, University of Nebraska College of Nursing, Lincoln.

Rheumatology, news release.

Menopause may speed physical decline in women with rheumatoid arthritis (RA), a new study suggests.

While rheumatoid arthritis rates in women are three times higher than in men, and women with RA have more severe physical decline and disability, sex-based differences in RA are poorly understood, the researchers said.

Background

Rheumatoid arthritis is an autoimmune disorder that causes inflammation and pain in the joints.

Other research has shown that rheumatoid arthritis in women is influenced by childbirth and other reproductive and hormonal changes. For example, the study authors pointed out that women with early menopause are more likely to develop RA than those with normal or late menopause.

"Further study is needed as to why women with rheumatoid arthritis are suffering a greater decline in function after menopause," said study lead author Elizabeth Mollard PhD, APRN-NP. She's an assistant professor of nursing at the University of Nebraska College of Nursing in Lincoln.

The Study

To learn more, Dr. Mollard and her colleagues looked at nearly 8,200 women with rheumatoid arthritis. Those women whose periods had not yet stopped had slower physical decline than those who were postmenopausal, the study found.

While only an association was seen, the results suggest menopause has a significant impact on the degree and rate of physical decline in women with rheumatoid arthritis and is linked to worsening disease.

The study was published in the journal *Rheumatology*.

Implications

"Not only is this decline causing suffering for women, it is costly to both individuals and the health care system as a whole," said Dr. Mollard.

"Research is specifically needed on the mechanism connecting these variables with the eventual goal of identifying interventions that can maintain or improve function in postmenopausal women with rheumatoid arthritis," she said.

The website of American Academy of Family Physicians has more information on rheumatoid arthritis at FamilyDoctor.org/condition/rheumatoid-arthritis.

Fish Eases Arthritis

Eating fish has many health benefits, including reducing inflammation.

New finding: In a study of the diets of 176 patients with rheumatoid arthritis, those who ate non-fried fish two or more times a week had less rheumatoid arthritis activity—as measured by a combination of swollen and tender joints and a blood marker for inflammation—than those who ate fish once a month or never.

Sara K. Tedeschi, MD, MPH, rheumatologist, Brigham and Women's Hospital, Boston.

Topical Treatments for Chronic Pain Can Beat Opioids

Topical treatments for chronic pain can be as effective as opioids and prescription nonsteroidal anti-inflammatory drugs (NSAIDs) for some patients. Prescription topical treatments, such as *diclofenac* and *keto-*

profen, may work for the pain of moderately severe arthritis, neuropathic conditions and musculoskeletal disorders. Treated patients for whom the topical approach worked said that they favored topical treatments for their convenience.

Jeffrey Gudin, MD, director of pain management and palliative care, Englewood Hospital and Medical Center, New Jersey, and leader of a study published in *Journal of Pain Research*.

Joint-Friendly Advice

How can you avoid overusing arthritic joints to minimize pain and stiffness?

Don't engage in exercise that involves your hands when the joints are inflamed. *Also helpful...*

- **Lift items with both hands** even if you're strong enough to use one.
- **Avoid carrying items with your fingers.** *Example*: Loop handles of shopping bags over your forearm instead of carrying them with your fingers.
- **Opt for "joint-friendly" tools**—a brush for washing dishes (it's easier on hands than a dishcloth)...large nail clippers (easier to grip than small ones)...and spring-loaded scissors.
- **Rest your hands periodically when typing, working in the yard, etc.** Also, avoid repetitive motions and switch tasks often.

Anjum Lone, OTR/L, CHT, PM&R manager, occupational therapy, Phelps Memorial Hospital Center, Sleepy Hollow, New York.

Women Who Receive Joint Replacements with Metal Implants Suffer More Pain

In a study involving 2,600 men and women who had received total hip and/or knee replacements, women were significantly more likely to have immune sensitivity (a hypersensitive reaction causing inflammation and pain) to the metals used in the artificial joints.

If you'll be undergoing joint replacement: Ask your surgeon what materials will be used. If you have a history of metal allergies, consider a metal- sensitivity test (such as a metal-LTT, a blood test) before surgery.

Nadim Hallab, PhD, professor of orthopedic surgery, Rush University Medical Center, Chicago.

The Best Way to Recover from Total Knee Replacement

"A Comprehensive Behavioral and Exercise Intervention Improves Physical Function and Activity Participation After Total Knee Replacement—a Pilot Randomized Study" by Sara R. Piva, PT, PhD, University of Pittsburgh Medical Center–Rehabilitation Institute, and colleagues, published in *Arthritis Care and Research*.

Every year, more than 700,000 Americans get a new knee (or two)—a number that's expected to rise to 3.5 million per year by 2030. And the doctors who perform these total knee-replacement surgeries say they're remarkably successful, with more than 90% of patients experiencing a "dramatic reduction" in knee pain and a "significant improvement" in the ability to perform activities of daily living, according to the American Academy of Orthopaedic Surgeons.

Yet...even after a successful total knee replacement, many people continue to have knee and mobility problems—in fact, one-third still have difficulty climbing stairs or even walking.

No wonder many people with new knees still get way too little exercise—and, perhaps as a result, gain weight—even after a "successful" procedure. The problem? A new study tells us that the physical therapy that knee replacement patients get is too limited in scope—and it stops too early.

The study also shows how much more successful recovery can be if patients get the right kind of exercise at the right time.

Joint Pain and Rain

Is it a myth that joint pain worsens when it rains?

Perhaps. An analysis of more than 10 million Medicare physician office visits found no increase in office visits for joint or back pain on rainy versus nonrainy days.

But that doesn't mean that there's no connection between rain and achy joints. Some researchers theorize that changes in barometric pressure affect the ligaments and nerves within joints, causing pain. Since the research counted doctor visits, it could be that some people managed pain with self-care. Regardless of the weather, stretching, warm compresses and over-the-counter pain relievers can help your pain.

Anupam B. Jena, MD, PhD, Ruth L. Newhouse Associate Professor, Harvard Medical School, Boston.

Background: Standard physical therapy after knee replacement focuses on range of motion, muscle strength and endurance exercises. That's all well and good. But most people who need total knee replacement also have problems—both before and after surgery—with getting up from a sitting position, climbing stairs and keeping their balance while walking.

Physical therapy researchers tested a program that starts after the knee has had time to heal, so more intensive exercises are possible, to see whether they could help people overcome these limitations.

New study: A research team at University of Pittsburgh Medical Center-Rehabilitation Institute compared a type of therapy called comprehensive behavioral intervention, or CBI, against a standard less intense exercise program in 44 people age 50 and older who had had knee replacements at least three months earlier. Both groups got 12 supervised 75-minute sessions with a physical therapist over 12 weeks, followed by a 12-week at-home exercise program. Both groups had a warmup, endurance exercise (treadmill walking) and strength training focused on the legs. *But the CBI group got a different mix of exercises...*

- **A shorter warmup**
- **Higher intensity endurance exercises**
- **Higher intensity strength training**
- **A set of "functional" exercises** (walking in place, mini-squats, chair rises)
- **Balance exercises** (side stepping, walking backward, changing direction, standing on unstable surfaces)
- **Mini-lectures on fitness and nutrition** to encourage a healthy lifestyle after recovery.

Results: After six months, the CBI group, compared to the standard care group, had less pain and rated higher on a scale of "physical function"—the ability to do everyday actions such as standing up from a chair and climbing stairs. They also did better on balance tests and were more physically active.

Bottom line: If you're planning on total knee replacement, talk to your surgeon and primary care doctor about getting physical therapy not just immediately afterward but also three months or more later, when you're able to exercise more easily and more intensely and can make even more progress. You may need to get another referral from your doctor for insurance to pay for this "additional" physical therapy. Talk to your physical therapist about including exercises for functional fitness and balance, too—and work together to plan how you'll stay active after this second round of rehab.

How to Relieve Shoulder Pain Without Surgery

Beth E. Shubin Stein, MD, associate attending orthopedic surgeon and a member of the Sports Medicine Service at Hospital for Special Surgery in New York City.

The shoulder is the most movable and complex joint in the human body. And it's basically unstable.

Imagine a golf ball perched on a tee. That's your shoulder. The humerus (upper arm bone) is the ball and the scapula (shoulder blade) is the tee. It doesn't take much to knock them apart.

So it's no wonder that as you get older, normal wear and tear often leads to shoulder pain. You might notice the discomfort while serving a tennis ball, reaching for a jar on a shelf, carrying a heavy suitcase or simply putting on a sweater or fastening a bra. *The most likely culprits...*

Impingement: The rotator cuff, a collection of muscles and tendons surrounding the humerus, gets pinched between that bone and the scapula.

Frozen shoulder: Tissue around the shoulder joint gets inflamed and stiff.

Tendinitis: Rotator cuff tendons become inflamed or irritated.

Bursitis: Tiny fluid-filled sacs (called bursa) that act as a gliding surface to reduce friction between shoulder tissues become inflamed.

Each condition is caused by inflammation, often as a response to tiny injuries that you didn't notice when they happened. Each can get so painful that surgery seems like a good idea. But why go through that discomfort, recuperation and expense if you can avoid it?

Surprising truth: With pain management and physical therapy, two-thirds of patients get better on their own.

But if your shoulder is bothering you, that doesn't mean you can just do nothing. Your pain will continue and even may intensify the next time you overstress the shoulder. Worse yet, you could get a rotator cuff tear, which definitely requires surgery and then four to six months of recovery.

To learn the best way to avoid shoulder surgery, we interviewed orthopedic surgeon Beth E. Shubin Stein, MD. *Her advice...*

If you feel pain in a shoulder and your movement is restricted, see an orthopedist right away to rule out a rotator cuff tear. As long as your rotator cuff is intact, you have a very good chance of making your shoulder feel better and avoiding surgery if you, in consultation with your doctor, follow these steps.

Manage Your Pain

The first step is to manage your pain so that you can start physical therapy. Ice your shoulder for 20 minutes at a time, two or three times a day. Also, take a nonsteroidal anti-inflammatory drug (NSAID), either over-the-counter or prescription, to reduce inflammation and pain (don't exceed the recommended dosage).

If that's not enough to ease pain and allow exercise, your doctor can give you a cortisone shot. It's a potent anti-inflammatory, but repeated shots can limit a tendon's healing ability.

My protocol: If a first cortisone shot works for two months or more and you can exercise, I typically recommend a second shot and continuing physical therapy.

But if the first cortisone shot doesn't ease pain and allow exercise, I offer patients platelet-rich plasma (PRP) injections ($1,000 to $2,500). It's experimental and generally not covered by insurance. If PRP doesn't work, another option is to use donor stem cells from amniotic membranes to help regenerate tendon tissues. This can be about twice as expensive as PRP, and insurance most likely won't cover it either. These treatments don't work for everyone, but if they do, shoulder discomfort should subside within three days to a week.

Tip: You also may want to consider acupuncture as a complement to any of the above approaches.

Once pain isn't holding you back, it's time to get your shoulder moving. You can complete this stretching/strengthening program in 15 minutes. Do it twice a week. It's also great for anyone who wants to avoid shoulder problems.

Important: You should never feel pain when doing either stretching or strengthening exercises.

These exercises might sound like a lot of work, especially if you've become accustomed to avoiding using your shoulder because of pain. But take it from someone who both performs necessary shoulder surgery and does my best to help patients avoid it—it's well worth the effort to avoid the knife. I do these exercises myself two or three times a week—I've had shoulder pain in the past, but these exercises let me stay strong and pain-free.

***EXERCISE STEP 1*: Get Limber**

Much of the work of supporting the shoulder falls to the rotator cuff. *These stretches improve rotator cuff flexibility and support normal range of motion…*

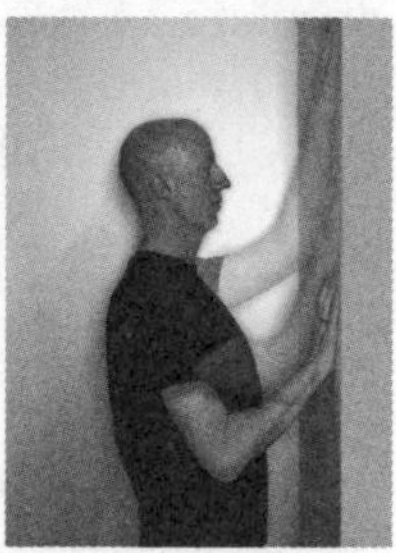

• **Wall crawl.** Stand facing a wall. Place the palm of one hand in front of your chest and "walk" it upward along the wall. Go as high as you can without feeling pain, hold for three to five seconds, and walk your hand back down. Do five to 10 repetitions. Switch hands and repeat.

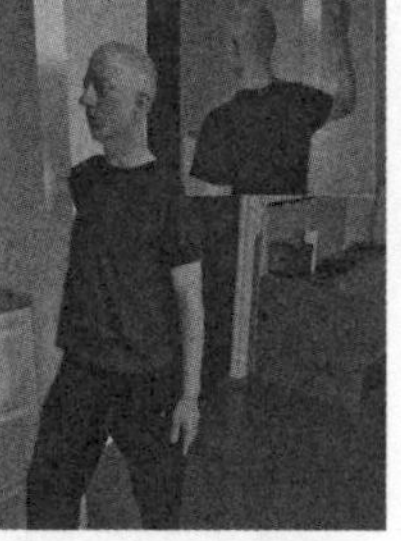

• **Doorway stretch.** Stand in an open doorway, and place your right hand flat against the wall next to the right side of the doorway frame at shoulder height, with your elbow bent. Keeping your right hand in place, step forward with your right foot, bending your right knee (as in a lunge), with your left leg stretched behind you. You should feel a stretch in your shoulder but not any pain. Hold for three to five seconds, and do five to 10 repetitions. Repeat with the left arm on the left side of the doorway and left foot stepping forward.

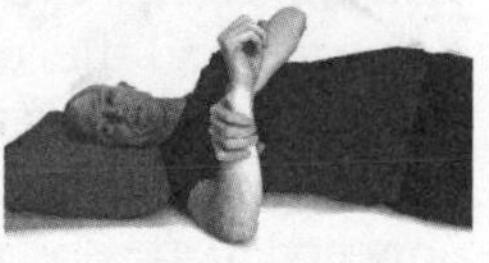

• **Side stretch.** Lie on your side on the floor (on an exercise mat or rug), your painful shoulder on the floor and your head supported on a pillow or bolster so that your spine is in a straight line. Bend the arm that's on the floor at the elbow, with the forearm and hand raised and palm facing your feet. Now use your other hand to gently push the wrist of the bent arm toward the floor. Hold for three seconds and release. Do a total of 10 reps. Repeat with your other arm.

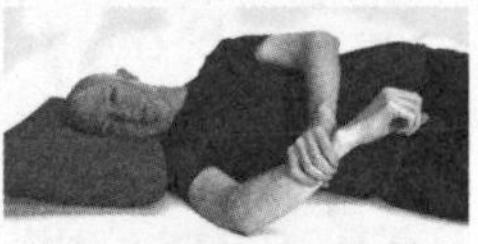

***STEP 2*: Strengthen the Right Muscles**

While impingement, frozen shoulder, tendinitis and bursitis often are referred to as overuse issues, I prefer to call them "understrength" issues. The problem isn't the 100 times you serve during a typical tennis match—it's that your muscles aren't strong enough to handle the stress you're placing on them. Even people who lift weights often focus on the biceps and triceps and ignore the rotator cuff.

Caution: Stay away from military presses and other exercises that require you to lift weights overhead—that can injure your shoulder. Skip kettle bells, too—they require swinging that can inflame your shoulder.

My recommendation: To build the strength of your rotator cuffs, use resistance bands, which do the job and are safer. *Try these three stability builders…*

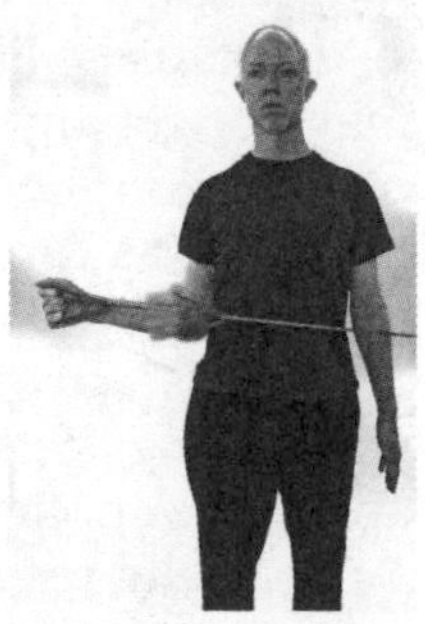

• **External rotation.** Loop a resistance band at waist height around a secure anchor such as the base of equipment at a gym or a strong door handle of a locked door at home. Standing sideways to the anchor, grab both ends of the band with one hand so it's taut. Keep your elbow bent and against your side and your hand near your stomach. Now pull the band away from your stomach, keeping your elbow against your side, until you feel light tension on the outside of the shoulder. *Hint*: Your shoulder blade should move toward your spine. Hold for one second. Do a total of 10 reps. Repeat with your other arm.

• **Internal rotation.** This is the reverse of the external rotation. Keep the resistance band looped around a secure anchor, and stand in the same position as above. But this time, grab the band with the hand that is closest to where it's anchored. Keeping your elbow bent and at or near your side, pull the band across your torso toward your belly button. Hold for one second. Do a total of 10 reps. Repeat with your other arm.

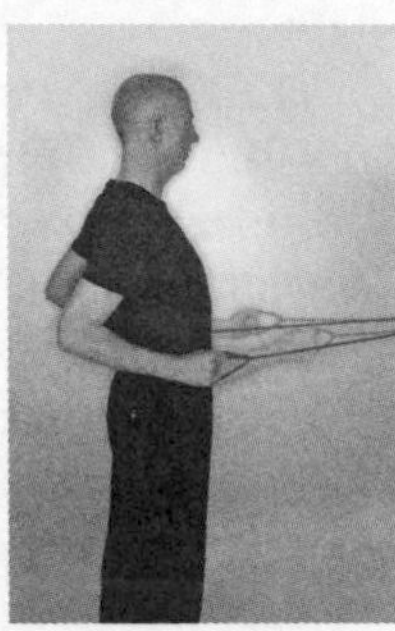

• **Rowing.** With the elastic band securely anchored as above, grab one end of the band in each hand so it's taut. Pull both arms back, bending your elbows and keeping them close to your sides. Hold for one second. Do a total of 10 reps. Repeat with your other arm.

Is Surgery a Must When You Have a Hernia?

Hien Tan Nguyen, MD, assistant professor of surgery, Johns Hopkins University School of Medicine, director, Johns Hopkins Comprehensive Hernia Center and assistant professor of biomedical engineering and associate medical director, Johns Hopkins Center for Bioengineering Innovation and Design, all in Baltimore.

A hernia can be a serious problem—or not. For example, the average hernia causes little or no discomfort…and may not get any worse. Nevertheless, doctors often recommend surgery due to the risks that hernias can pose.

When is a hernia about to change from "harmless" to "extremely dangerous?" Are you getting the latest and most effective therapies? We spoke with Hien Tan Nguyen, MD, a nationally recognized expert on hernias.

What Is a Hernia?

A hernia is a protrusion of tissue, such as intestine, through a weak spot in the abdominal muscles. *Types of hernias…*

Both inguinal and umbilical hernias are easy to diagnose and rarely require an imaging test because your doctor can see and feel them. The bulge can cause discomfort or even severe pain.

Where to look: Inguinal hernias appear on either side of the groin or, in men, within the scrotum. Umbilical hernias appear near the belly button. Both types tend to get larger and more tender during activities that increase abdominal pressure, such as while straining with a bowel movement, during a sneezing or coughing fit or just from standing up.

A special warning for women: Women are more prone than men to occult (hidden) hernias—too small to be seen or felt by touch—that can press on nerves and cause pain. Often, these hernias get misdiagnosed as endometriosis or another gynecological problem. A woman with pelvic pain should start by consulting with her gynecologist and make sure to ask whether a hernia could be the cause.

What you can do: The size and discomfort of inguinal or umbilical hernias can vary over time. *What helps…*

• **A cold compress.** Encourage protruding tissue to retreat back into the abdomen or groin, thus "reducing" a hernia, by lying down and applying a cold compress for about 10 minutes. Use gentle pressure to slowly press downward on the bulge.

• **Wear a truss.** Some people wear a truss (hernia belt). While this may help, it isn't a cure, and wearing a truss can cause the wearer to forget about the hernia and overexert, making a small hernia larger.

• **Try yoga.** A study found that men with reducible inguinal hernias (they readily retract) who practiced a daily one-hour program of yoga followed by relaxation for three months rated their pain up to five points lower on a 10-point scale compared with before starting yoga. Yoga and other gentle workouts won't cure a hernia but can help to minimize symptoms, such as pain and cramps.

Hernias tend to get bigger over time, so to avoid possible future complications, many doctors recommend surgery to minimize the risk for complications. But painless inguinal or umbilical hernias are unlikely to need emergency surgery.

My advice: Consult your doctor if you are concerned that you have a hernia. Don't delay too long—you'll have fewer surgical complications when a hernia is repaired before the symptoms are severe.

Latest treatment options: Most surgeries for inguinal or umbilical hernias can be performed on an outpatient basis with minimally invasive surgery, using small incisions that allow for faster recovery and less pain following surgery. You'll be sore for about two weeks, and able to resume normal activities in about a month.

Caution: Hernias can come back. Reduce risk by maintaining a healthy weight, not smoking and exercising to strengthen abdominal muscles.

Best exercise: Cardio helps manage weight, especially abdominal weight.

With a hiatal hernia, the upper part of the stomach pushes through an opening in the diaphragm. You can't see or feel a bulge, but you might notice heartburn—or have no discomfort at all.

Most people only discover their hiatal hernia from an imaging test done for another condition. In severe cases, the hernia protrudes into the chest and interferes with normal function of the lungs or heart, causing symptoms that include shortness of breath.

If your doctor suspects a hiatal hernia, he/she will order an upper endoscopy to check your stomach and esophagus for inflammation and/or ulcers. He/she may also order a manometry test to measure pressure inside the esophagus...an esophogram to look for abnormalities...a pH test to measure the amount of acid flowing into your esophagus...or a CT scan to see how much of the stomach protrudes into the chest cavity also may be done.

What you can do: If you have heartburn that is mild/occasional and your hiatal hernia is small, your doctor is likely to prescribe medication rather than recommend surgery. Acid-blocking drugs such as *omeprazole* (Prilosec) or *cimetidine* (Tagamet) can reduce discomfort. Lifestyle changes, such as eating smaller, more frequent meals, not lying down immediately after eating and avoiding foods that trigger heartburn, won't heal the hernia but can alleviate symptoms.

Caution: Acid-suppressing drugs can have side effects such as increased risk for pneumonia and nutritional deficiencies, including vitamin B-12. Your doctor should supervise your use of these drugs.

Hiatal hernias that require surgery usually can be repaired with a minimally invasive procedure, but larger incisions may be needed in some cases. Surgery commonly involves pulling the stomach down through the diaphragm and narrowing the esophageal opening...and wrapping the stomach around the lower end of the esophagus, a procedure called *Nissen fundoplication*. The tighter fit keeps the stomach where it belongs and increases pressure on the esophagus—important for relieving heartburn. Most patients spend a night in the hospital and resume their regular activities within a few weeks.

When Any Hernia "Goes Bad"

Whether it's an inguinal, umbilical or hiatal hernia, if your doctor believes that there is a risk for strangulation (twisting), in which the protruding tissue gets trapped between the muscle layers, you'll need surgery. With strangulation, the blood supply to the twisted tissue is cut off, causing it to become damaged or to die, leading to sepsis or gangrene—both life-threatening complications.

Critical symptoms: With an inguinal or umbilical hernia, sudden, worsening pain, nausea, vomiting, fever, inability to move bowels or pass gas...with a hiatal hernia, hoarseness or difficulty breathing.

A "Cinematic" Way to Beat Pain

Brennan Spiegel, MD, professor of medicine, director of Health Services Research and director of the master's degree program in health delivery science, all at Cedars-Sinai Health System in Los Angeles.

Imagine this: You are lying in a hospital bed after surgery when you begin to feel a stabbing pain. Desperate for relief, you look for your daily dose of pain medication. Not so fast. Soon, you may reach instead for a set of virtual-reality goggles.

Using virtual reality (VR) for pain is not some sci-fi snake oil. This high-tech therapy, which immerses you in a three-dimensional, multisensory world of cinematic grandeur, is on the cutting-edge of pain relief approaches.

Scientific evidence: New research shows that VR significantly reduces many types of pain and may lessen (or, in some cases, replace) the need for pain medication—a well-timed breakthrough given the addiction epidemic that's being fueled by pain medicine such as opioids.

What you need to know about this exciting new advance...

Virtual Reality in Action

So what's it like to experience VR? Once you slip on the somewhat clunky-looking headset or even a simpler pair of special goggles, you'll be ready to watch three-dimensional, 360-degree streaming video complete with sound that depicts a wide variety of vibrantly colored realistic scenes—either photographed or animated. You'll hear the sounds associated with that scene and even experience vibrations or other sensations for a completely immersive experience.

Depending on the purpose of the VR therapy—whether you need to focus your mind to distract yourself from pain, for example, or you need relief from anxiety—you may view scenes that give you the feeling of swimming with dolphins in the ocean...lobbing snowballs while hurtling through an animated snowscape...or relishing the splendor of a gushing waterfall.

VR therapy has been used successfully by scientists for years to help treat the symptoms of conditions such as stroke, post-traumatic stress disorder, social phobia and burns. In hospitals, VR therapy is used as needed with children to distract them from painful or scary procedures, such as getting blood drawn.

Until recently, however, VR therapy was too expensive and not widely available. That's now changing.

New Scientific Evidence

To learn more about the effects of VR, researchers at Cedars-Sinai Medical Center in Los Angeles recently studied 100 patients experiencing pain from many different causes, including cancer, bone breaks and other ailments. In this study, published in *JMIR Mental Health*, half of the study participants received 10 minutes of VR therapy once a day, and half watched a two-dimensional nature video with calming music on a high-definition computer screen.

Result: While both groups reported less pain, those undergoing VR experienced a significant 24% drop in pain compared with a 13% decrease in the relaxing video group. The period of pain relief varied but generally lasted at least an hour.

While this study did not identify the exact mechanism behind VR's effectiveness against pain, it is an example of the spotlight attention theory. According to this theory, the human mind is able to track only a certain amount of information at one time—the eyes focus on what is in a "spotlight" and not the areas in the background. With VR, the brain is overwhelmed with positive imagery that engages the mind so that other signals, such as pain, are not perceptible (or not as perceptible) at the same time.

Reducing Pain Medication

Many people who use VR continue to have pain reduction even after discontinuing the therapy. Scientists theorize that VR may somehow reset the brain, making some people less susceptible to peripheral pain signals for a period of time.

Scientists are also investigating whether VR can reduce the use of painkillers after an acute injury, such as a broken leg, or postoperatively—for example, after hip- or knee-replacement surgery.

Sobering statistics: A one-day prescription of an opioid painkiller results in a 6% risk for use of the drug one year later. And when treated for at least 31 days with opioids, nearly 30% of patients were still taking the painkillers a year later.

VR Equipment

Cedars-Sinai and other medical centers use a VR kit provided by the company AppliedVR (go to AppliedVR.io). This kit consists of a Samsung headset and Galaxy phone at a cost of $800. A subscription to access the library of visualizations is extra.

But do not let that cost overwhelm you. You can use your own smartphone to access VR therapy by buying a headset (available on Amazon.com for about $20 to $100) and then streaming VR content by buying an app or going to YouTube.com. Look online for lists of highly rated VR apps.

Important: The VR therapy used in hospitals is prescribed for specific conditions. When using VR therapy on your own, try it on a trial-and-error basis. For example, if you are looking to relax or alleviate anxiety, you can search "VR and beach" or "VR and relax," and try out different scenes. There may be minor side effects, such as dizziness. People with dementia, epilepsy, nausea and certain other conditions should not use VR therapy without checking with their doctors.

How to Access VR Therapy

Several hospitals across the country are conducting clinical trials on the use of VR therapy for pain management (including neuropathic pain and phantom limb pain) and other conditions such as attention deficit hyperactivity disorder (ADHD), traumatic brain injury, fear of heights and more.

To find a VR trial near you: Go to ClinicalTrials.gov, type in "virtual reality" and choose your state or a nearby state.

Could Fish Oil and Vitamin D Help Ease Lupus?

See pg 194

Michelle Petri, MD, PhD, director, Hopkins Lupus Center, Johns Hopkins University, Baltimore

Stacy Ardoin, MD, assistant professor, department of medicine, Ohio State University and Nationwide Children's Hospital, Columbus, and member, Lupus Foundation of America Medical-Scientific Advisory Council

Prae Charoenwoodhipong, MS, graduate student, department of nutrition science, University of Michigan, Ann Arbor

American College of Rheumatology annual meeting, San Diego

People with lupus may fare better if they have enough vitamin D and omega-3 fats in their diet, preliminary research suggests.

In separate studies, researchers linked the two nutrients—or lack thereof—to higher risks of certain lupus symptoms and complications.

In one, lupus patients with low blood levels of vitamin D faced a higher risk of kidney damage than those with sufficient levels.

In the other, people who ate more omega-3 fats—mainly found in oily fish—tended to have less severe symptom flare-ups and better sleep quality.

"Questions about diet are some of the most common ones I get from patients with lupus," said Stacy Ardoin, MD, a member of the Lupus Foundation of America's Medical-Scientific Advisory Council. "And it's an area where we have little evidence."

Despite some Internet claims, there is no such thing as a lupus-defeating diet, said Dr. Ardoin, an assistant professor at Ohio State University.

But the new studies looked into whether certain nutrients are related to the risks of certain symptoms and complications. Both were reported at the annual meeting of the American College of Rheumatology in San Diego this week.

About Lupus

Lupus has several forms, with the most common called *systemic lupus erythematosus.* In

SLE, the immune system mistakenly produces antibodies against the body's own tissue. The onslaught can have widespread effects, damaging the skin, joints, heart, lungs, kidneys and brain.

At least 1.5 million Americans have the disease, according to the Lupus Foundation of America. It mostly strikes women, usually starting in their 20s or 30s.

Vitamin D Study

The vitamin D study involved nearly 1,400 patients with SLE who had their blood levels of the nutrient measured in 2009-10. Slightly more than 27% had low levels—defined as less than 20 nanograms per milliliter.

The researchers looked at the patients' rates of organ damage over the following years, and estimated their lifetime risks of those complications.

On average, they found, patients with low vitamin D had a 66% higher risk of severe kidney damage, versus those with normal levels. The nutrient was not linked to damage in other specific organs.

Michelle Petri, MD, PhD, of Johns Hopkins University in Baltimore, led the study.

It's known, she said, that vitamin D helps reduce protein in the urine, which is a predictor of future kidney damage. So that might explain why low vitamin D was specifically tied to that risk.

Implications

While the study was not a clinical trial, Dr. Petri said, vitamin D can be safely prescribed to lupus patients who need it.

According to Dr. Ardoin, many rheumatologists already screen lupus patients for low vitamin D, because it is a common problem for people with the condition.

"If you haven't been screened," she said, "you can ask your doctor about it."

Omega-3 Study

The omega-3 study involved 456 SLE patients who completed a detailed diet survey. In general, researchers found, the more omega-3 fats people consumed, the better their sleep quality.

And when they ate plenty of omega-3, and tempered their intake of omega-6 fats, they typically had lower scores on a measure of lupus "disease activity."

Omega-6 fats are largely found in vegetable oils like corn, sunflower and safflower oils. Omega-3s come mainly from fish like salmon, mackerel and tuna, plus certain seeds and nuts—such as flaxseed, chia seeds and black walnuts.

The average US diet is high in omega-6, according to the researchers, led by Prae Charoenwoodhipong, MS, a graduate student in the department of nutrition science at the University of Michigan. In contrast, a better balance of omega-6 and omega-3 might quiet inflammation.

Implications

Again, Dr. Ardoin said, the findings do not prove that omega-3 will ease any lupus symptoms. And even if there is a benefit, she added, it's not clear how much omega-3 is necessary to achieve it.

That said, Dr. Ardoin noted, paying attention to diet—including getting enough healthy fats—is generally a wise move.

The Lupus Foundation of America has more information on treating lupus, Lupus.org.

Tai Chi for Fibromyalgia

When 226 adults with the chronic pain condition fibromyalgia were randomly assigned to twice-weekly aerobic classes or tai chi classes, those in the tai chi group reported significantly more improvement in pain intensity, fatigue, depression and overall well-being after 24 weeks.

Theory: The gentle movements and emotion-regulating effects of tai chi are especially effective for fibromyalgia.

Chenchen Wang, MD, director, Center for Complementary and Integrative Medicine, Tufts Medical Center, Boston.

The Big Mistake Most MS Patients Make

Allen C. Bowling, MD, PhD, a neurologist specializing in multiple sclerosis (MS) and a physician associate at Colorado Neurological Institute in Englewood, Colorado, and clinical professor of neurology at University of Colorado in Denver. He is author of five books on MS, including *Optimal Health with Multiple Sclerosis*. NeurologyCare.net

Medications are often a must for the roughly 400,000 Americans with multiple sclerosis (MS). Powerful disease-modifying drugs (DMDs) can reduce the development of new brain and spinal cord lesions that lead to symptoms...prevent relapses...slow the disease's progression...and delay disability.

The big mistake: For the majority of patients with MS, drugs are the only therapy used.

In my own experience treating thousands of people with MS, I have found that an integrative approach—a treatment plan that combines conventional medicine with science-supported nondrug strategies such as diet, nutritional supplements and exercise—is a much more effective way to manage symptoms and improve quality of life than medications alone.

New evidence: In a one-year study published in *Journal of the American College of Nutrition*, an integrative approach including a healthy diet, stretching, meditation and self-massage eased depression, anxiety and fatigue in people with MS and helped prevent mental decline.

Additionally, starting a healthy lifestyle when MS is diagnosed (typically between the ages of 20 and 50) can help prevent chronic, lifestyle-associated medical problems, such as obesity, arthritis, heart disease and diabetes, that may worsen disability and quality of life in those with MS.

Here are the most reliable, safest and cost-effective integrative treatments for MS patients...

Diet

I advise my MS patients to stay away from (or at least minimize) processed foods...avoid overeating...and consume a plant-based diet. This simple advice may make a huge difference in their health, especially over the long-term.

What not to do: I find that extreme diets—for example, a strict Paleolithic diet or strict gluten-free diet—may be difficult to follow and may not actually be healthy for people with MS. They don't provide the variety of foods that support good health.

Bottom line: There is no one diet that is best for MS. But the worst diet for MS is the standard American diet, loaded with processed foods, fatty meats and sugar. Eliminating those foods and ingredients goes a long way toward maintaining good health.

Nutritional Supplements

There are two common nutritional deficiencies that I have found in people who have MS—vitamin B-12 and vitamin D. I test my patients for these two deficiencies and advise supplements if necessary, customizing the dose to the patient. A multivitamin may be considered for those with an unhealthy diet, but it is preferable to change the diet.

Recent scientific research: Dozens of studies show that low vitamin D levels or low vitamin D intake increases the risk for MS and, in those with MS, increases risk for attacks, disability progression and new brain lesions. Also, there are studies that a subgroup of people with MS are at risk for vitamin B-12 deficiency—this is of concern because many of the symptoms of vitamin B-12 deficiency are the same as those of MS.

Beware: There is a lot of hype about nutritional supplements for MS. Watch out for products asserting that a single nutritional supplement can treat many different diseases, including MS...touting one or more "secret" ingredients...or relying heavily on customer testimonials as evidence of effectiveness.

Exercise

Research shows that regular exercise can reduce the fatigue, muscle weakness and walking difficulties common with MS. Other symptoms that exercise may ease include anxiety, anger, depression, bowel and bladder difficulties (such as constipation, incontinence, urgency and frequency), pain, sleeping difficulties, stiffness in the arms or legs (spasticity) and cognitive decline. Exercise may even slow the progression of the disease.

New scientific research: In a six-month study of 35 people, published in *Multiple Sclerosis Journal*, researchers found that twice-a-week resistance-training slowed the rapid shrinking of the brain common in MS. Some areas of the brain even started to grow.

My advice: In addition to twice-weekly strength training (such as wall squats with or without hand weights, lunges and wall push-ups), I urge my patients to do aerobic exercise (30 minutes of medium-intensity exercise, such as stationary cycling, dancing or walking, twice weekly). Aerobic exercise has many benefits for MS patients including improved cardiovascular fitness...better bowel and bladder control...and less fatigue and depression.

Also helpful: Hydrotherapy (water exercise such as swimming and water aerobics) may be especially well-suited for people with MS who have leg weakness. And yoga is particularly good for easing spasticity. In a recent study published in the journal *Medicine & Science in Sports & Exercise*, eight weeks of water exercise or yoga improved fatigue, depression and tingling and numbness in women with MS, compared with a group that didn't exercise.

Emotional Well-Being

Emotional health is a crucial but often-neglected component in the treatment of MS.

New scientific research: In a study of more than 1,000 people with MS, published in *Neurology*, 44% reported their emotional well-being was worsening due to fatigue, trouble concentrating and bladder/urinary problems.

What I recommend: To improve emotional well-being, I counsel my MS patients to identify their difficult emotions—and to talk about those feelings with a spouse or friend. I have found that patients who do this not only feel happier but also dramatically reduce their feelings of stress.

Also helpful: Listening, creating or moving to music stimulates feelings and facilitates emotional processing. A professional music therapist can suggest an approach geared to your specific situation. A study published in the journal *Expert Review of Neurotherapeutics* found that music therapy improved self-acceptance and eased depression and anxiety in MS patients. To find a music therapist near you, consult the American Music Therapy Association at MusicTherapy.org.

Low Thyroid: The Diagnosis That Doctors Miss

Jacqueline Jonklaas, MD, PhD, MPH, professor of medicine, division of endocrinology and metabolism, specializing in thyroid disorders at Georgetown University Medical Center in Washington, DC.

Do you have memory loss...fatigue...weight gain...constipation? If you're in your 60s or older, your doctor might dismiss these symptoms as normal aspects of aging. But they could be caused by a very treatable condition that doctors often miss in older people.

These symptoms can be a result of trouble with the thyroid gland—specifically, hypothyroidism, in which the thyroid gland doesn't produce enough thyroid hormone. Typically, when a blood test shows a thyroid-stimulating hormone (TSH) level around 4.0 milli-international units per liter (mlU/L), it suggests hypothyroidism—but after age 60 or so, you can have a TSH level well above 4 even with a healthy thyroid.

Your doctor might think you have hypothyroidism and prescribe hormone treatment when you don't have it. And that's just as bad as missing it.

What to do: If your doctor dismisses your symptoms as normal aspects of aging, ask whether he/she has considered hypothyroidism—especially if your symptoms developed relatively rapidly.

If your doctor conducts a TSH blood test and then prescribes synthetic thyroid hormone, ask, "What's my TSH level?" If it is above 10, treatment is almost certainly justified. *But if it is between 4 and 10 and you are past age 60, ask…*

- **"Are we sure that my TSH level is above range for my age?"** Your doctor's response should indicate that he understands that older people can have healthy thyroids even with levels above 4 mlU/L.
- **"Can we do a second TSH test to confirm that finding?"** A single TSH test can produce a misleading result.
- **"Do I have hypothyroidism or 'subclinical' hypothyroidism?"** Subclinical hypothyroidism means that your TSH level is a bit high, but your level of thyroxine (T4, another thyroid hormone) is fine. Doctors sometimes prescribe synthetic thyroid hormone in these situations, but a study published earlier this year in *The New England Journal of Medicine* found no benefit to doing so, at least among people age 65 and up.
- **"Did I test positive for anti-thyroid antibodies?"** If the answer is yes, you may have Hashimoto's thyroiditis, an autoimmune condition that causes a gradual loss of thyroid function. That would strongly support your doctor's decision to prescribe hormones (or to monitor your TSH levels closely).

Deadly, Daily Hormone Disrupters

Holly Lucille, ND, RN, naturopathic doctor in West Hollywood, California. She is author of *Creating and Maintaining Balance: A Woman's Guide to Safe, Natural Hormone Health.* DrHollyLucille.com

Ok, deadly might be a strong word. But I got your attention, didn't I? Women dealing with symptoms associated with perimenopause or menopause, such as hot flashes, night sweats, fatigue, achiness, irritability and weight gain, are familiar with the idea of hormonal imbalances or deficiencies—but *disruption*? Not so much.

These disruptors can indeed lead to diseases that most certainly can be deadly.

Many of the everyday things we come in contact with are a source of endocrine disruptors, also known as hormone disruptors. These troublesome agents can contribute to altering normal hormone function. They can be absorbed through your skin, so that over time they accumulate and get stored in body fat—wreaking havoc with natural hormone balance. They are among the more than 85,000 manufactured chemicals in the US, lurking in things we touch and consume every day.

Hormone disruptors, often derived from petrochemicals, make their way into our lives disguised inconspicuously as "harmless" household cleaners, air fresheners, plastic toys, food containers, cosmetics, perfumes and health and beauty aids. Exposure also comes from industrial chemicals and persistent pesticides that are pervasive in our modern day environment, processed foods and car exhaust.

They were once dismissed as unimportant because they were emitted in very small quantities, but research now shows that even tiny amounts of these hormone disruptors can have overwhelming effects on our health and hormone balance.

Here are three examples of endocrine disruptors that you need to know about…

• **BPA, which stands for bisphenol A,** is an industrial chemical used to make two common synthetics—polycarbonate and epoxy resin. Epoxy is used to line the majority of the more than 130 billion food and beverage cans made in the US every year. Sidestep BPA by skipping the cans and choosing fresh or frozen food whenever possible. BPA is also found in 40% of the receipts that you grab without a thought from the store clerk. Say "no" to receipts when possible, or take it with a tissue if saving it is necessary. "BPA free" is getting a lot of attention, but be a wise consumer. Some companies are replacing BPA with bisphenol 5 (BPS). While this allows them to claim that a product is "BPA free," recent research suggests that BPS also disrupts hormones.

• **Phthalates.** This chemical plastic softener is often found in cosmetics. It's used to keep nail polish from cracking...in hair spray to maintain flexibility...and as a solvent and fixative in synthetic fragrances. Phthalates are easily absorbed by the skin and make their way to the bloodstream. How do you know if a product harbors phthalates? Since manufacturers aren't required to list them, look for the term "perfume" or "fragrance" on cosmetic and personal-care product ingredient labels. You'll also find phthalates in many plastics, including food containers, toys, and medical devices such as IV tubes and catheters. When possible, check labels for DBP, DNOP, DiNP, DEP, BBzP, DEHP, DiDP, DMP, DnOP—that's your clue that phthalates are part of the product.

• **PFCs or perfluorinated chemicals.** Love that nonstick pan? Well, PFCs that prevent food from sticking to your cookware can leach into your food and stick to you! In fact, these endocrine disruptors are so widespread that researchers believe 99% of Americans now have PFCs as part of their chemical body burden. They don't break down—ever—so every one that has ever been here is still here. Time to refresh your cooking style. Skip nonstick pans, and choose alternatives such as glass, ceramic or cast iron. Beware of coatings that promise fewer stains and water resistance on your clothes, furniture, and carpeting. PFCs are also used to coat the inside of microwave popcorn bags and fast food containers.

With the tenet of "prevention is the cure" in mind, let's learn to reduce exposure where we can! The more you learn, the better equipped you'll be to lessen the threat these hormone disruptors pose and make your personal environmental and hormone system as healthy as possible.

Tips to Avoid Endocrine Disruptors

• **Get rid of plastics** (including water bottles) and use glass.

• **Buy organic food whenever possible.**

• **Make your own household cleaners.**

• **Opt for chemical-free cosmetics and personal care products.**

• **Always read product labels.**

• **Do not microwave food in plastic containers.**

• **Use unbleached paper products and feminine protection** (if you still need it).

• **Trade in garden pesticides and herbicides for organic alternatives.**

• **Visit helpful websites such as EWG.org,** a nonprofit, nonpartisan organization dedicated to protecting human health and the environment.

A Foot Problem That Gets Misdiagnosed

Mitchell Yass, DPT, a specialist in diagnosing and resolving the cause of pain and creator of the Yass Method for treating chronic pain. He is the author of *Overpower Pain: The Strength Training Program That Stops Pain Without Drugs or Surgery* and *The Pain Cure Rx: The Yass Method for Diagnosing and Resolving Chronic Pain.*

If you're age 50 or older, overweight and have recently experienced pain, tingling or numbness in one or both feet, you fit the classic profile of a person with diabetic neuropathy (DN).

This condition occurs when diabetes leads to nerve damage, which most often affects the feet. Sometimes DN hurts, while other times it creates an inability to feel pain, heat or cold. This loss of sensation is serious, because a sore or ulcer can go unnoticed, become infected and sometimes lead to a foot or leg amputation—so your doctor diagnoses you with DN.

Here's the kicker: You may not have DN—or diabetes. Even though people who are overweight are at much greater risk for type 2 diabetes, you may not have the disease.

Still, when doctors see a heavy patient with foot pain, tingling and/or numbness, many are quick to assume that it's DN. Add to that the widespread advertising for *pregabalin* (Lyrica), an antiseizure medication often used to treat the nerve pain of DN, and you can see how many doctors would jump to this treatment. Lyrica can be effective when properly prescribed, but it's a powerful drug with side effects, including dizziness, blurred vision, weight gain, difficulty concentrating and, in rare cases, suicidal thoughts. If you take this drug but don't actually have DN, you put yourself at risk for these side effects...while failing to address the real cause of your foot troubles.

What Else Could It Be?

If your doctor has diagnosed you with DN, make sure that your blood tests (such as a fasting blood glucose test) confirm that you actually have diabetes. If you are not diabetic but your physician has diagnosed DN, it's time to find a new doctor. But if you don't have DN, then what's causing your foot problems?

Unraveling the Clues

Based on my experience treating hundreds of patients with foot pain who were misdiagnosed with DN, I recommend special exercises.

To ensure that you're doing the most effective exercises, it's crucial to isolate where you're experiencing pain or numbness in your foot—is it all over...on top...or on the bottom? *What the location may mean...**

If your entire foot is affected—it could be sciatica. This condition, characterized by shooting pain that travels down one or both legs, can occur when the piriformis muscle in the buttocks compresses the sciatic nerve, which runs down the leg before branching off in the foot. The result can be gluteal pain, as well as pain, numbness or a "pins and needles" feeling in the foot. Sciatica often occurs when the gluteus medius muscle above the hip joint is weak, leading the piriformis muscle to compensate.**

Self-test for a weak gluteus medius muscle: Look at yourself in a mirror while standing casually. Does one hip naturally sit higher than the other? A higher hip indicates that the lower back muscle on that side is overworked and shortened, pulling the hip higher. This points to sciatica—not DN—as the cause of your foot discomfort.

To strengthen the muscles of the weaker hip, do these two exercises...

- **Hip abduction.** Lie on your side, with your bottom leg bent at the knee and your top leg (the weaker one) extended in a straight line. Rotate the foot of your extended leg slightly so that your toes point down and your heel is the first to rise. Raise your top leg several inches keeping it parallel with the floor, then lower it, keeping movements controlled.

Perform two to three sets of 10 repetitions, two or three times a week. If doing 10 repetitions is easy, add a weighted ankle cuff (available online). Begin with a one-pound weight and increase weight when the exercise becomes too easy. Do the exercise on your weak leg only.

- **Dorsiflexion.** Slip one end of an elastic resistance band around a sturdy table leg. While wearing sneakers, sit on the floor facing the table. Extend your weak leg, bend

*If your foot pain, regardless of location, isn't eliminated by these exercises in four weeks, see a neurologist.

**If sciatica causes severe pain or you have trouble controlling your bowels or bladder, see a doctor right away.

your knee and slip the other end of the resistance band over your instep. Point and flex, keeping the heel stationary and movements slow and controlled. Perform two to three sets of 10 repetitions, two or three times a week, on your weak leg only.

If just the top of the foot is affected—you may have a pinched peroneal nerve. This happens more frequently in people with strained hip muscles. Symptoms are similar to those of weak gluteal muscles. Unlike sciatica, however, there's no gluteal pain, and the altered foot sensation is on the top of the foot only—not all over. *To strengthen hip muscles, perform the two exercises above, plus this exercise…*

• **Inversion.** Knot a resistance band on one end, and place the knotted end behind a closed door. Sit in a chair, parallel to the door. Loop the other end of the resistance band around your instep. Angle your toes slightly to the outside of the heel, then stretch the band until toes are in line with the heel. Perform two to three sets of 10 repetitions, two or three times a week, on your weak leg only, using slow and controlled motions.

If pain is in the sole of your foot—you may have a collapsed arch.

What can happen: If the gluteus medius or the muscles that support the arch are weak, your arch may flatten. When this occurs, the sole of your mid-foot will be flat on the floor when you stand or walk, compressing nerves in the bottom of the foot. This triggers tingling and/or numbness in the sole.

Self-test for a collapsed arch: Wet the sole of your foot, shake off any excess water, then step on a brown paper bag. If the arch side of your footprint is filled in, you may have a collapsed arch.

To alleviate pain, do all three of the exercises above.

Chapter 11

EMOTIONAL HEALING

Overcoming the Pain of Sexual Abuse Memories

A new social movement, in which women (and some men) bravely come forth to tell their stories of sexual harassment, abuse and violence, has felled the careers of some of the most powerful men in business, politics, media and entertainment—even as it empowers the abused to stand up for their rights.

For many people, however, these stories, while inspiring, can trigger very painful memories—even bring new ones to light that you may have suppressed. To learn how to deal with these, we spoke with Wendy Maltz, LCSW, DST, a psychotherapist, lecturer and sex therapist. (*Note:* These recommendations apply to anyone—including men—who has been a victim of sexual abuse.)

The truth is, there are many paths to healing. *Here is how to find the ones that are a good fit for you...*

• **Honor your experiences.** Don't minimize your experiences or compare them with someone else's experiences that seem even worse. Each event of sexual harassment, abuse or violence—from catcalls to crude remarks to groping and beyond—is an invasion of your privacy and an attempt to diminish your dignity that can make you feel vulnerable, violated and humiliated. The appropriate response to yourself to each experience is compassion and understanding.

• **Don't overshare on social media.** The #MeToo hashtag allows anyone to make a valuable public statement without getting into the details of what happened. But sharing specifics or naming names is riskier because what goes online stays there forever, and you can't control how others might respond to your story or use it against you in the future. If your goal is to push the problem of sexual abuse out into the sunshine by saying more than "me, too" and you're willing to face potential personal consequences of that, then sharing specifics of your #MeToo experience is an option you can be proud of. But I think it's counterproductive to expect that you'll find healing on social media.

• **Use your memories to heal.** It's upsetting to remember the painful past, but the resurfacing of old memories provides an op-

Wendy Maltz, LCSW, DST, psychotherapist, lecturer and sex therapist based in Eugene, Oregon, who has written six books on sexuality including *The Sexual Healing Journey: A Guide for Survivors of Sexual Abuse.* HealthySex.com

portunity for deeper healing. It's a chance to recognize how strong you are. Even if you feel you haven't fully resolved what happened, focus on the extent to which you withstood the incident and moved forward in spite of it.

• **Talk to someone you know who is sympathetic.** Not everyone wants to share his/her story—it's OK to stay silent forever or until you feel ready to talk—but if you do, decide how much you want to disclose and to whom. Disclosure can help dispel feelings of isolation and shame. It can feel freeing to finally receive the validation and comfort you deserve. Choose someone carefully—whether a spouse, friend, relative, clergy member or family doctor—who you know understands the prevalence and significance of sexual violence. Such a person is most likely to provide helpful support.

One way to gauge whether someone is a good person to talk to: Begin by bringing up sexual abuse in general or via a news story. Pay attention to how the person responds. Does he express sympathy with abuse victims or, instead, challenge or doubt their stories? Then you might talk in general about your own experience without going into specifics ("This kind of thing happened to me, too") and feel out the response before saying more. Remember that once you share details, you can't take them back. That's why it's wiser to reveal small amounts of general information at first and then more only if it feels important and right to do so. Keep in mind that friends, family members and others are not therapists and may have difficulty hearing specifics and explicit information. You don't need to share a lot to receive some understanding and caring from people you know.

• **Find strength in numbers.** If confiding in one person isn't for you or if you feel you could benefit from joining with others in an active healing process, there are a number of support groups for survivors of sexual abuse or violence. Find local groups and resources on RAINN—the Rape, Abuse & Incest National Network (Rainn.org/statistics/victims-sexual-violence—just type in your zip code).

• **Read helpful books or listen to podcasts.** Reading about or listening to other survivors' stories can show you there's a light at the end of the tunnel. If you find the details too upsetting, you can skim over those parts to get to the recommendations. Some books to try include *The Courage to Heal* and my book *The Sexual Healing Journey*. Sometimes just listening to others' stories is therapeutic. Safe Space Radio features conversations on sex abuse and related topics.

• **Seek counseling.** I'm not a fan of digging up the past for no reason. But if the abuse you suffered in the past is affecting your mental and physical health or harming your ability to be intimate—or if you want to understand better how it has influenced your life—find a therapist. Sex abuse recovery therapists can help you undo negative thinking patterns and develop skills for self-care, self-compassion and speaking up for yourself. Ask your doctor or a rape crisis center for therapists who have worked with sex abuse survivors. It's also OK to make trial appointments with two or three therapists and see which one is the best fit.

Should I Confront the Abuser?

Counseling can be particularly helpful if the person who abused or harassed you has resurfaced or somehow still is a part of your life. A therapist can help you work out whether you want to call out this person's behavior. There's no single right answer—unless you believe that someone else, especially a child, is in danger. Then it's your responsibility to do whatever is necessary, including calling the police, to avert future abuse.

Choosing to confront an abuser depends on your emotional strength, what you want to accomplish and who else is involved, including other potential victims, and how cooperative and safe they are. The best scenario is to confront the person with the guidance and presence of a trained professional. When therapists facilitate such conversations, they can help you prepare well and move the discussion along to a resolution. But if that's not possible, it may be appropriate to enlist a supportive friend to be there. Remember, confrontations are not always necessary or advised.

As an alternative, you may decide to confront your abuser through a letter or a phone call or by e-mail. These, too, are best accomplished with a therapist's guidance. Focus on the power of asserting your truth, rather than making the success of the interaction whether you receive a specific response.

Figure out beforehand how you'll handle your abuser's reaction. Many offenders will deny the extent of the abuse, minimize it or blame the survivor in some way. And all of that can be really upsetting, so you want to be emotionally prepared and supported.

Healing Our Culture

Finally, it's important to realize that sexual violence is a cultural problem. I challenge anyone to turn on the TV and not find a program on some channel where a woman has been or is about to be sexually intimidated in some form. Sexual aggression against women is a common feature in popular pornography, as well. It's become entertainment, and we've become desensitized to it.

We can't keep role-modeling negative behaviors and expect change or expect the victims to mop up the mess. Instead, we must change our behavior in terms of what we tolerate in the media and as bystanders. When something that is meant "as a joke" is demeaning, say so. When you see abuse, call it out—if necessary, to the authorities.

Many New Moms Hide Postpartum Depression

More than one in five women with postpartum mood disorders (PPMDs) don't discuss depression or other symptoms with their doctors. Between 10% and 20% of new mothers suffer from PPMDs.

What this means: More needs to be done to create social networks for new mothers.

Maternal and Child Health Journal.

You Can Be Surrounded by People and Still Be Lonely

Julianne Holt-Lunstad, PhD, professor of psychology and neuroscience at Brigham Young University, Provo, Utah. Her research focuses on the long-term health effects of social connections and includes a meta-analysis on the effects of loneliness and social isolation on mortality.

We tend to think of loneliness as a negative feeling of being disconnected and alone.

But here's some good news: Loneliness also can be a powerful motivator—even a biological urge—to reconnect. We are social animals, after all, and the urge to have strong bonds with others is a powerful one.

You don't have to be lonely. And neither do any of your loved ones.

Loneliness is such an epidemic in the US that social scientists have been digging deep to find ways to help people overcome it.

Unfortunate fact: The prevalence of loneliness has more than doubled in the US since the 1970s. It now affects an estimated 42 million Americans over age 45.

The truth is, what helps one person leave loneliness behind may be different from what helps another. It may take trial and error to stop feeling lonely or to help someone do so. But there are now evidence-backed approaches that can help many people feel less lonely—and improve their health. To find out more, we spoke with Julianne Holt-Lunstad, PhD, a professor of psychology and neuroscience at Brigham Young University.

Lonely in a Crowd

What is loneliness? It's a gap—between the kind of social relations you want and what you actually have. It's a perception of social isolation that doesn't always have to do with how many people surround you. You can be lonely with colleagues, with friends...and in a marriage. If most of our dealings with our friends and relatives are superficial or filled with conflict, we will feel disconnected no matter how big our social network is.

Conversely, you can feel just fine even when you are totally alone—that's the positive experience called solitude. That's why, to transcend loneliness, you need to have people who you can trust and who understand you—people who you are working with to manage life's challenges and truly thrive.

As Unhealthy as Obesity

Loneliness is a hot topic in social science these days because of growing scientific evidence that a lonely life is an unhealthy one. It's truly a killer.

Sobering finding: A meta-analysis of 70 studies found that loneliness increases the risk for an early death by 26%. That makes it about as great a public health threat as obesity.

Feeling isolated increases the risk for chronic body-wide inflammation, which can lead to a host of diseases including high blood pressure, diabetes and cancer. Loneliness also is strongly linked to increased risk for cognitive decline and, for people with Alzheimer's, a faster progression of the disease. It's not just biology, either. Good relationships improve our satisfaction with life and enhance a sense of meaning and purpose—and that in turn makes it more likely we'll take good care of ourselves. Close bonds also help us cope with stress and minimize the risk for depression.

The Path Toward Lonely

If we have such a strong drive to be socially connected, why are so many people becoming lonely? Research has revealed a common psychological trap that many people fall into.

People don't start to become lonely voluntarily. Rather, there may be some kind of disruption—moving away, retiring, a death or divorce or even a new marriage—that takes you away from most or all of your social support system. Health issues, such as hearing loss or vision loss, can make it hard to hold a conversation, and injury or poor health can make it hard to get out of the house. And while we tend to associate older people with these risk factors and more isolation, studies show that loneliness powerfully affects all age groups, even college students who are literally surrounded by peers their own age. Faced with isolation, many people feel a strong need to connect with others.

Problem: Loneliness that is deep enough also makes people so desperate for connection—and makes the stakes of social interaction so high—that they become hypersensitive to people around them. Of course, social sensitivity can be a strength, making you more empathetic, which draws people to you. But social hypersensitivity can make you more likely to misinterpret offhand remarks or behavior or worry too much about how other people see you, causing you to feel anxious, act awkwardly and withdraw from social situations. That can turn into a vicious cycle—less connection, more hypersensitivity and therefore even less connection.

Worship for a Longer Life

Men and women who attended church or other places of worship had a mortality risk that was 55% lower over an 18-year period than nonworshippers.

Theory: Attendance at religious services may have a stress-fighting effect that extends longevity.

PLOS ONE.

Solutions for Lonely

If you see yourself in some of what's described above, consider all of the following suggestions...

• **Reframe your thinking.** If you find yourself feeling lonely despite being around others, your first step should be to reframe/replace negative thoughts that you have about and in social situations—*He really doesn't like me if he walked right past me without saying hello!*—with nonjudgmental interpretations such as, *He might have been in a rush, so not saying hello doesn't necessarily mean* *he doesn't like me*. Reframing your thoughts takes practice—indeed, it's a key part of the popular and effective talk therapy called cognitive behavioral therapy, or CBT. There are many highly qualified therapists who use CBT, so if you want a professional to guide you, consider one-on-one visits or group sessions for people with social anxiety.

• **Visit people face-to-face.** There is robust evidence that visiting with people in person is particularly powerful—so do what's needed to make it happen! Using social media isn't nearly the same thing.

Exception: Digital connections can deter loneliness if they help you get together with friends or find like-minded groups to join—especially if these groups meet in the "real" world.

• **Lend a hand.** When you hear, "It's better to give than to receive," whom do you think it's better for? The answer is—the giver. Evidence shows that volunteering, with the focus on helping others rather than oneself, makes people feel less lonely. It bolsters both social connections and a sense of purpose—you're helping people, and they're depending on you.

• **Renew bonds that already exist.** The friends and family members we're emotionally closest to have the greatest influence on our health, research shows. Make a special effort to nurture those relationships. Set a reminder on your phone to call those folks regularly, and make concrete plans to get together. If you've had a falling out with a friend or family member and think the relationship could be retrievable without too much stress, see what you can do to make amends.

• **If you are in a relationship, be more responsive to your partner's needs.** There is a lot of loneliness within marriages—even reasonably good marriages. You may feel a distance between what you want your relationship to be and what it actually is. A love relationship is complicated, no doubt, but one thing that can make a lonely partner less lonely is for that partner to increase his/her responsiveness to the other partner. That means, for example, that you not only listen when your spouse is venting about a looming work deadline, but you also offer to lighten her load at home so she can meet it—and then follow through even if you're both eating takeout for a week. When partners acknowledge each other's needs and desires, both of them are less likely to feel disconnected and frustrated with their marriage.

Healing Society

One reason loneliness has become a virtual epidemic is that there is shame and stigma attached to this emotion. We might not hesitate to tell others we are angry, for example, but many people refuse to admit—even to themselves—that they feel disconnected. The realization that loneliness is a health risk as serious as obesity can help change that. We can create a national dialogue around it. Students can learn about the health benefits of good relationships...doctors can talk to their patients about loneliness and do risk assessments...and perhaps workplaces could institute policies that would encourage a work-life balance. Even government policy can help.

Example: We now know that untreated hearing loss puts older people at greater risk of becoming isolated and lonely. And a new federal law allowing hearing aids to be sold over the counter rather than only by prescription—making them more affordable—was passed partly to address just that problem. It's too early to know whether this law will reduce isolation, but it aims to address one risk factor—and it's a start.

Sexual Bereavement

Alice Radosh, PhD, research psychologist and coauthor of the study "Acknowledging Sexual Bereavement: A Path Out of Disenfranchised Grief," published in *Reproductive Health Matters*.

The death of a spouse is not just the loss of a life partner. It also is the loss of a sexual partner. Unfortunately, most widows and widowers must cope with the emotional impact of that loss of sexual intimacy alone, and the isolation only deepens their suffering. Cultural taboos and personal embarrassment often prevent them from raising their feelings of what is called "sexual bereavement." But there's a way to help yourself psychologically if you are in this situation...or help a loved one who is.

Recent finding: A survey of 104 partnered women age 55 and older published in *Reproductive Health Matters* found that 72% anticipated missing sex with their partners after their partners died, and most said that they would want to discuss this feeling of loss with a friend. But the majority reported that they would feel more comfortable about the conversation if the friend raised the subject.

The problem: Most of the women surveyed also admitted that they would not raise this topic if it were one of their friends who had been widowed.

What to do: If you are the close friend of someone who has been widowed, raise the topic of the loss of sexual intimacy. If it makes you uncomfortable to ask your friend about his/her sex life, you could mention that you would grieve the loss of your sex life if you were widowed...or you could say that someone else you know who was widowed experienced these feelings. Don't assume that your recently widowed friend is too old to have had an active sex life—many couples remain sexually active into their 80s.

If you are recently widowed and are experiencing sexual bereavement, understand that these feelings are perfectly normal. Raise the topic with a friend or relative without shame. If you are not comfortable doing this, you could raise the topic with a therapist or support group...or with a friend by mentioning a recent sexual-bereavement article you read about (such as this one).

Depression Common in US, Women Hit Hardest

Debra Brody, MPH, division of Health and Nutrition Examination Surveys, National Center for Health Statistics (NCHS), U.S. Centers for Disease Control and Prevention, Atlanta, Georgia.

David Roane, MD, chairman, psychiatry, Lenox Hill Hospital, New York City.

U.S. Centers for Disease Control and Prevention's NCHS Data Brief, online.

Nearly one in 10 US adults has depression, and the rate is almost twice as high for women as men, health officials say.

National survey data showed that more than 8% of adults aged 20 and older suffer from low mood, according to a new report from the US Centers for Disease Control and Prevention.

Among women, slightly more than 10% have depression, versus 5.5% of men. And the mood disorder affects everyday life for a majority of these people, the 2013–2016 questionnaires show.

"One of the findings that surprised us the most was that for both men and women, about 80% of adults with depression had at least some difficulty with functioning with daily life," said lead author Debra Brody, MPH.

These include going to work, completing daily activities at home and getting along with other people, said Brody, of the CDC's National Center for Health Statistics (NCHS).

Report Details

According to the report, depression is most prevalent among blacks (9%) and least so among Asians (3%). Among whites and Hispanics, the rate is about 8%.

Also, as income levels fall, depression rises. Poor Americans are four times more likely to have depression than middle class or rich people—about 16% versus 4%, respectively.

Data for the report were gathered from the US National Health and Nutrition Examination Surveys. The findings were published online in the CDC's *NCHS Data Brief.*

Diagnosis and Treatment

According to David Roane, MD, chairman of psychiatry at Lenox Hill Hospital in New York City, "The biggest issues with depression are diagnosis and treatment."

In most cases, primary care doctors are able to diagnose depression, he noted. "But people often don't get adequate treatment in terms of both medication and psychotherapy," Dr. Roane said.

He stressed that anyone with depression should be monitored by a doctor or mental health professional, such as a social worker, nurse or therapist.

Effective treatment includes antidepressant medications and talk therapy, Dr. Roane explained.

However, there are obstacles to treatment, he said. For one thing, people often don't realize they are depressed, even if they have mood problems and changes in thinking.

Also, mental health problems are still often considered taboo.

"The stigma related to depression has decreased somewhat, but it's still a major issue for someone to be diagnosed with a mental health disorder," he said. In addition, many cases of mild depression will resolve over time, so some patients don't want treatment.

"The problem is that if you are having functional impairment, it can be highly disruptive to your life," he said. "Six months is a long time to suffer from depression, and I don't recommend that."

Anyone with recurrent depression, suicidal thoughts or manic and depressive swings should be under the care of a mental health professional, Dr. Roane advised.

Implications

He said that depression affects all aspects of life, including physical well-being.

When people are depressed, they don't sleep or eat well. They are sad and have a negative view of life and feelings of hopelessness, he explained.

The researchers reported that the percentage of American adults who suffered from depression in a given two-week period remained steady from 2007 to 2016.

The study authors also pointed out that major depression is associated with high societal costs and greater functional impairment than other chronic diseases, such as diabetes and arthritis.

"This report should make people aware how serious depression is, and that it impacts everyday life," Brody added.

It has been shown before that women are more prone to depression than men, but the reasons are not known, Dr. Roane said.

For more about depression, visit the website of the National Institute of Mental Health, NIMH.NIH.gov, and search "depression."

Antidepressants Do Work, Some Better Than Others

John P.A. Ioannidis, MD, DSc, professor, disease prevention, and professor, statistics and biomedical data science, Stanford University, Stanford, California.

Richard Catanzaro, MD, chairman of psychiatry, Northern Westchester Hospital, Mount Kisco, New York.

The Lancet, online.

Antidepressant drugs actually do help ease depression, countering debate over whether the medications do what they're supposed to, a large research review has found.

Some antidepressants, though, are more effective and better tolerated than others, the findings showed.

Study Findings

The researchers analyzed data from 522 trials—published and unpublished—that included more than 116,000 participants. Of the 21 antidepressants studied, all of them worked better than a placebo.

"In the short-term, for acute depression, antidepressants seem to work modestly," said study author John P. A. Ioannidis, MD, DSC. He's a professor of disease prevention at Stanford University in California. "They do have some benefit, on average, but they are not a panacea. Clearly, we need more effective interventions."

Antidepressants sold in the United States that the study found to be most effective included...

- *amitriptyline* (Elavil)
- *venlafaxine* (Effexor)
- *escitalopram* (Lexapro)
- *paroxetine* (Paxil)
- *mirtazapine* (Remeron)
- *vortioxetine* (Trintellix)

Those that made the least-effective list of antidepressant drugs sold in the United States included...

- *fluvoxamine* (Luvox)
- *trazodone* (Oleptro)
- *fluoxetine* (Prozac)

When the researchers checked which depression drugs were tolerated the best, these topped the list...

- *citalopram* (Celexa)
- *escitalopram* (Lexapro)
- *fluoxetine* (Prozac)
- *vortioxetine* (Trintellix)
- *sertraline* (Zoloft)

The drugs that were found to be less well-tolerated included...

- *amitriptyline* (Elavil)
- *clomipramine* (Anafranil)
- *duloxetine* (Cymbalta)
- *venlafaxine* (Effexor)
- *fluvoxamine* (Luvox)
- *trazadone* (Oleptro)

Implications

According to the study authors, there's been "a long-lasting debate and concern about [antidepressants'] efficacy and effectiveness, because short-term benefits are, on average, modest and because long-term balance of benefits and harms is often understudied."

However, Richard Catanzaro, MD, chairman of psychiatry at Northern Westchester Hospital in Mount Kisco, New York, said this review shows that "all of these medications can be effective in treating depression."

He explained that "all distinguish themselves from placebo, but there's no hands-down winner."

And, Dr. Catanzaro said, if you're looking for the most tolerable and the most effective, you're left with Lexapro and Trintellix.

In addition, Dr. Catanzaro noted that while amitriptyline was on the most-effective list, it was also on the least-tolerated list, and he said it's generally not considered a first-line drug for depression treatment.

Dr. Ioannidis said that the differences between the medications were small, so even medications on the less-effective list might work very well for some people.

Both experts noted that this study looked only at responses after eight weeks of treatment. How these medications might work for people taking them for years was not assessed.

The study was published in *The Lancet.*

Hormonal Birth Control Linked to Depression

Women who used birth-control pills, hormonal patches or IUDs containing progestin were from 23% to twice as likely to start taking an antidepressant, compared with women using nonhormonal birth control. The likelihood was even greater for teenagers ages 15 to 19.

Self-defense: Women with a history of depression should talk to their doctors about nonhormonal birth control.

Study by researchers at University of Copenhagen, Denmark, published in *JAMA Psychiatry.*

Expert Advice

That's another issue with antidepressant medications, Dr. Catanzaro explained: What works well for one person doesn't always work well for another, so there may be some trial and error involved in finding the right medication for you.

It's also important to be sure you're getting the right dose of medicine and that you take the drug long enough to give it time to work well, Dr. Catanzaro said. That can be as long as four to six weeks.

Both Dr. Ioannidis and Dr. Catanzaro said that people with depression shouldn't rely on medications alone, whenever possible.

"I would never advocate that antidepressants are the only way to approach this major problem," Dr. Ioannidis said, recommending psychotherapy with medications.

Dr. Catanzaro said that he, too, recommends therapy along with medication. "But in many areas it can be hard to get good-quality therapy. Medications are often the only treatment people have access to, and if the alternative is nothing, then that's certainly preferable," he advised.

The National Institute of Mental Health has more information about depression at NIMH.NIH.gov. Search "depression."

Prevent Depression Without Breaking a Sweat

Study titled "Exercise and the Prevention of Depression: Results of the HUNT Cohort Study," by an international team of researchers lead by the Black Dog Institute in Australia, published in *American Journal of Psychiatry*.

Exercise is proven to help prevent depression. But the issue of how much exercise is needed...and how intense that exercise must be...has not been very clear. Now, there's research that helps answer both these questions—and it could help protect you (and millions of others) from depression's heavy burden.

Are you getting enough exercise to ward off depression?

Background: Exercise is a powerful and well-established short-term mood booster. And decades of studies have found that getting regular activity is one of the most effective and reliable ways to treat clinical depression. But research on exercise to prevent depression in healthy people has been more mixed. Many studies have lumped together depression with anxiety, but they are different disorders. Nor has there been good evidence to identify the optimal duration or intensity needed to prevent the onset of depression.

Study: An international team of researchers led by the Black Dog Institute, a nonprofit mental health organization in Australia, analyzed the exercise levels and the symptoms of depression and anxiety in about 34,000 mentally and physically healthy Norwegian adults (average age 45) over a span of 11 years. This work is part of one of the largest and longest health studies ever conducted. At the beginning of the study, the participants were asked to report how often they exercised and how hard they worked out—for example, without becoming breathless or sweating...to the point of becoming breathless and sweating...or to exhaustion. At the end of the study, participants completed a questionnaire designed to identify signs of depression or anxiety.

Results: Not exercising at all was the big depression risk—people who didn't exercise had a 44% increased chance of becoming depressed over 11 years compared with those who exercised just an hour or two per week. Then the researchers delved deeper into the duration question. It turned out that there was no additional benefit to exercising two hours per week compared with one. Nor was there any benefit to intensity such as breaking a sweat. In short, just one hour a week of moderate-intensity exercise, the kind you can get by walking or with easy biking, was enough to significantly reduce the risk of becoming depressed.

The findings were the same regardless of a range of variables—age (under age 50 or over age 50), gender, socioeconomic and demographic factors, use of alcohol or other substances, body mass index, physical health and social support.

Put another way, according to the researchers, 12% of depression cases could have been prevented with just one hour of moderate physical activity once per week. While the study couldn't pinpoint how exercise protects, they believe that it's a combination of physical effects on the brain, such as stimulating serotonin levels and brain-protective chemicals such as brain-derived neurotrophic factor, psychological benefits such as increased self-esteem and general improvements in physical health.

Surprising finding: Despite the significant effect exercise had on the risk for depression, it had no effect on preventing anxiety. That is, people who exercised a little, a moderate amount or a lot were all about as likely to experience an anxiety disorder. (*Editor's note:* While exercise levels may not affect overall risk, other studies have found that a single bout of aerobic exercise, such as going for a run, can help reduce acute episodes of anxiety.)

Bottom line: Getting people who are sedentary to become moderately active just an hour or more a week could be one of the most effective ways to reduce the burden of depression in society...and if you are sedentary, it could be one of the most effective ways for you to shield yourself from the onset of depression.

To be clear, though, that's not enough exercise for optimal health. To protect your heart and help prevent other chronic ills, aim for 150 minutes of moderately intense exercise a week, or 75 minutes of intense exercise a week, or a combination of the two.

But it does underscore the good news that it doesn't take superintense or superlong workouts to get the mood-stabilizing benefits of regular activity. Virtually anyone should be able to incorporate enough activity in their weekly schedule to potentially ward off depression. In other words, beating the blues may be, literally, a walk in the park.

Use "Nostalgia" for Emotional Healing

Krystine Batcho, PhD, professor of psychology at Le Moyne College, Syracuse, New York. She has studied nostalgia since 1995.

We all know people who seem to dwell on the past. They are constantly bringing up memories from years or decades ago. Sometime we're tempted to shake them and yell, "Live in the present, not the past!"

Maybe it would be better to emulate them. We now know from science—not conjecture—that nostalgia is good for you. It can improve your mood, help you become more resilient and increase your motivation to tackle new challenges.

What Nostalgia Really Is

At its core, nostalgia is a sentimental affection...a yearning...for the past. We associate it with being older, but young adults often are intensely nostalgic, too—for their childhoods.

Are you nostalgic? The way researchers identify this is to ask volunteers to rate, on a scale of one to five, how much they miss things from when they were younger such as their parents and siblings...having heroes or heroines...being carefree...particular friends...school/college...a previous home... TV shows...music...pets...trips/vacations... the "way people were." The more "fours" and "fives" you record, the more sensitive you are to triggers of nostalgia. *Here's why that's a good thing...*

The Benefits of Nostalgia

Connecting your present and past selves can strengthen your sense of personal identity—remembering how you experienced unconditional love as a child, for example, can be reassuring during difficult times. In my research, a clear picture of nostalgic individuals has emerged, and it's largely positive.

People who score high on measures of nostalgia, compared with those who score low, tend to be…

• **Empathetic.** They feel things deeply—and other people are a high priority.

• **Resilient.** They use healthy coping strategies in stressful times, including getting emotional support from others and expressing their emotions rather than burying them.

• **Stronger in their sense of self.** They have a keener sense of who they are inside while remaining respectful of other people's standards.

• **Less anxious.** The sense of continuity from connecting to the past can have a grounding effect, helping to ease stress.

• **More connected.** When lonely, nostalgic memories encourage people to reach out to others and stay socially connected. That counteracts loneliness and may help prevent depression.

• **Better at reaching goals and solving problems.** They are more likely to employ approaches such as planning, strategizing and reframing a situation more positively—and then take action to improve the situation.

• **More positive.** A study in *Psychology & Health* found that people who were asked to write about a nostalgic event rather than an ordinary event scored higher immediately afterward on measures of health optimism…and got more exercise over the next two weeks.

Nostalgia even can change how you feel physically—making you feel warmer in a cold environment.

Evoking the Good Old Days

You don't have to wait for random events to trigger nostalgic memories. *You can make it happen any time you want to…*

• **Listen to songs from your early days.** Songs we loved as teenagers or young adults retain their emotional power throughout our lives. Listen to your favorites—and remember how you felt back then. And watch old movies you enjoyed when you were younger, especially those with great sound tracks.

• **Flip through your past.** Look through boxes of old family pictures. Dig out your yearbooks or souvenirs.

• **Reminisce with others.** Getting together with old friends or family can provide opportunities to bring up crazy old memories…and sometimes share stories of someone who has died.

• **Recruit your senses of smell and taste.** These olfactory cues are particularly effective at triggering autobiographical memories, studies show. Breathe in a scent you loved… cook your favorite childhood dish.

• **Anticipate future nostalgic moments.** The next time you spend joyful time with friends or family and something memorable happens, call attention to it. Say something such as, "Let's remember this moment!" This is called "anticipatory nostalgia." You're storing up future nostalgia recollections.

Staying on the Right Side of the Past

Is there ever a downside to thinking about the past? Yes, there can be. Brooding about past negative experiences (injuries, rejections, mistakes)—what psychologists call rumination—can contribute to depression. Most nostalgia, in contrast, evokes a positive feeling.

Some forms of nostalgia can be problematic, too, especially historical nostalgia—a longing for a past era. The desire to escape into an idealized world of yesteryear, say Edwardian elegance or 1960s free-spiritedness, can sometimes lead to becoming more isolated as you spend more time alone. If so, consider whether you're neglecting people or issues in your life, and work to restore healthy relationships by reaching out to others.

Personal nostalgia is more positive. It's often joyous, although it can be bittersweet and poignant. But that's good, too—it can help you integrate negative feelings, such as grief over the loss of a loved one, with positive feelings, such as memories of good times spent together.

Yet personal nostalgia can become unhealthy if it traps you in repetitive memories of the past without attempts to seek fresh positive experiences. Ask yourself, *How am I building on my past? How can the love, knowledge and skills I once enjoyed help me move forward?* At its best, revisiting a happy or healthy period from the past can help you gain strength and optimism to handle the challenges of the present.

When Nostalgia Was a Disease

Fond memories of the past haven't always had a good reputation. The term "nostalgia" was invented in 1688 by Johannes Hofer, a Swiss physician who combined the ancient Greek words for "home" (nostos) and "pain" (algos) to make "nostalgia." He considered the phenomenon a debilitating form of homesickness, which was weakening the troops. In 1733, a Russian general whose soldiers came down with the nostalgia bug punished a few by burying them alive. Over the following centuries—even into the early-20th century—nostalgia was considered a psychiatric disorder, a form of depression or melancholia. Over the years, treatments have included leeches, stomach purges and shaming.

More Evidence That Depression Shortens Lives

Stephen Gilman, ScD, acting chief, health behavior branch, U.S. National Institute of Child Health and Human Development, Bethesda, Maryland.

Aaron Pinkhasov, MD, chairman, behavioral health, NYU Winthrop Hospital, Mineola, New York, and associate professor, clinical psychiatry, Stony Brook University School of Medicine, Stony Brook, New York.

John Hamilton, LMFT, LADC, chief clinical outreach officer, Mountainside Treatment Center, Canaan, Connecticut.

CMAJ, online.

People with depression tend to die earlier than expected—a pattern that has grown stronger among women in recent years, new research finds.

The study followed thousands of Canadian adults between 1952 and 2011. Overall, it found people with depression had a higher death rate versus those without the mood disorder.

The link only emerged among women starting in the 1990s. Yet by the end of the study, depression was affecting men's and women's longevity equally.

The findings do not prove that depression itself shaves years off people's lives, said lead researcher Stephen Gilman, ScD.

The study could not account for the effects of physical health conditions, for example.

"So one explanation could be that people with depression were more likely to have a chronic condition," continued Dr. Gilman, of the U.S. National Institute of Child Health and Human Development.

But even if that were true, he added, it would not mean that depression bears no blame—because depression can take a toll on physical health.

"Many studies have found that people with depression have higher risks of heart disease and stroke, for example," Dr. Gilman said.

Study Details

The findings are based on 3,410 Canadian adults who were followed for up to several decades. The first wave of participants was interviewed in 1952, the next in 1970, and the final in 1992.

At each wave, roughly 6% of adults had depression, based on a standard evaluation.

And on average, those people had a shorter life span. For example, a 25-year-old man who was depressed in 1952 could expect to live another 39 years, on average. That compared with 51 years for a man without depression.

Men with depression at any point had a higher risk of dying over the coming years, versus those free of the disorder.

The picture was different for women, though. The connection between depression and mortality only surfaced in the 1990s.

Women with depression at that point were 51% more likely to die by 2011, compared with other women. That brought their risk on par with depressed men.

The results were published in the journal *CMAJ*.

Possible Explanations

The reasons are unclear. "Why would depression be less toxic to women at one time point than another?" Dr. Gilman said.

He speculated that societal shifts have some role. Women in recent decades have been much more likely to juggle work and home life, or be single mothers, for example.

Another possibility, Dr. Gilman said, is that women tend to suffer more severe depression these days.

There was some evidence that the impact of depression lessened over time. Men with depression in 1952 no longer showed a higher death risk after 1968, for example—unless they also had depression at the later interviews, too.

As for causes of death, there was no evidence that suicides explained the risks among people with depression.

"There were actually few suicides," Dr. Gilman said. "People with depression died of the same causes that other people did—like cardiovascular disease and cancer."

Aaron Pinkhasov, MD, is chairman of behavioral health at NYU Winthrop Hospital in Mineola, New York.

He said depression can indirectly shorten life span in a number of ways. Depressed people are less able to maintain a healthy lifestyle, and are more vulnerable to smoking and drinking. They may also be less equipped to manage any physical health conditions.

"Once depression sets in, you may not have the motivation or energy," said Dr. Pinkhasov, who was not involved with the research.

Advice

Dr. Gilman said his study can't say whether treating depression erases the higher death risk associated with it.

But, Dr. Pinkhasov said, there is evidence that depression treatment can help people better control high blood pressure and diabetes, for example. He stressed that there are various effective treatments—from "talk therapy" to medication.

"Don't blame yourself for being 'weak,' or tell yourself you should just snap out of it," Dr. Pinkhasov said.

John Hamilton, LMFT, LADC, a counselor at Mountainside Treatment Center in Canaan, Connecticut, agreed.

He said that women, in particular, can have a "sense of shame" over mental health symptoms in part because they feel they need to be the rock of the family. "They might even have people around them saying, 'Snap out of it, you have kids,'" said Hamilton, who also had no role in the study.

"But depression is no different from any other chronic disease," he said. "We need to have a compassionate, nonjudgmental approach to it."

For more information about depression, visit the website of the National Institute of Mental Health at NIMH.NIH.gov and search "depression."

With Stress and Trauma Come Excess Weight

Michelle Albert, MD, professor of medicine and cardiology, and founding director, Center for the Study of Adversity and Cardiovascular Disease, University of California, San Francisco.

American Heart Association, news release.

As if weathering a stressful event isn't tough enough, new research shows these episodes might even widen a woman's waistline.

The Study

Researchers analyzed data on nearly 22,000 middle-aged and older women.

The goal: to assess the relationship between obesity and traumatic events—such as the death of a child or being a victim of a serious physical attack—as well as negative events, for example, long-term unemployment or burglary.

About 23% of the women included in the study were obese.

Findings

Study participants who reported more than one traumatic life event were 11% more likely to be obese than those who did not experience a traumatic event, the findings showed.

In addition, women who reported four or more negative life events within the previous five years were 36% more likely to be obese than those who reported no negative events.

The link between stressful events and obesity was stronger among women with high levels of physical activity, but the reason for this was unclear, the study authors said.

The report was presented at the American Heart Association (AHA) annual meeting, in Anaheim, California.

Implications

"Little is known about how negative and traumatic life events affect obesity in women," said senior author Michelle Albert, MD.

"We know that stress affects behavior, including whether people under-eat or overeat, as well as neuro-hormonal activity by, in part, increasing cortisol production, which is related to weight gain," she added.

Dr. Albert is a professor of medicine and cardiology, and founding director of the Center for the Study of Adversity and Cardiovascular Disease at the University of California, San Francisco.

"Our findings suggest that psychological stress in the form of negative and traumatic life events might represent an important risk factor for weight changes and, therefore, we should consider including assessment and treatment of psychosocial stress in approaches to weight management," she said.

This line of research is important "because women are living longer and are more at risk for chronic illnesses, such as cardiovascular disease," Dr. Albert said. "The potential public health impact is large, as obesity is related to increased risks of heart attack, stroke, diabetes and cancer, and contributes to spiraling health care costs."

More than one-third of US adults are obese, according to the US National Institutes of Health.

The National Heart, Lung, and Blood Institute has more on obesity at NIMH.NIH.gov (search "Overweight and Obesity").

---

1 in 5 Young Women Who Tan Indoors Gets Addicted

Darren Mays, PhD, MPH, assistant professor, oncology, Georgetown University Medical Center, Washington, DC.

Doris Day, MD, dermatologist, Lenox Hill Hospital, New York City.

Joseph Levy, scientific advisor, American Suntanning Association.

Cancer Epidemiology, Biomarkers & Prevention.

More than 20% of young white women who've been to a tanning salon become addicted to tanning—even though doing so raises their risk of deadly skin cancer and premature skin aging, a new study reports.

These women seem to depend on tanning to feel attractive and often show symptoms of depression, the researchers said.

"Indoor tanning remains a public health concern for skin cancer prevention," said lead researcher Darren Mays, PhD, MPH, an assistant professor of oncology at Georgetown University Medical Center in Washington, DC.

"Our study indicates a substantial proportion of young women who indoor tan may become dependent, putting this group at especially high risk for skin cancer later in life," he said.

Risks of Indoor Tanning

Indoor tanning is dangerous. It increases the risk of melanoma, the most deadly cancer, by 20% and increases the risk of other skin cancers as well, Dr. Mays said.

The Study

Dr. Mays and his colleagues studied tanning addiction among nearly 400 white women between 18 and 30 years old. White women were chosen for the study because they're the ones most likely to use indoor tanning.

The participants completed online questionnaires and had used an indoor tanning device one or more times in the past year. Nearly 47% of the women were college students.

The researchers measured tanning dependence based on two questionnaires. The participants were considered tanning-dependent if they tested positive for addictive behavior on both questionnaires.

The Findings

In total, nearly 23% of the women tested positive for indoor tanning dependence, the researchers found.

Women who were dependent were more likely to have begun tanning at an earlier age, to be concerned about their appearance and to have depressive symptoms, compared with women who weren't dependent, Dr. Mays said.

As beliefs about the importance of appearance grew stronger, young women were 73% more likely to be addicted to indoor tanning.

In addition, women who were depressed were nearly four times more likely to have a tanning addiction, compared with women who weren't depressed, Dr. Mays said.

The report was published in the journal *Cancer Epidemiology, Biomarkers & Prevention.*

Possible Explanation

It's not yet clear why some women become addicted to tanning. Some scientists believe that tanning produces a by-product that has an opioid drug-like effect on some people.

Expert Commentary

Joseph Levy is scientific adviser to the American Suntanning Association, which represents the tanning salon industry. He disagreed that tanning can be addictive.

"It is imprudent to characterize our natural and intended attraction to sunlight as addictive," he said. "Ultraviolet exposure is a natural attraction, and humans get less regular sunlight today than at any point in human history."

At least one medical specialist disagreed with Levy. Doris Day, MD, a dermatologist at Lenox Hill Hospital in New York City, said she sees women who are addicted to tanning every day.

"Tanning is not safe and it's not healthy," she said. Dr. Day tells women who are addicted to tanning about the risk for skin cancer and premature skin aging.

In addition, she helps them reduce their need to tan and gradually reduce the amount they tan.

Advice

Dr. Day advises using sunscreen, and if you absolutely need to have that suntanned look, to use a bronzer instead.

"I tell them to perfect their pale or go with their own glow," she said.

Dr. Mays said women need to understand not only the risks of tanning but to be on the lookout for signs of tanning addiction, such as symptoms of depression.

However, getting people to change this behavior may be tough, he added.

"We do not yet have resources available to help young women who may be tanning-dependent to change their behavior to reduce their risk," Dr. Mays said.

For more on skin cancer, visit the American Cancer Society website at Cancer.org/cancer/skin-cancer.

Opiod Use After Nose Jobs

Sagar Patel, MD, ear, nose and throat specialist, Facial Plastic Surgery Associates, Houston.

JAMA Facial Plastic Surgery, news release.

Could some patients recovering from a nose job get a problem they didn't bargain for?

After these operations, patients are often sent home with more opioid pain pills than they need, increasing the risk for misuse, researchers say.

About 218,000 cosmetic nose surgeries were performed in the United States in 2015. In fact, "rhinoplasty" is one of the most common plastic surgery procedures in the United States, which is experiencing an opioid epidemic.

The Study

The new study included 62 patients at two private practices and an academic health center who underwent rhinoplasty. The patients were prescribed the opioid painkiller *hydrocodone/acetaminophen* (Vicodin) for pain relief after surgery.

On average, patients used nine of the 20 to 30 tablets they were prescribed. Seventy-four percent used 15 or fewer tablets, and only three patients needed refills. The number of tablets used was not associated with gender, age or surgical factors.

The study was published in the journal *JAMA Facial Plastic Surgery*.

Implications

Most people who misuse opioids for nonmedical use get them from friends and family who have leftover medication.

"To mitigate the misuse or diversion of physician-prescribed opioid medications, surgeons must be steadfast in prescribing an appropriate amount of pain medication after surgery," according to Sagar Patel, MD. Dr. Patel is an ear, nose and throat specialist with Facial Plastic Surgery Associates in Houston.

The U.S. Food and Drug Administration has more information on opioids at FDA.gov. Search "opioids."

The Dangers of "Feel Good" Sedatives

Cara Tannenbaum, MD, professor in the faculties of medicine and pharmacy at Université de Montréal and the Michel Saucier Endowed Chair in Geriatric Pharmacology, Health and Aging at Centre de Recherche de l'Institut Universitaire de Gériatrie de Montréal, both in Canada.

Imagine that you've had a particularly bad year. Maybe you've lost a close friend...suffered from financial problems...or struggled with frequent insomnia.

A doctor—maybe a psychiatrist, but more likely an internist or a family physician—might suggest that a sedative will help you get through the rough patch. The drug will probably be a benzodiazepine, a class of "sedative hypnotics" that includes popular medications like *alprazolam* (Xanax), *lorazepam* (Ativan) and many others. Or it could be a related "Z" drug, such as *zolpidem* (Ambien) and *zaleplon* (Sonata).

You'll immediately start to sleep better and worry less. But every day that you take it, the risk for side effects—including addiction—increases. Experts now believe that the risks are so high that "benzos" should never be the first choice for insomnia and/or anxiety...and that their use should be limited to four weeks or less.

Dangerous Drugs

Benzodiazepines are among the most popular drugs ever developed. A recent study found that more than 5% of American adults took at least one of these drugs during a one-year period. Shockingly, the majority of these prescriptions were written for patients age 65 and older.

The same study found that about one-third of the older patients who took a benzodiazepine did so for months, years or even decades—even though these drugs are intended for short-term use.

Why it's a problem: Benzodiazepines and the related "Z" drugs bind to brain receptors that cause sedation. They're highly addictive in patients of all ages...but the risk for side effects is much higher in older adults because of an age-related decline in kidney function and an increase in fat mass, both of which cause the drugs to accumulate in the body. A dose that would quickly be metabolized and excreted in a younger adult might stay active for days in older adults.

Older patients who take these drugs are at increased risk for a number of health issues. For example, they are five times more likely to suffer from memory/concentration problems...four times more likely to experience daytime fatigue...and twice as likely to fall, suffer hip or wrist fractures or have car accidents. There's even some evidence that benzodiazepines may increase the risk of developing Alzheimer's or other forms of dementia.

Important: When benzodiazepines are taken with opioid painkillers, the risk for opioid overdose increases significantly.

Too Many Prescriptions

Doctors know that benzodiazepines are inherently risky but continue to prescribe them freely. It's estimated that 20% to 25% of all inappropriate prescriptions (that is, medications for which harms outweigh the benefits and safer alternatives exist) in older adults involve one or more of these drugs...and about half of doctors will continue to renew prescriptions (citing patient resistance to tapering, among other factors) despite the risks.

It's common in medicine to prescribe potentially risky drugs when the benefits clearly outweigh the risks. But for most patients, benzodiazepines do not pass this simple test. It's estimated that 13 patients would have to take one of these drugs for one patient to benefit (the "number needed to treat").

Put another way, for every 13 patients taking these drugs, 12 are not gaining benefit. Conversely, about one in five patients who takes benzodiazepines suffers from serious impairments (the "number needed to harm"), such as memory problems, lack of concentration and daytime drowsiness, that interfere with function.

Why do doctors continue to prescribe them? It's partly because patients demand these drugs. They believe that benzodiazepines help them, and doctors don't want to deprive their patients of well-being. There's also a financial aspect—insurance companies and HMOs that routinely pay for drug prescriptions often don't cover long-term, nondrug treatments for insomnia and/or anxiety.

For about 10% of patients, benzodiazepines are essential treatments. They're used, in some cases long-term, for seizures and some mental disorders, including disabling anxiety. They can be lifesavers when used short-term for patients who are withdrawing from alcohol or other drugs. But the vast majority of prescriptions are written for patients who would do just as well—or better—with nondrug treatments.

Going Drug-Free

When I meet with patients who take these drugs, many say that they would like to stop because of side effects, such as fatigue, memory loss, incontinence, etc. But the drugs are addictive. People who try to quit often experience intense insomnia, anxiety and other symptoms during the withdrawal period, which typically lasts one to four weeks.

Good news: We conducted a study that looked at 261 patients who were taking these drugs for at least three months. After six months, 62% of those in an intervention group (who were given a patient-education brochure that discussed drug risks, nondrug treatments and advice on discontinuing drugs) had asked their doctors/pharmacists for advice about stopping...and 27% did stop, compared with 5% in a control group.

Some of these patients had been taking benzodiazepines for 40 years and then stopped within six months because of the brochure! A few of the patients started using cognitive behavioral techniques to help them sleep, and eight patients began taking an antidepressant because underlying depression was unmasked.

Caution: If you've taken a benzodiazepine for months or years and have developed a physical dependence, don't quit "cold turkey." (After two to four weeks, everyone develops a physical dependence.) Abruptly stopping the drug can cause confusion, heart palpitations, nausea and sometimes mental disturbances, including hallucinations.

About half of patients who quit a benzodiazepine will experience at least some side effects. To make the process easier (and safer), experts recommend gradually decreasing the dose—under the supervision of a doctor—over several months. Some patients might go four to five months before they're completely drug-free. *How it works...*

- **During the first two weeks,** a patient might be advised to take a half dose on Monday and Friday. The other days, he/she will take the same dose as before.

- **For the next two weeks,** the "half-dose" days might expand to include Wednesday, Saturday and Sunday. During subsequent weeks, patients will reduce their doses still more. The exact amounts will depend on the patient, the degree of side effects, etc.

- **Anticipate discomfort.** When you start reducing doses, you will experience withdrawal. I warn patients that they'll feel like they have jet lag for a week or two. Stick it out! If you absolutely can't function while you're tapering, it's OK to take the same dose for a while longer—but never go back to a higher dose.

- **To deal with daytime sleepiness,** I advise patients to avoid taking a nap and to keep active. Expose yourself to bright light (either outside or with bright indoor lamps). The goal is to get back on a natural energy and day–night wake cycle. This includes not going to bed until you're ready to sleep.

- **If you're taking one of these drugs to deal with anxiety,** talk to a health-care professional or a therapist to identify the root cause of your discomfort and to help you get through stressful situations.

Support groups for anxiety-related disorders can help you learn to manage stress more effectively.

Relaxation techniques, such as stretching, yoga, massage or tai chi, can be worthwhile, too.

- **To deal with insomnia,** consider cognitive behavioral therapy for insomnia (CBT-I) and the use of a sleep diary. These are the most effective nondrug therapies for insomnia.

For more information on tapering off a benzodiazepine, go to DeprescribingNetwork.ca.

Smartphone Addiction Is Real

Smartphone addiction changes the brain. Teenagers considered to be addicted to their phones and the Internet—based on a test of their usage habits—had an imbalance of brain chemicals similar to that seen in people experiencing anxiety and depression. They tended to say that Internet and smartphone addiction interfered with their daily activities, productivity, sleep and social lives...and they had significantly higher scores on scales of depression, anxiety, insomnia and impulsivity than teens whose test scores did not indicate addiction. The addicted teens had an overabundance of the neurotransmitter *gamma-aminobutyric acid* (GABA) in their brains' emotional control center. Addictive substances such as alcohol are already known to alter GABA levels.

Hyung Suk Seo, MD, professor of neuroradiology, Korea University, Seoul, and leader of a study presented at a recent meeting of the Radiological Society of North America.

Group Singing Beats the Blues

Adults with mental health conditions, including anxiety and depression, who participated in free, weekly singing workshops for six months reported improvement or maintenance of their mental health—regardless of other therapies or medications.

Why it worked: Singers of any skill level could participate, making the group inclusive and stress-free. The social aspect of the activity along with structure and peer support were also cited as important.

What to do: If you can't find a just-for-fun singing group in your community or through Meetup.com, consider starting one.

Tom Shakespeare, PhD, professor of disability research, University of East Anglia, Norwich Medical School, Norwich, UK.

Common Gynecologic Condition Linked to Mental Health Issues

Aled Rees, MD, PhD, Neurosciences and Mental Health Research Institute, Cardiff University, Wales.

Journal of Clinical Endocrinology and Metabolism, news release.

Could women with polycystic ovary syndrome (PCOS) be at increased risk for mental health problems? And are their children more likely to have autism and attention deficit hyperactivity disorder (ADHD)?

That's the suggestion of a new British study that hints at a connection between the gynecologic condition and mental health issues, but does not prove cause and effect.

About PCOS

"PCOS is one of the most common conditions affecting young women today, and the effect on mental health is still underappreciated," said study author Aled Rees, MD, PhD, who's with the Neurosciences and Mental Health Research Institute at Cardiff University in Wales.

The findings suggest that women with PCOS should be screened for mental health disorders, the study authors said.

In PCOS, a woman produces more male hormones than normal. Symptoms include pelvic pain, irregular menstrual periods, excess hair growth, weight gain and infertility.

It affects 7% to 10% of women of childbearing age.

Study Findings

For the study, the researchers examined data from nearly 17,000 women in the United Kingdom with PCOS. These women were more likely to be diagnosed with conditions such as depression, anxiety, bipolar disorder and eating disorders than women without PCOS, the study found.

Children of mothers with PCOS were found to be at higher risk of developing ADHD and autism than other children, according to the study. It was published in the *Journal of Clinical Endocrinology and Metabolism*.

Implications

Dr. Rees noted that further research is needed to confirm the findings, since the investigators only found an association between PCOS and mental health issues.

"This is one of the largest studies to have examined the adverse mental health and neurodevelopmental outcomes associated with PCOS, and we hope the results will lead to increased awareness, earlier detection and new treatments," said Dr. Rees.

The U.S. Office on Women's Health has more on information on polycystic ovary syndrome at WomensHealth.gov. Search "PCOS."

Easy, Everyday Way to Get Happier...and Healthier!

Rebecca Shannonhouse, editor, *Bottom Line Health*.

If you're like most people, taking all the steps that are needed to get and stay healthy may feel a little overwhelming at times. Wouldn't it be great if there were a health-promoting strategy that's easy and quick? Well, there is.

People who cultivate everyday interactions that make them feel connected to the world around them tend to be healthier and happier, according to research published in *Psychology & Health* and elsewhere.

Scientifically known as micro-moments of positive connections, these interactions help fight stress and depression...and promote metabolic and cardiovascular health.

These feel-good moments create a positive spiral of behaviors that help us flourish—both physically and psychologically. *How to cultivate micro-moments...*

• **Connect.** Not just with your loved ones, but with everyone you can.

What you can do: Let a pregnant shopper go ahead of you in line...offer to watch your neighbor's house when his/her family is out of town...chat with the dog walker you see every day.

• **Appreciate the details.** A lovely flower in your garden catches your eye—think how lucky you are to have such beauty in your life. Appreciate a gentle breeze...the luxury of a hot bath...and the miracle of a sunset.

• **Reflect.** Take a moment each day to think about the warm feelings you had when talking with a friendly cashier...while smiling at a cute child...or when enjoying a moment of particular closeness with a loved one.

Our days are filled with possibilities for micro-moments. All we have to do is seize them!

Chapter 12

FOOD AND FITNESS

Dairy Foods Might Help You Delay Menopause

Early menopause—before age 45—is associated with a slew of health problems. Until now, there wasn't much a woman could do to prevent it—at least not easily.

But there may be a kind of food that can help protect you from starting down the menopause path too soon.

It's probably already in your refrigerator.

Background: Women who go through early menopause (before age 45) are more likely to suffer osteoporosis, cardiovascular disease and cognitive decline than women who continue to produce estrogen for more years. Unfortunately, the known factors that affect the time of menopause aren't easily modified—they include a woman's age when she had her first period, how many children she's had and, if she breastfed, for how long.

But some studies have suggested that vitamin D may play a role. So investigators decided to plumb a major database of women and diet to learn more.

Study: Researchers used data from the Nurses' Health Study II, which began collecting information from 116,000 female nurses who were between the ages of 25 and 42 in 1989. Information about medical conditions and lifestyle behaviors was collected every other year, and dietary questionnaires were completed every four years. In this study, only the 86,234 women who had not started menopause before completing their first food questionnaires were included.

The researchers divided the women into five groups based on their cumulative average intake of vitamin D and calcium over 20 years. They broke down results by dairy foods only...all dietary sources...and all dietary sources-plus-supplements.

Results: After adjusting for age, body mass index, smoking and other factors, women with the highest dietary intake of vitamin D had 17% reduced risk for early menopause compared with women with the lowest dietary intake. Similarly, dietary calcium was associated with a 13% reduction in risk. And, both associations were stronger for dairy sources of vitamin D and calcium than for nondairy dietary sources.

Surprising finding: While taking vitamin D supplements was not associated with early menopause risk at all, taking calcium supple-

Study titled "Vitamin D and Calcium Intake and Risk of Early Menopause" by researchers at University of Massachusetts Amherst et al., published in *American Journal of Clinical Nutrition.*

ments was linked to a slightly higher risk for early menopause. However, the researchers note, this result may just reflect women who were taking calcium supplements due to other health concerns—such as a family history of osteoporosis. It's possible that these other issues may be behind the early menopause in these cases.

Bottom line: Foods rich in calcium and vitamin D—especially dairy foods—might help women stave off going into menopause too early. It's an observational study, so it doesn't prove cause and effect. But it's one more reason—potentially a big reason for some women—to choose whole foods rich in calcium and vitamin D, which we already know are healthful for a bunch of other reasons. Besides dairy sources, you can find vitamin D in eggs and fish, and calcium in leafy greens, almonds and canned salmon and sardines (eaten with the bones).

Flexitarian: The Vegetarian Diet for Meat Eaters

Emma Derbyshire, PhD, registered public health nutritionist, Nutritional Insight Limited consultancy, a company that undertakes evidence-based research for food and health-care companies, government organizations and other organizations, Surrey, England, lead author of study titled "Flexitarian Diets and Health: A Review of the Evidence-Based Literature," published in *Frontiers in Nutrition.*

You keep hearing how healthy it is to eat vegetarian, not to mention that it's better for the planet—but it seems so extreme! Besides, how bad can an occasional hamburger, grilled chicken breast or seared salmon steak be? We have a healthy-eating solution for you—go "flexitarian"!

As you might have guessed, the term "flexitarian" is a newly coined combination of the words "flexible" and "vegetarian." Also called "semi-vegetarian," a flexitarian diet reduces meat but doesn't cut it out entirely—and can be an easier way for people who are daunted by strict vegetarian diets to get into a healthier eating pattern.

Background: While the concept seems simple, in real life exactly what constitutes a flexitarian diet is harder to pin down. Eating meat just on some days of the week is vague. Although definitions vary, one common description is a diet that significantly reduces meat consumption on at least three days of the week.

The philosophy behind a flexitarian diet is an attempt to find a balance among conflicting health, environmental and ethical concerns—namely, that meat (which, in this context, includes fish and poultry) is an important source of protein, fat and micronutrients...the need to improve animal welfare and be more judicious with our use of global resources...evidence that long-term consumption of large amounts of red meat and certain processed meat may increase the risk for cardiovascular disease, type 2 diabetes, certain forms of cancer, especially colon cancer, and premature death from other causes.

Study review: Using a large national database, British researchers looked at specific markers for health in 25 studies related to meat-reducing diets, 12 of which focused on body weight and diet quality, published between 2000 and 2016.

Finding: Flexitarian diets improved body weight, metabolic health and blood pressure and reduced risk for type 2 diabetes. Men were less likely than women to embrace flexitarian eating patterns—and more likely to overconsume meat. The researchers also speculated that flexitarian diets may help ease symptoms of inflammatory bowel diseases such as Crohn's disease, since there is evidence that plant-based diets are effective for calming gut inflammation.

Bottom line: A consistent definition for flexitarian diets is needed before they can be clinically recommended or effectively studied. But why wait for an official definition to take advantage of this easy way to do great things for your health and the health of the planet? Just cut back! Eat meat, poultry and fish in moderation—and include meat-free days while you enjoy delicious veggie-based meals. (Men, this means you, too!)

Better Than Drugs: Berries Are So Powerful Even Scientists Are Stunned

Bill Gottlieb, CHC, a health coach certified by the American Association of Drugless Practitioners. He is author of 15 health books that have sold three million copies and been translated into 10 languages, including *Speed Healing* (Bottom Line Books).

If you were asked to make a list of "superfoods"—nutrient-loaded foods that effectively fight disease—you'd probably include items such as kale, beans, walnuts, broccoli, green tea, wild-caught salmon...and berries.

What few people realize: As a superfood, berries—blueberries, strawberries, raspberries, blackberries, cranberries and the like—are in a class by themselves. They can be more health-giving than medications or supplements, according to experts at Harvard Medical School and Harvard T.H. Chan School of Public Health. The antioxidants in berries—*anthocyanins*, the compounds that give these fruits their lustrous colors—deliver a pure dose of prevention and healing to the brain, heart and every other system and cell in the body. And you don't have to eat a bushelful to get the benefits.

Here's what you need to know about the amazing power of berries...

Berries and Your Brain

For more than a decade, scientists at the Jean Mayer USDA Human Nutrition Research Center on Aging at Tufts University have been studying the effect of berries on the brain—in cells and in laboratory animals. They have found that regular ingestion of blueberries, strawberries and/or blackberries can help improve "plasticity," the ability of brain cells to form new connections with one another...generate new brain cells...stop inflammation and oxidation from damaging brain cells...ease the destructive effect of stress on the brain...prevent and reverse age-related memory loss, particularly short-term, or "working," memory...and protect against amyloid-beta, the plaques in the brain that cause Alzheimer's disease. *Now research has shown that blueberries can help rejuvenate the aging human brain...*

Startling new findings: The researchers from Tufts studied 37 people, ages 60 to 75, dividing them into two groups—one group consumed one ounce of freeze-dried blueberries every day (the equivalent of one cup of fresh blueberries)...the other a blueberry placebo. At the beginning, middle and end of the three-month study, the participants took tests measuring learning and memory. By the end of the study, those in the blueberry group had a 20% improvement in their scores on a memory test compared with those in a placebo group.

Strawberries are good, too. The Tufts researchers gave participants either freeze-dried strawberry powder (the equivalent of two cups of fresh strawberries) or a placebo. After three months of daily intake, the strawberry group had much greater improvements in memory than the placebo group.

What to do: Eat one cup of blueberries or strawberries daily, either fresh or frozen. Choose organic. Every year, the Environmental Working Group announces its "Dirty Dozen," a list of the produce with the most pesticides. In 2017, strawberries topped the list and blueberries ranked number 17.

Berries and Your Heart

Hundreds of studies show that anthocyanins battle oxidation and inflammation, the evil twins of chronic disease—including heart disease. *Berries can...*

- **Reduce high blood pressure**—the number-one risk factor for heart attack and stroke. Researchers from Florida State University studied 48 postmenopausal women with high blood pressure, giving them either one-third cup of freeze-dried blueberry powder daily or a placebo. After two months, the women getting the blueberry powder had a drop in systolic blood pressure (the upper number in a blood pressure reading) of 5.1% and a drop in diastolic blood pressure (the lower reading) of 6.3%—decreasing the risk for heart attack and stroke. Their arteries were also more flexible. There were no changes in the placebo group.

• **Reduce other risk factors for heart disease.** The cranberry is no slouch when it comes to guarding the heart. Scientists from the USDA's Human Nutrition Research Center studied 56 people, average age 50. Half drank two eight-ounce glasses of no-sugar-added cranberry juice daily...the other half made no changes to their diets. After two weeks, the scientists measured several risk factors for heart disease. Those drinking the juice had lower levels of C-reactive protein (CRP), a biomarker for heart-damaging inflammation...lower levels of triglycerides, a heart-hurting blood fat...and lower levels of blood sugar.

Bottom line: More berries, fewer heart attacks. In a study published in *Circulation,* researchers examined 18 years of health data from 93,600 women and found that those who ate three or more servings of blueberries and strawberries per week (one serving is one-half cup) had a 34% lower risk for heart attack, compared with women who ate them less than three times weekly.

What to do: If you have heart disease or any risk factors for heart disease (high blood pressure, high LDL cholesterol, high blood sugar, high CRP, a family history of heart disease), eat three cups of blueberries or strawberries per week.

Berries and Cancer

Cellular research and animal research have shown that berries can fight just about every kind of cancer.

Example: A scientific paper recently published by researchers from the Medical College of Wisconsin in *Antioxidants* shows that cranberries can help fight 17 different cancers, including bladder, blood, brain, breast, colon, esophageal, oral, prostate and stomach cancers.

But the real test of berries' anticancer power is whether berries can help people with cancer. *Research published in 2016 shows that they can...*

• **Oral cancer.** Researchers at The Ohio State University Comprehensive Cancer Center gave lozenges of freeze-dried black raspberry powder (which contains very high levels of anthocyanins) to people with oral cancer for two weeks. Analyzing the tumors, they found that several genetic markers of cancer severity—prosurvival genes and proinflammatory genes—were significantly reduced by up to 21%.

In an earlier study, researchers at University of North Carolina and three other universities gave a "bioadhesive" black raspberry gel or a placebo to 40 people with premalignant oral lesions (neoplasia), which often progress to oral cancer. After four months, the lesions of those using black raspberry had shrunk in size and were less likely to advance to cancer.

• **Colon cancer.** In several studies on colon cancer at the National Cancer Institute and other institutions, daily intake of 60 grams of black raspberry powder (the equivalent of 15 servings of black raspberries) reversed dozens of biomarkers of the disease. These studies showed that the powder can kill cancer cells, block the growth of new blood vessels to tumors (angiogenesis), kill cancer cells (apoptosis) and stop cancer cells from dividing and growing (proliferation).

What to do: If you are at risk for oral or colon cancer...or are being treated for one of those diseases...or are a survivor of any of them—talk with your doctor about adding black raspberry powder to a daily smoothie. (You could never eat enough black raspberries to get the cancer-reversing effect.)

Good product: Freeze-dried black raspberry powder from BerriHealth (BerriHealth.com).

For preventing cancer, eat five or more servings of fruits and vegetables every day—including berries.

The Best "Forgotten" Greens

Michael T. Murray, ND, a licensed naturopathic physician based in Paradise Valley, Arizona. Dr. Murray has published more than 30 books, including *Bottom Line's Encyclopedia of Healing Foods,* with coauthor Joseph Pizzorno, ND. DoctorMurray.com

Leafy greens are the superstars of the vegetable brigade. Kale, widely considered the reigning king, is unusually high in calcium, magnesium and vitamin K...and, like other greens, is loaded with disease-fighting phytochemicals, such as lutein and vitamin C.

But let's be honest—kale's somewhat bitter taste isn't for everyone...and even if you love this veggie, you're probably not going to eat it every day. What other disease-fighting greens do you need in your diet?

Targeted Nutrition

Basic nutrition is just one reason that experts advise Americans to eat at least five servings of greens and other vegetables daily. But if you're concerned about specific medical conditions, research has shown that some leafy greens are particularly effective. *For example...*

- **Arugula and cancer.** Arugula is a peppery green with a sharp taste that adds a distinctive zip to otherwise bland salads. The pungent flavor has earned it the nickname "salad rocket."

The zesty flavor of arugula is largely due to its high concentration of sulfur-containing compounds. We think of arugula as a salad green, but it's actually a crucifer—in the same plant family as superfoods such as broccoli, cabbage and kale. Like other crucifers, it contains a group of anticancer compounds known as glucosinolates, which have detoxifying effects.

How arugula helps: Compounds in arugula, including *sulforaphane* and *indole-3-carbinol,* increase the body's excretion of a form of estrogen that has been linked to breast cancer. A Chinese study found that women who regularly ate a daily serving of cruciferous vegetables were 50% less likely to develop breast cancer. Another study found that just one weekly serving was enough to reduce cancer risk (including oral, colorectal and kidney malignancies).

Bonus: The sulforaphane in arugula has another benefit. It appears to help the body eliminate *H. pylori,* a bacterium that causes most peptic ulcers and greatly increases the risk for gastric cancer.

- **Spinach and macular degeneration.** As the US population ages, there's been a dramatic increase in age-related macular degeneration, a leading cause of blindness. Could a few weekly servings of spinach make a difference? There's good evidence that it might.

How spinach helps: Spinach is exceptionally high in lutein, a plant pigment that concentrates in the eyes and deflects damaging light from sunshine. Studies have found that people who consumed 6 mg of lutein daily—the amount in about one-half cup of cooked spinach—were 43% less likely to develop macular degeneration. Research published in *JAMA Ophthalmology* shows that people who consume generous amounts of lutein are also less likely to develop cataracts than those who eat less.

Important: Whether you prefer your spinach raw or cooked, be sure to have it with a little bit of oil or fat—a drizzle of olive oil is plenty—or a small amount of some other fat such as chopped nuts or avocado. Lutein is a fat-soluble nutrient, which means it is absorbed more efficiently when it's consumed with a little fat.

- **Parsley and UTIs.** Most people think of parsley as a colorful garnish—pretty to look at, but not much of a food. But around the world, parsley is found in tabbouleh, pesto (with or without basil) and other fragrant dishes…and it's a good green to eat if you get frequent urinary tract infections (UTIs).

About half of all women will eventually get a UTI…men get them, too, but less often. Patients with recurrent UTIs (defined as two separate infections within six months or three within one year) often depend on antibiotics—and resign themselves to the likely side effects of these drugs, such as diarrhea.

How parsley helps: It contains *apigenin,* a compound that acts as a diuretic and also has anti-inflammatory effects. According to a report in the journal *Case Reports in Medicine,* women who combined parsley with other herbal treatments (such as garlic) had an impressive decrease in urinary frequency and other symptoms—by 80%, in one case. Parsley's UTI-fighting effect is presumably because of apigenin's diuretic effect.

Another benefit: Reduced risk for cancer. Chlorophyll and other compounds in parsley have anticancer effects—including the ability to help inhibit the cancer-causing effects of fried foods.

Since parsley is so concentrated in nutrition and phytochemicals, just a few sprigs (or about one-quarter cup) consumed whenever possible provides exceptional health benefits. Chopped parsley can be added to salads, sauces, soups and grilled fish.

- **Kale and osteoporosis.** Kale's reputation as the king of veggies is based, in part, on its ability to promote bone health. People often think that milk is a great calcium source, but the absorption of calcium from kale and other leafy greens is actually higher—between 40% to 64%, compared with about 32% from milk.

And that's not all. In addition to being rich in calcium, kale also is an excellent source of vitamin K, a critical nutrient that helps anchor calcium into bone. One cup of raw kale supplies more than 600% of the recommended daily vitamin K intake. If you're concerned about bone health, you should definitely make an effort to eat more kale.

Another benefit: Improved heart health. Kale and other greens, as well as beets and celery, have been found to improve blood pressure and blood flow. While a high intake of fruit and vegetables is associated with healthy blood pressure and reduces risk for heart disease and stroke, kale and cruciferous vegetables are linked to even greater protection.

A good goal: Three to four servings of kale and other greens a week.

Important caveat: In normal amounts, kale is among the healthiest foods you can eat. But some people go overboard. Too much kale, like other cruciferous vegetables, can cause flatulence (gas) for many people. Eating too much raw kale (for example, more than three servings a week) can also interfere with the production of thyroid hormone, leading to the formation of a goiter. And because kale is such a rich source of vitamin K, anyone taking *warfarin* (Coumadin), an important anticlotting drug that interacts with this vitamin, should consult a doctor before eating kale or any leafy greens.

Soy: Superfood or Scapegoat?

Janet Bond Brill, PhD, RDN, FAND, a registered dietitian nutritionist, a fellow of the Academy of Nutrition and Dietetics and a nationally recognized nutrition, health and fitness expert who specializes in cardiovascular disease prevention. Based in Allentown, Pennsylvania, Dr. Brill is author of *Blood Pressure DOWN, Cholesterol DOWN* and *Prevent a Second Heart Attack.* DrJanet.com

Over the last decade or so, soy has gone from superfood to scapegoat as health pros debate its potential health benefits, including heart disease prevention. Given all this back and forth, you may wonder if this food is still worth eating.

The short answer: Yes, as long as you stick to largely unprocessed whole foods, such as tofu, edamame, tempeh, soy nuts and soy milk, and skip the more highly processed ones—think soy hot dogs, burgers and protein bars. The problem with highly processed soy foods is that they contain additives such as sodium, fillers and preservatives used to extend shelf life. Others contain only isolated soy protein, so you lose the benefits of whole soy. *Here's why soy should still be part of your diet...*

• **It's a healthy alternative to red meat.** All beans provide protein, but soybeans are exceptional. One-half cup of cooked soybeans provides 15 g of high-quality protein—double the amount found in other legumes. Like animal protein, soy contains all the essential amino acids in just the right proportion. It's also packed with fiber, phytochemicals, good fats such as omega-3s and lots of vitamins and minerals—ingredients that are often lacking in some animal proteins. You can toss soybeans in a salad to add crunch, use them instead of chickpeas for hummus or add them to quinoa as a tasty side dish.

• **It contributes to heart health.** While no single food can reduce your risk, eating a mostly plant-based diet that includes healthy fat and is rich in fiber and phytochemicals (this could include soy, copious amounts of fresh fruits and vegetables, nuts and extra-virgin olive oil)...working out at least 30 minutes a day...and not smoking can improve your cardiovascular health.

• **It is widely consumed in countries with lower rates of chronic disease.** No matter what the studies say, many scientists believe that high soy consumption explains why many Asian countries, where soy has long been a major staple, have lower rates of heart disease, cancer, stroke, osteoporosis and diabetes compared with the US.

So do your heart a favor and keep eating soy—starting with this recipe...

Curried Roasted Cauliflower and Tofu over Brown Rice

This quick and easy recipe is a perfect way to incorporate soy into a delicious heart-healthy dish...

1 container extra-firm tofu (14 ounces), drained and cut into one-inch cubes
1 fresh head cauliflower, cut into small pieces
3 Tablespoons extra-virgin olive oil
3 Tablespoons curry powder
1 teaspoon ground ginger
1 teaspoon ground cumin
1 teaspoon salt
1 large Vidalia onion, halved and sliced
2 Tablespoons currants
2 cups cooked brown rice (or quinoa)

What to do: Preheat the oven to 400°F. In a large bowl, combine the tofu with the cauliflower and one tablespoon of olive oil. Heat two tablespoons of olive oil in a skillet over medium-high heat. Add the curry, ginger, cumin and salt and stir until blended. Add the onion and stir until light brown. Add the currants and onion mixture to the large bowl and toss with the tofu and cauliflower until they are well coated. Spread the mixture on a baking sheet. Bake, stirring occasionally, for 40 minutes. Serve over brown rice or quinoa. *Yield:* 4 servings.

Vegetables: Cooked vs. Raw

All forms of cooking can destroy some nutrients (such as vitamin C and B vitamins) in vegetables. But the flip side is that some nutrients actually become more bioavailable after cooking, since cooking helps release the nutrients from the cell walls of the plant. These include lycopene (in tomatoes and red peppers) and beta-carotene (in carrots, spinach and kale). Mushrooms, asparagus and cabbage all supply more antioxidant compounds when cooked.

Vitamin B-6 and folate in broccoli and the polyphenols in onions that help protect against cancer and cardiovascular disease are better preserved in raw vegetables.

Sharon Palmer, RDN, author of ***Plant-Powered for Life,*** Duarte, California. SharonPalmer.com

---

What's the Best Diet? Experts Rate Them

Angela Haupt, assistant managing editor, health at *U.S. News & World Report.*

Kelly Hogan, RD, CDN, clinical nutrition and wellness manager, Mount Sinai Hospital's Dubin Breast Center, New York City.

U.S. News & World Report's Best Diets 2018.

Your diet should be based on a well-balanced eating plan that fits your lifestyle, rather than a weird fad replete with food restrictions.

That's according to *U.S. News & World Report's* best diet rankings for 2018. The two diets that tied for the top spot—the Mediterranean Diet and the DASH Diet—fit that bill because they feature real food and reasonable, flexible guidelines, experts said.

"It's tasty, it's sensible, nutritionally sound, and there's great research that it can help ward off or control a whole host of chronic diseases," Angela Haupt, assistant managing editor of health at *U.S. News & World Report,* said of the Mediterranean Diet.

On the other hand, you should avoid fad diets that require you to adopt severe restrictions. The hot new Keto Diet got a raspberry from the *U.S. News'* panel of nutrition experts, tying for last on the list.

The Keto Diet requires people to severely restrict their carbohydrate intake while indulging in high-fat foods, a plan that is simply not sustainable, Haupt said.

"It really is the diet of the moment, but it can be a pretty extreme plan. There's a very strict carb limit. Our experts say it's not necessary to be so extreme or restrictive," Haupt said.

Expert Findings

The rankings come from an expert panel of the country's top nutritionists, dietary consultants and physicians, which evaluated 40 different diets across nine categories. The categories included ease of compliance, likelihood of short- and long-term weight loss, and effectiveness against chronic conditions like heart disease and diabetes.

Both the DASH and Mediterranean diets allow people the flexibility to choose from a wide variety of healthy foods, so they can eat what best suits them, said Kelly Hogan, RD, CDN, clinical nutrition and wellness manager of the Mount Sinai Hospital's Dubin Breast Center in New York City.

The diets share a number of similar themes, Hogan said—lots of colorful fruits and vegetables, whole grains, healthy fats, lean proteins, low-fat dairy, and avoidance of foods that are processed, packaged or high in saturated fats.

"The DASH and Mediterranean diets are not excluding any foods or food groups or restricting anything," Hogan said. "I think that's really important when it comes to how a normal person eats in general."

The diets also are both backed by a lot of scientific data that show they can help people lose weight and avoid heart disease and diabetes, Haupt said.

"There's a lack of good solid research on nutrition and diets in general, so it says something when a plan like the Mediterranean Diet is backed up with good solid research," Haupt said.

Fads like the Keto Diet can cause quick weight loss, but a person can't maintain such eating restrictions, Haupt and Hogan noted.

Weight Watchers scored high in the *U.S. News* rankings, coming in first as the best commercial diet and the best weight-loss diet.

"Weight Watchers offers the flexibility to shape your own diet," Haupt said.

The plan also benefited from the amount of encouragement and accountability Weight Watchers provides its members, Haupt added.

"We know that having that support, having people to talk to and staying accountable to a plan is really important," Haupt said.

Hogan said Weight Watchers is great for people who've never really taken stock of their regular eating patterns.

"For someone who is just starting to pay more attention to what they're eating, something like a Weight Watchers can be helpful for them to start to understand things like that," Hogan said.

Diet Advice

Hogan believes that people need to move on and find their own path eventually, after learning what they can from a commercial plan.

"What I don't like about any commercial diet is that the focus is not on your actual food choices," Hogan said. "It's about calories or points or numbers, and that really takes away from your ability to be in tune with your hunger cues and your fullness cues and what you're really craving. If we become more in tune with those things, we naturally consume how much the body needs. Paying too much attention to numbers takes away from that."

For more on the DASH diet, visit the National Heart, Lung, and Blood Institute, NHLBI.NIH.gov. Search "DASH Eating Plan."

Mediterranean Diet Mistakes You're Probably Making

Kelly Toups, MLA, RD, LDN, director of nutrition at Oldways, a nonprofit dedicated to improving public health through healthy cultural food traditions, Boston. Oldwayspt.org

In some ways, the famously good-for-you Mediterranean diet is a victim of its own success. It's got such a healthy glow that promoters selling diets that are radically different—even diametrically opposed—try to bask in it. But even people who are doing their level best to eat the real thing often misunderstand the diet and make mistakes that can substantially undermine its enormous potential.

That matters because there is more scientific evidence for the health benefits of the real Mediterranean diet than for any other diet in the world. Eating the Mediterranean way—the real Mediterranean way—has been shown to protect people from heart disease and stroke, as well as obesity, diabetes, dementia and colon cancer.

People who eat this way also have healthier DNA and live longer, on average, than people who don't.

Latest finding: Adults age 60 and older who most closely followed the diet over an average of four years were 38% less likely to experience frailty such as muscle weakness and fatigue, compared with those who followed it less closely.

One reason: The diet is rich in antioxidants and anti-inflammatory nutrients that help keep muscles strong as we age.

So let's get introduced to the Mediterranean diet right—as if it were for the first time—and get all the benefits...

What Is the Real Mediterranean Diet?

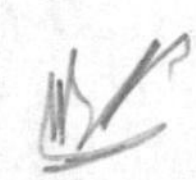

The diet evolved in olive oil–producing regions near the Mediterranean Sea. At its most basic, it's mostly vegetables, legumes, fruit, nuts and seeds ("plant" foods), olive oil and seafood...some poultry and dairy...and very little red meat, sweets or processed foods. The Mediterranean Diet Pyramid, developed 25 years ago by researchers at Harvard School of Public Health and Oldways, a nonprofit that promotes healthy food traditions and lifestyles, remains an excellent guide today...

Eat every day: Fruits, vegetables, grains (mostly whole grains), olive oil, legumes (such as beans and lentils), nuts and peanuts, seeds, herbs and spices.

Eat often—at least twice a week: Fish and other seafood.

Eat often—daily or a few times a week, in moderate portions: Fermented dairy (yogurt, cheese) and eggs.

Eat less often, such as weekly: Poultry.

Eat infrequently—once or or twice a month: Red meats and sweets.

Drink: Water, and if you drink alcohol, only wine in moderation.

- **Get plenty of physical activity.**
- **Make meals relaxed and enjoyable.** A less stressful eating experience is part of the healthy Mediterranean way, too.

That's Not Mediterranean!

Easy-peasy, right? You'd think so. But it's surprisingly easy to deceive yourself. Here are some things that the true Mediterranean diet is not...

• **It's not low-fat.** It's easy to find low-fat "Mediterranean" cookbooks. But the real Mediterranean diet includes plenty of fat. The truth is, all that delicious olive oil is one reason why it's so easy to eat all those vegetables. And yet studies show that sticking to the real thing—fat and all—helps people lose weight and keep it off. One reason is that the vegetables are so rich in fiber that they're very filling.

• **It's not low-carb.** The book *The Pioppi Diet: A 21-Day Lifestyle Plan* is promoted as a "take on the Mediterranean diet," yet it is essentially a very-low-carb diet that also calls for periodic fasting days and recommends coconut oil. None of these attributes are part of the traditional Mediterranean diet, which includes plenty of grains, including moderate portions of refined pasta mixed with olive oil and veggies, fish or beans—and whole grains including bulgur wheat, farro (an ancient form of wheat) and barley.

• **Pizza?** Think again. Despite its Italian name, American-style pizza is fast food and generally not good for you. It's one of the biggest sources of calories, sodium and saturated fat in the American diet. To make it healthier, make the crust whole-grain and top it with vegetables (not meat) and only a little cheese.

• **It's not vegetarian and certainly not vegan.** Beef, pork and lamb traditionally were considered luxuries and were reserved for special occasions, maybe a few times a month. But the Mediterranean diet is not a vegetarian diet and certainly not a vegan one. Seafood is key, but it's fine to eat moderate amounts of poultry, eggs and dairy—especially fermented dairy foods such as yogurt and cheese.

• **It's not about superfoods.** No single food—not even olive oil—explains this diet's power. It's an eating pattern. Just adding one or two components—washing down your rib roast with a Barolo—won't do much. It's about shifting your overall approach and maintaining it for many years.

• **It's not a license to drink.** Alcohol plays a part in the Mediterranean diet, but again, it's the pattern that counts—moderate drinking (up to one drink a day for women, two for men), mostly wine, almost always with meals. Beer isn't unhealthy—it's just not a big part of this dietary pattern. And drinking heavily, especially without eating—such as the cocktail hour—is the opposite of the Mediterranean way.

Now that you can spot Mediterranean-diet mistakes, you can get closer to the real thing—with its enormous health benefits, not to mention sheer deliciousness. Nobody's perfect, and your diet doesn't need to be either. But you can get close to this way of eating by taking a series of small steps—replace chips with nuts or fruit for snacks...choose beans or seafood over beef...replace soda and juice with water...drink wine at meals rather than booze on an empty stomach...switch to fresh fruit for dessert and save baked sweets and ice cream for special occasions.

Best Mediterranean Diet Cookbooks

We asked Kelly Toups for her favorite Mediterranean cookbooks. *Her choices include a classic, a newer book and one from the Oldways collection...*

• ***Mediterranean Cookery* by Claudia Roden.** Well before Greek yogurt and olive oil were kitchen staples in the US, there was Claudia Roden, one of the foremost authorities on Mediterranean cuisine. Her simple-yet-elegant recipes have stood the test of time.

• ***The Complete Mediterranean Cookbook* by America's Test Kitchen.** This colorful collection of more than 500 recipes is a wonderful way to immerse yourself in the bold flavors of the diet.

• ***The Oldways 4-Week Mediterranean Diet Menu Plan.*** The menu plan takes you on a 28-day journey through many of the delicious and satisfying tastes of the Mediterranean diet. It includes plans for each day.

Foods That Boost Your Energy

Lisa Young, PhD, RD, CDN, a nutritionist in private practice and an adjunct professor of nutrition at New York University in New York City. She is the author of *The Portion Teller Plan.*

Hitting a wall at 3 pm—even though you had a full night's sleep? Your first instinct may be to reach for a cup o' joe or a sugary treat just to keep you going.

Why this is a mistake: It's common for our blood sugar levels to drop in the late afternoon, making us feel tired and hungry. But the mind-buzzing, heart-racing effects of so-called quick fixes soon lead to a crash-and-burn, putting us right back where we started.

What Works Better

Once you accept that quick fixes are really nothing more than "fool's gold," you can embrace the true source of sustained vitality—energy-producing real foods.

What you need to know: Often it is not a single ingredient itself that invigorates but how that powerhouse is combined with flavorful and nutritionally satisfying add-ons.

Rule of thumb: The best foods for natural all-day vibrancy typically balance a complex carbohydrate with a healthy fat and a punch of protein—a combination that takes longer to digest and stabilizes blood sugar levels for hours.

For advice on the best foods to eat for all-day energy, we spoke with leading nutritionist Lisa Young, PhD, RD, CDN, to learn about her top choices for maintaining day-long vim and vigor…

Avocado

Avocado contains heart-healthy monounsaturated fat and provides nearly 20 vitamins and minerals.

My favorite way to eat avocado: Sliced or smashed on whole-grain toast. In addition to being a perfect base for creamy avocado, whole-grain toast boasts its own benefits and makes for a great energy-boosting combo—it fills you up with fiber and is low in saturated fat.

Canned Salmon

What's easier than peeling back the lid on a ready-to-serve portion of this versatile, tasty fish? Especially when two ounces of canned salmon contain just 90 calories and only 1 g of saturated fat in a convenient protein source.

Note: To reduce possible toxins, I recommend wild salmon sold in a BPA-free can.

My favorite way to eat canned salmon: On salad greens topped with heart-smart olive oil and a side of polenta. Cornmeal-based polenta, which is loaded with complex carbs to keep blood sugar levels stable for hours, even comes in ready-made refrigerated tubes. You can cook up a slice or two in just minutes on the stove or in the oven!

Farmer's Cheese

Protein-packed foods such as farmer's cheese —born from farmers' efforts to use milk left over after cream is skimmed for butter—can help you stay on top of your game. Two tablespoons of farmer's cheese offer 4 g of protein with only 2.5 g of fat and 40 calories.

My favorite way to eat farmer's cheese: On Ezekiel 4:9 bread with cinnamon and/or fresh walnuts on top. You can spread farmer's cheese, with its ricotta-like texture, on Ezekiel bread—itself an efficient protein source as well as a unique blend of six grains and legumes. A dash of cinnamon not only adds the yin-yang of sweet and savory, but also helps control blood sugar levels. A few diced walnuts provide satisfying crunch and omega-3 fats that promote cardiovascular health.

Quinoa

Quinoa (pronounced "keen-wah") contains iron, B vitamins, magnesium, calcium, potassium and other nutrients, boasting zero saturated or trans fats. Even better, it takes only about 15 minutes to prepare.

My favorite way to eat quinoa: With chopped veggies and garnished with chickpeas. By topping with chickpeas, you'll boost the overall protein, vitamin and mineral content—and stay fuller longer. Or you can try a quinoa-based hot cereal.

Sorghum

Sorghum, a substantial source of protein and dietary fiber, is a versatile, gluten-free grain that keeps your belly full and your energy levels high.

My favorite way to eat sorghum: In a tomato and red pepper slaw.

To prepare: After simmering and draining your desired amount of sorghum, add some color by folding in a julienned slaw of tomatoes and red peppers.

Tomatoes, with their energy-boosting carbs and fiber, are also a major source of the anticancer nutrient lycopene…while red peppers aid in the absorption of iron from food, which boosts energy by promoting optimal blood oxygen levels.

Tasty Fixes for Food Cravings!

Janet Bond Brill, PhD, RDN, FAND, registered dietitian nutritionist. Based in Allentown, Pennsylvania, Dr. Brill is the author of *Blood Pressure DOWN, Cholesterol DOWN* and *Prevent a Second Heart Attack*. DrJanet.com

It's been a long, hectic day, when all of a sudden you pass your local bakery and simply must have that gooey fudge brownie.

Translation: Lots of butter, sugar, chocolate…and calories. You gobble it down, lick the fudge off your fingers, then proceed to feel guilty about indulging in such a decadent treat and resolve to forgo sugar. Smart idea? Not really. A better approach would be to analyze when and where these cravings tend to occur. Once you determine your vulnerable times, you can plan ahead and have healthy treats at hand. *Simple substitutions to reach for the next time you have that insatiable urge to splurge on something that is…*

- **Sweet.** If you're in the mood for something sinfully delicious, chocolate may be your guilty pleasure. If so, have some emergency backups around such as a 60-calorie chocolate pudding cup, topped with fat-free whipped topping. Or how about a rich dark chocolate peppermint patty? It's got 70% less fat than candy bars and only 140 calories. Be sure to buy the single patties and not a huge bag of minis, or you may not be able to stop at just one! Maybe you're yearning for a slice of strawberry shortcake smothered in real whipped cream (to the tune of about 400 calories). Instead, you'd be much better off having a slice of low-calorie angel food cake, topped with thawed Lite Cool Whip, fresh strawberries and a fresh raspberry purée. This version offers all the deliciousness for half the calories, along with the nutrition from the fresh berries (fiber, antioxidants and many vitamins and minerals—especially vitamin C and potassium).

- **Salty and crunchy.** If you find yourself eating out and need some crunch with your sandwich, you don't have to give yourself a big hit of sodium by grabbing a bag of chips. Instead, head to the salad bar and have some thick carrot slices to satisfy that urge to crunch. If you feel you must have some chips during your favorite miniseries, you can make your own healthy version of potato chips by using extra-thin sliced potatoes (coat with olive oil, season and bake at 400°F for about 30 minutes). Dying for fatty, salty movie popcorn? Try buying popcorn kernels and popping them up in a microwave popper. Add your own seasoning and a spray oil, and you avoid the added calories, bad fat and sodium found in the commercial brands. Or you can munch on seaweed snacks, the latest nutrition trend that's delicious, not fishy at all, and truly addicting. Most seaweed snacks, available at many major supermarket chains such as Walmart, Whole Foods and Trader Joe's, house a cocktail of nutrients, including vitamins A and C, calcium, iodine, potassium, iron and magnesium. And all this for a measly 50 calories a pack!

• **Fast food.** If a juicy burger with the works is on your mind, make your own veggie burger or portobello mushroom burger at home and add on all the toppings (this satisfies your craving for a fraction of the fat and calories). It's not fast food, but definitely a tasty substitute. Or what if you just have to have that gooey, cheesy slice or two of pizza? Make your own by using a whole-wheat pita or tortilla topped with tomato sauce and lots of melted low-fat mozzarella cheese. In the mood for Chinese fried rice? Try making your own using cauliflower rice (chop florets in a blender to make the "rice," then fry in extra-virgin olive oil and season with a touch of low-sodium soy sauce and pepper).

The truth is, it's OK to splurge on unhealthy foods once in a while. It's when these indulgences become a daily habit that these less-than-nutritious choices can harm your health and lead to weight gain. If you try these healthy and satisfying swaps, you can (occasionally) have your cake and eat it, too!

Stop Emotional Eating

Break emotional eating patterns by figuring out what triggers them and finding alternative responses to those stimuli. Chew sugarless gum so you have the sensation of chewing. Relax when emotional cravings strike—try a hot shower, a soak in a tub or listening to music. Become mindful by learning meditation-based mindfulness, which helps you become more aware of eating triggers and behaviors. Exercise when emotions start to take over—go for a walk or jog, or do yoga or tai chi. Distract yourself by playing a game on your phone, doing a hobby, organizing a messy closet or spending time on social media.

NutritionLetter.Tufts.edu

It's Not Your Imagination: You're Hungrier After Losing Weight

Catia Martins, PhD, associate professor, faculty of medicine, Norwegian University of Science and Technology, Trondheim, Norway.

Lona Sandon, RD, assistant professor, clinical nutrition, and program director, department of clinical nutrition, School of Health Professions, University of Texas Southwestern Medical Center at Dallas.

American Journal of Physiology-Endocrinology and Metabolism.

If you find yourself famished after you've managed to diet away a sizable number of pounds, you're not alone.

Cutting back on calorie consumption is likely to spark changes that permanently boost appetite among obese men and women, Norwegian researchers report.

The Hunger Hormone

Blame it on the hunger hormone ghrelin, which spikes when you suddenly lower your food intake. It's a phenomenon that harkens back to when early humans had to survive bouts of famine, the researchers said.

Now, that ancestral hormonal swing may undermine long-term efforts to keep the weight off, judging by what happened to 35 morbidly obese patients as they spent two years on a highly structured weight-loss program.

"It is extremely important that both patients with obesity and health professionals working with them are aware of the expected increase in hunger with weight loss," said study author Catia Martins, PhD. "This can explain why it is so difficult, at least for some individuals with obesity, to comply with energy-restricted diets, and why so many give up."

Dr. Martins is an associate professor with the faculty of medicine at the Norwegian University of Science and Technology.

The statistics can be disheartening: The researchers noted that only 1 in 5 obese dieters is able to keep off the weight he or she sheds.

Study Details

The study focused on 22 women and 13 men in Norway who weighed about 275 pounds, on average, and characterized as "severely obese," before embarking on a highly supportive weight-loss program.

First, all underwent a three-week inpatient program that offered nutritional education, psychological counseling and routine exercise activities. Four more three-week sessions were completed over the course of the program.

Throughout, all participants were placed on a "moderately restricted" diet. This meant consuming about 500 calories per day less than otherwise needed to maintain a status quo weight. Food breakdown was set at 50% carbs, 30% fat and 20% protein.

On average, the patients lost about 11 pounds within the first three weeks of the program, and an average of 24 pounds by the two-year mark.

Risk for Regaining Weight Explained

But at both the one- and two-year marks all the patients also reported feeling increasing hunger following their weight loss.

Why? On the one hand, as weight went down, ghrelin levels went up and stayed up. On the other, as the participants' weight dropped their energy needs for basic functions—such as breathing, sleeping, walking and eating—also dropped.

And the result is strong pressure towards regaining lost weight over time, turning weight loss maintenance into a lifelong daily struggle, the researchers said.

The findings were published recently in the *American Journal of Physiology-Endocrinology and Metabolism*.

Expert Recommendations

Lona Sandon, RD, is program director of the department of clinical nutrition with the School of Health Professions at the University of Texas Southwestern Medical Center at Dallas. The study "supports what is already known," she said.

"And the authors make a great point in regards to obesity treatment/management," said Sandon, who wasn't involved with the study. "People need long-term support, and the standard care or payment methods [health insurance] for obesity management are short-term, despite the oodles of evidence for long-term support and support beyond the physician setting."

Insurance, for example, rarely kicks in to cover the services of a registered dietitian or personal trainer, Sandon noted.

But for those anxious to minimize the hunger hormone trap, Sandon says slow and steady weight loss is the way to go.

"It may take months, six or more, of consistent daily exercise combined with mild calorie restriction, decreasing 200 to 300 calories per day, to reach a lower [hormonal] 'set point,'" she said.

But, "the slower the weight loss, and the more modest the calorie restriction to obtain weight loss, the more likely someone might keep the lost weight off," she said.

An hour a day of exercise can also help to lower a set point, Sandon added, whether that be time spent on a treadmill or time spent dancing, playing basketball or soccer, swimming or even roller-skating.

There's more on the importance of achieving a healthy weight at the National Heart, Lung, and Blood Institute website, NHLBI.NIH.gov. Search "healthy weight."

Menopause, Stress…and Weight Gain

Penny Kendall-Reed, ND, naturopathic doctor, director of natural therapies, Urban Wellness Clinic, Toronto, Canada. She is coauthor of several books, including *The No Crave Diet* and *The Complete Doctor's Stress Solution*. *Disclosure*: She receives a royalty from Douglas Laboratories on sales of Serenitin Plus.

During perimenopause and menopause—the late 40s and early 50s for most women—not only do levels of estrogen, progesterone, growth hormone and testosterone start to drop, but the level of the stress hormone cortisol *rises*.

And cortisol has a surprisingly direct effect on your metabolism. Elevated cortisol boosts your body's insulin response (how much insulin your body pumps out) when you eat carbohydrate-rich grains, starchy vegetables, fruits, sweets and alcohol. That increase in insulin shifts how we metabolize food so that more calories are stored as fat—especially around the abdomen.

Cortisol also affects appetite. It influences how our bodies handle adiponectin and leptin, the two main hormones that regulate food cravings and satiety (the sense of having eaten enough). Cortisol contributes to leptin resistance, for instance, so the amount of leptin your body produces has less of an effect. That leads to an increased desire to consume more food. So even though you're not aware of it, you may be feeling more cravings and eating more.

Sure, you can—and should—counter this effect by upping your commitment to eating right and exercising. But you'll also want to tackle the cortisol connection.

The Cortisol Breakdown

After menopause, women are more susceptible to stress than at any other time in their lives.

Here's why: They secrete a greater amount of cortisol for each stressor than when they were younger.

The irony here is that many women have less stress in their lives at this age...for example, many have fewer financial worries and are no longer taking care of their now-grown children. But their bodies have become more sensitive to stress, whether it comes from smaller hassles such as traffic, moderate issues such as loss of sleep or major traumas such as an illness or a death in the family. The adrenal glands (which produce cortisol) start to lose proper communication with the hypothalamus (the part of the brain that controls the production of cortisol) to a point where the body begins to produce cortisol all day long independent of the presence of a stressor.

Without changing the way our bodies handle cortisol—its production and the feedback loop with the hypothalamus—weight loss is extremely difficult.

Changing the Feedback Loop

The goal isn't simply to produce less cortisol but also to re-establish normal control of the adrenal glands by the brain so that cortisol (and other stress-related hormones such as adrenaline and noradrenaline) are produced when they are needed and not produced when they are not needed.

Good news—you don't have to take drugs or do anything extreme to accomplish this. Mind-body practices including yoga, meditation and tai chi—even for just a few minute a day—can help restore the normal feedback loop and make it easier to lose weight, especially around your middle. Indeed, women who practice yoga regularly are less susceptible to post-menopausal weight gain. Deep breathing and meditation work very well, too. So does any exercise that you enjoy—walking, dancing and running all reduce cortisol levels. But if you don't enjoy the kind of exercise you do, and are doing it only because you think you should, that could create stress and backfire, increasing cortisol.

Diet matters, too. Balancing your blood sugar by consuming adequate protein and little sugar will help moderate cortisol levels.

The Supplement Approach

Supplements can help. There are several products that reduce cortisol production such as magnolia bark extract, *gamma-aminobutyric acid* (GABA) and the Ayurvedic herb ashwagandha. One compound that I have found to be very effective is an amino-acid sequence isolated from dairy milk (*casein decapeptide*) that helps reduce the chronic secretion of cortisol and has antianxiety and sleep-promoting properties. Another helpful supplement is theanine—a green tea extract that can take one out of beta wave brain activity (the kind accompanying racing thoughts) into alpha wave activity (the kind accompanying calming thoughts). For my patients, I often prescribe a supplement called Sereniten Plus that I developed for Douglas Laboratories—it contains both casein decapeptide and theanine. In my experience, it's effective at resetting stress-hormone production. (Check with your doctor before taking any of these supplements, however—especially if you are taking antidepressants or antianxiety medications.)

If your body has been in cortisol overdrive, besides gaining weight, you might be experiencing a number of cortisol-related conditions that call for the care of a health-care practitioner—these may include high blood pressure, skin ailments, diabetes and/or irritable bowel syndrome.

One final thought: We often get so consumed with "doing" things to treat ourselves that we forget about the simple things like laughter and learning to say "no." Those can be some of the most powerful stress management tools.

9 New Ways to Lose the Last 10 Pounds

Torey Armul, MS, RD, CSSD, LD, a spokesperson for the Academy of Nutrition and Dietetics. She counsels clients on weight management, sports nutrition, pregnancy and family nutrition through her private practice in Columbus, Ohio.

You've changed your diet. You've exercised. And it worked—you lost weight. But not that last 10 pounds. Sound familiar?

Those last few pounds really are more difficult to lose. One reason, ironically, is that you weigh less now—so you need fewer calories to maintain your weight. Your body also fights back, resisting further weight loss through hormonal and metabolic means. Your resting metabolic rate falls, so you burn fewer calories at rest. Hormones kick in to increase your appetite. The result may be a weight plateau—or even weight regain.

What to do? If you can't bear the thought of cutting more calories or spending more time exercising, here are some unconventional methods to get you over the finish line...

Drink Green Tea

A green tea habit may help you lose weight.

One reason: Gut bacteria. A recent study showed that mice that received green and black tea extracts had fewer gut microbes linked to obesity and more linked to lean body mass. Green tea is particularly rich in gut-friendly polyphenols. In a study published in *Clinical Nutrition,* women who consumed green tea extract every day for 12 weeks lost an average of 2.5 pounds—without following a reduced-calorie diet.

Get Outside—and Go High

Do you exercise mostly indoors? Head out! Exercising outside burns more calories, due to harder terrain and wind resistance, and can improve your mood and increase your enjoyment of the workout.

Fun fact: Gardeners weigh less than nongardeners, according to research—11 pounds less for women, 16 for men.

To really jump-start your weight loss, though, book your next vacation in the mountains. Research published in *Obesity* found that spending one week at a high altitude (8,700 feet) led study participants to eat less than those at sea level and to lose an average of three pounds. Both metabolic rate and levels of leptin (the "satiety" hormone) were higher.

Go Beyond Calories

Counting calories still is the primary way most people approach weight loss—but different foods with the same calorie counts can have very different effects on satiety levels and weight.

Case in point: Plant-based proteins—beans, legumes, nuts, seeds, soy and grains such as quinoa—help you feel more full than animal-based proteins. Fiber is one reason. In one study, participants who ate a plant-based rather than an animal-based breakfast spontaneously ate about 100 fewer calories at lunch.

Share a Selfie

If you've kept your weight goals to yourself, it's time to share them aloud. Make a public commitment. It will increase accountability and help build a community of support. That comes in handy when you need motivation or experience a setback.

One study from Northwestern University found that people in an online weight-loss group who "friended" others in the group and posted photos of their progress lost more weight than those who were less active online. In another study, those who shared goals with friends were more likely than those who didn't to meet them (62% versus 43%). Social-media outlets such as Twitter and Facebook can help, too, studies show—just be sure to unfollow people who don't support you or who make fun of your goals.

Intense Exercise Maintains Significant Weight Loss

In a study of former contestants on *The Biggest Loser* TV show, only those who did at least 80 minutes a day of moderate activity such as walking, or 35 minutes a day of vigorous exercise such as running, did not regain weight within six years. Significant weight loss causes the body's metabolism to slow down, so additional exercise is needed to compensate for the lower caloric needs. To keep weight off after losing it, it is necessary to increase physical activity well beyond what is recommended for people who are trying to maintain their weight without having lost a lot of it. Ask your doctor for details.

Jennifer C. Kerns, MD, hospitalist and co-director of bariatric surgery, Washington DC Veterans Affairs Medical Center, former contestant on *The Biggest Loser*, and lead author of a study of 14 contestants, published in *Obesity*.

Add Some Weight on Purpose—Muscle Weight

Building strength may not have been your focus in the initial stages of your weight loss, but it's crucial now. As you lost weight, your metabolic rate decreased. Strength training helps bring it back up. In one study, for example, a 26-week strength-training program increased resting metabolic rate by 7%.

Muscles are not miracle calorie burners, though. Their ability to radically change metabolism often is hyped in the media. The average actually is about 50 calories a day, according to a research review—not much if you're seeking a big weight loss. But adding muscle is great if you want a little edge to lose those last few pounds, since 50 calories per day translates to losing five extra pounds a year.

Don't Let Another Night Go By

You know that sleep is essential for health, but you might not realize how even a little sleep deprivation can drive cravings and slow metabolism.

Amazing statistic: After a single night of poor sleep, study subjects ate an average of 385 extra calories the next day, according to statistical analysis of multiple studies. In fact, just two consecutive sleep-deprived nights (four hours each night) may be enough to alter your metabolism, according to research published in *Endocrine Development*. It increases the body's level of the hunger-stimulating hormone ghrelin and decreased hunger-reducing leptin. To lose those last 10 pounds, commit to healthier sleep habits.

Time-Restricted Daytime Eating

"Time-restricted eating," in which you consume all of your calories each day within a 10- or 12-hour window, is a new fad with potential weight-loss benefits. But to make it work best, eat your calories relatively early in the day. One two-month study from the University of Pennsylvania's Perelman School of Medicine found that participants who ate all their calories between 8 am and 7 pm weighed less than those who did so between noon and 11 pm—and they all consumed the same number of calories. For the daytime eaters, ghrelin peaked earlier and leptin peaked later. That helps deter late-night cravings.

If you're truly hungry late in the evening, don't be a martyr! Instead, choose a snack with fiber and protein, such as a handful of nuts…or fruit with Greek yogurt.

Redefine Yourself

One of the greatest predictors of weight-loss success is in your own head. A study published in *International Journal of Obesity* found that regardless of actual weight status, people who perceived themselves as overweight were significantly more likely to gain weight. It may not be easy, but give yourself credit for the weight you have lost (even if you haven't hit your goal), and try to think positively about yourself and your weight. Love and respect yourself just as you are.

Take a Break

Dieting all the time is exhausting—and can be self-defeating. Research published in *International Journal for Obesity* found that men who took a two-week break from dieting lost more weight than those who dieted continuously. During their dieting break, the men ate simply to maintain their weight. So take a break when you feel you need it, be kind to yourself and envision yourself meeting your goals.

Are Women Naturally Fitter Than Men?

Thomas Beltrame, PhD, kinesiology graduate student, University of Waterloo, Ontario, Canada.

Richard Hughson, PhD, professor, faculty of applied health sciences, University of Waterloo, Ontario, Canada.

University of Waterloo, news release.

When it comes to getting and staying fit, women may have an aerobic edge over men, new research suggests.

The Study

In a small new study, investigators compared oxygen uptake and muscle oxygen extraction in 18 young men and women while they worked out on a treadmill. Oxygen uptake is an important measure of aerobic fitness.

Women consistently processed oxygen about 30% faster than men, according to researchers at the University of Waterloo in Ontario, Canada.

"The findings are contrary to the popular assumption that men's bodies are more naturally athletic," said study author Thomas Beltrame, PhD.

Another researcher put it this way—"We found that women's muscles extract oxygen from the blood faster, which, scientifically speaking, indicates a superior aerobic system," said Richard Hughson, PhD. He is a professor with the faculty of applied health sciences at Waterloo and is also an expert in vascular aging and brain health.

Because women process oxygen faster, women are less likely to accumulate molecules linked with muscle fatigue, effort perception and poor athletic performance, the researchers explained.

The findings were published in the journal *Applied Physiology, Nutrition, and Metabolism*.

Implication

"While we don't know why women have faster oxygen uptake, this study shakes up conventional wisdom," Dr. Beltrame said. "It could change the way we approach assessment and athletic training down the road."

The U.S. National Heart, Lung, and Blood Institute offers a guide to physical activity at NHLBI.NIH.gov. Search "physical activity guide."

For a Better Menopause, Exercise Just Three Hours a Week

Study titled, "Improvements in health-related quality of life, cardio-metabolic health, and fitness in postmenopausal women after a supervised, multicomponent, adapted exercise program in a suited health promotion intervention," by Nicolás Mendoza Ladrón de Guevara, PhD, University of Granada, Spain, and colleagues, published in *Menopause*.

It just makes sense that being in good shape will help you navigate the sometimes-turbulent waters of the menopause transition. But let's get real. If you're a couch potato and you start going to the gym, will it really make a difference?

Now we have the answer—yes. Definitely.

The best part—it doesn't take a big fitness commitment to cool down hot flashes, fight the battle of the bulge, enhance mood and make your quality of life better. That's especially good news for women who don't want to use hormones to ease symptoms.

Background: There is growing evidence that an active lifestyle reduces symptoms such as hot flashes and enhances health, quality of life and fitness in postmenopausal women. But there has been surprisingly little research to determine what benefits are realistic to expect from a modest exercise program.

Study: Researchers at the University of Granada in Spain recruited 166 women aged 45 to 64 (average age 56). Each woman had had her final menstrual period at least 12 months before—that is, she had hit menopause and was postmenopausal. None were using hormone therapy, and all had been sedentary for at least a year. About half of the women were asked to keep living their lives with no changes (the control group), while the other half were entered into a structured exercise program.

The exercise requirement wasn't huge—three one-hour sessions per week for 20 weeks. Each session included cardio/aerobic fitness, strength training and stretching.

But that was only part of the program. To help them stick with the fitness plan, the women also got 15 sessions of psychological counseling. They learned how to set goals, track progress, get social support and deal with setbacks.

Fitness levels, cardiovascular health and menopause-related symptoms were tested before and after the program—and one year later.

Results: Compared to the women who kept their sedentary ways, the active women improved in many ways. They had fewer hot flashes and better moods. They lost weight, reduced their blood pressure and heart rates, increased flexibility and could walk or run faster. While there was a little back-sliding after the program ended, they wound up keeping most of those positive changes a year later.

Bottom line: Three hours a week of cardio and strength training can make a significant difference in how you feel and how healthy you are in the menopausal transition. This is especially good news for women who are looking for safe, nonhormonal ways to manage menopausal symptoms. And while this study focused on one-hour gym sessions, there's plenty of evidence that breaking your workouts into smaller, more manageable time chunks as short as 10 minutes confers similar benefits.

But don't ignore the social and psychological support that helps you make healthy lifestyle changes—and sustain them. While you may not be able to afford a comprehensive psychosocial program such as this (or even find one), you can rely on your spouse or friends to get fitter together. One plus, note the authors, is that "the adoption of some healthy habits may encourage the practice of other healthy habits."

Neolithic Women Rocked

Prehistoric women were surprisingly strong. Neolithic women—from some 7,000 years ago—had arm bones 11% to 16% stronger than those of modern elite female athletes in their 20s. This means that the prehistoric women were nearly 30% stronger.

Alison Macintosh, PhD, anthropologist, Cambridge University, UK, and leader of a study published in *Science Advances.*

6 Common Stretching Mistakes That Can Hurt You

Karl Knopf, EdD, director of fitness therapy and senior fitness for the International Sports Sciences Association and retired director of adaptive fitness at Foothill College in Los Altos Hills, California. He is author of many fitness books including *Stretching for 50+.*

We now know that stretching is key to staying limber and flexible. But did you know that it also could be dangerous?

Many people stretch improperly, overstressing muscles and even tendons in ways that lead to strains and sprains. An injury can come on gradually as a result of cumulative "insults" from performing a stretch a certain way over and over again. You don't know you're hurting yourself...until you're really hurt.

Other people don't stretch wrong—they just don't stretch at all or only once in a while. Many people focus more on cardiovascular exercise and weight training, yet often neglect stretching—until they get hurt. To benefit from a flexibility program, you need to practice it regularly, ideally every day.

As we age, stretching becomes even more important. Our bodies undergo changes that result in lack of elasticity. Women tend to be more flexible than men, but starting in their 50s, both genders start to lose flexibility and range of motion, especially in the shoulders and low back, which can lead to shoulder and back issues. The good news is that this age-related decline can be slowed through a regular stretching program.

By learning to stretch properly, you'll maximize your mobility...greatly reduce the risk for pain and injury...perform better at any sport you engage in...and look younger. (*One caution:* If you've had a recent fracture, sprain, injury or surgery, or if you suspect that you have osteoporosis, speak to your doctor/physical therapist first.)

Here are common stretching mistakes that can hurt you—and how to steer clear of them...

Holding Your Breath

One common stretching mistake is holding your breath as you hold a stretch. Muscles need oxygen throughout a stretch—plus, holding your breath can elevate your blood pressure. Breathe slowly and consistently throughout each phase of a stretch—especially when you're holding one.

Simple stretches, such as shoulder rolls (see "Safe, Effective Stretches You Can Do Anywhere," on page 241), don't require that you hold them. But most do. These stretches should be held for at least 20 seconds—and recent studies suggest that for older adults, 60 seconds is even better. Breathe throughout.

Stretching Cold

Not that long ago, we were instructed to stretch before playing sports when our muscles were "cold." Now we know that's a bad idea. Think of your muscles and tendons as taffy. Then imagine trying to stretch and bend cold taffy. It can snap. On a micro level, that's like stretching a cold, tight muscle. Ouch!

Much better: Warm up for five minutes or more first, before you do any stretch that you hold. Try light running...a few minutes in a steam room or sauna...or, if you're home, a warm bath.

Getting Intense

Too many people follow the old paradigm that the more intense the exercise, the better. They overdo it with weights, aerobics—and stretching. In my opinion, no pain, no gain is...insane. If you feel sore a few hours after exercising, you overdid it.

Much better: When stretching, move slowly and gently, and stay within your comfort zone. You should feel mild tension in your muscles and joints. Don't push past it. Listen to your body, especially your neck, back, shoulders and knees. If you have tightness or joint pain, take some time off. If it continues, see your doctor or a physical therapist before it turns into a real issue.

Going Old School—Fast and Bouncy

If you played a sport in high school, it's time to unlearn some things you learned, including bouncing toe touches. These moves weren't safe then, and they are even riskier now that you're older. Those neck circles you started every gym class with? Terrible! They strain supporting ligaments and can lead to pinched nerves.

That hurdler stretch where you sit with one leg out in front of you and the other bent behind you? It stresses the meniscus and the medial collateral ligament of your knee—an injury in the making. Windmill toe touches? No! Bending and rotating at the same time is a recipe for trouble.

Red flag: Avoid stretches such as the hurdler that make your knees twist or move in an unnatural position. Be careful about back bends that call for you to raise both hands over your head and lean back. That can pinch the facet joints of the spine.

Much better: Always keep knees "soft" (slightly bent) when stretching. When turning, move your body slowly, as a unit, and pivot your feet.

Stretching Only When You Exercise

Chances are that if you stretch, you do so only before working out or playing a sport. Big mistake! To maintain flexibility, your muscles need to be worked just about every day.

Much better: Think of stretching as part of your daily routine, like brushing your teeth. You don't need a designated area or even to wear gym clothes. Spend a few minutes doing a body-flexibility session daily, especially in high-risk areas such as the hamstrings, shoulders and lower back.

Not Being Well-Balanced

The body is designed with opposing muscle groups, and each group needs to be worked equally. Weight training can unbalance muscles, so you need stretching to get you back into balance.

Example: If you do a movement such as a bench press that rolls your shoulders forward, you should do a stretch that pulls them back. My golden rule is, *Do unto the front as you do unto the back, and do unto the left as you do unto the right.*

Conversely, being too flexible can be a problem, especially if you don't have muscles that are strong enough to support your joints. I once taught a dancer who kept dislocating her shoulder joints because her muscles weren't strong enough to keep her shoulders in place. It's all about balance.

One final tip—enjoy your stretching session. It's a great time to integrate the mind and the body.

Safe, Effective Stretches You Can Do Anywhere

Here are two different kinds of stretches—no-hold stretches that you can do anywhere anytime and standard stretches for which you warm up for five minutes and then hold for at least 20 seconds, ideally 60.

Together, these stretches work on your upper and lower body. Repeat each one at least three times.

Upper-body no-hold stretches...

• **Elbow touches (for the chest).** Place your hands on your shoulders (left on left, right on right), elbows pointing forward as much as possible. Slowly move your elbows out to the side as far as is comfortable, pinching the shoulder blades together, and hold for just a few seconds. Bring your elbows back to the starting position and repeat.

• **Shoulder rolls (for the upper back).** With your arms hanging down naturally, shrug your shoulders up and squeeze them back, as if attempting to touch them together...then relax them.

• **Apple pickers (for the shoulders).** Place your hands on your shoulders (left hand on left, right on right). Then slowly raise your right hand as high up as is comfortable—reach for that apple! Return to the start position, and repeat with the left hand. Keep good posture throughout.

These are standard "hold 'em" stretches...

• **Chest stretch (for the chest and shoulders).** Stand facing a corner. Place one hand on each side wall, with your elbows in a push-up position. Lean gently into the corner until you feel a stretch across your upper chest. Hold for at least 20 seconds.

• **Seated knee to chest (for the lower back and gluteal muscles/butt).** Sit on a stable chair with your feet flat on the floor. Clasp your hands beneath your left leg. Pull your left knee toward your chest with your hands and hold for at least 20 seconds, feeling the stretch in the gluteal and low-back area. Return to start position, and repeat with other leg.

• **Rear calf stretch (for your calves).** Stand facing a wall, with both hands on the wall at shoulder height. Your knees should be slightly bent. Keeping the heel down, slide your right leg back until you feel the stretch in the calf area. Hold for at least 20 seconds. Switch sides and repeat.

Tai Chi May Aid Cardiac Rehab

More than 60% of heart attack victims refuse cardiac rehabilitation, often because of financial concerns or difficulty getting to a rehab center. But some refuse because they regard physical exercise as unpleasant, painful or impossible after a heart attack. For those patients, tai chi's slow, gentle movements may be an option. Researchers found tai chi to be safe, with no adverse effects except minor muscle pain, and well-liked by participants. Patients who went through an extended tai chi program involving three classes per week for 12 weeks (plus maintenance classes for 12 more weeks) engaged in greater weekly physical activity after three and six months than patients who did not do tai chi or who did a shorter tai chi program of two classes per week for 12 weeks.

Elena Salmoirago-Blotcher, MD, PhD, assistant professor of medicine, Brown University Alpert School of Medicine, Providence, and leader of a study published in *Journal of the American Heart Association.*

High-Intensity Exercise Delays Parkinson's

People with early-stage Parkinson's who exercised three times weekly at high intensity—80% to 85% of maximum heart rate—for six months had no worsening of their symptoms. The study showed that using a treadmill is effective, and other studies have shown that weight training also is beneficial.

Daniel M. Corcos, PhD, professor of physical therapy and human movement sciences at Feinberg School of Medicine, Northwestern University, Chicago, led a study published in *JAMA Neurology.*

Exercise in the Cold

While exercising in the cold weather can burn hundreds more calories per hour than exercising in warm weather, this effect primarily results from shivering. To burn extra calories, leave off a layer while keeping your hands, feet and head covered. If you have a heart or circulation issue, check with your doctor before exercising in the cold.

The downside of cold weather exercise is that your strength, power and endurance are all decreased, which often translates into shorter and less intense workouts.

Tom Holland, CPT, exercise physiologist, Darien, Connecticut. TeamHolland.com

The Ultimate Workout

Michael J. Joyner, MD, physician-researcher and leading expert on human performance and exercise physiology at the Mayo Clinic, Rochester, Minnesota. His research has focused on how humans respond to various forms of physical and mental stress. DrMichaelJoyner.com

If you're like most efficiency-minded Americans, you may be on the lookout for the exercise that's going to whip you into shape, keep you fit and slow down aging—with the least amount of time and fuss. For those of us looking to streamline our workouts to just the essentials, two simple exercises can do the job. They are challenging but worth the effort...and can be easily modified to suit your individual fitness level.

The Dynamic Duo

Burpees and jumping rope are the dynamic duo, in my opinion. Why burpees and jumping rope? Of all the exercise choices, these maintain high vigor while promoting strength, endurance, balance and coordination all at once—precisely the capabilities that tend to deteriorate as we age, increasing our risk for falls and other mishaps. *These exercises are also...*

- **Compact.** Both can be done almost anywhere—whether you're in a hotel room...in your family room...or in your backyard.

Note: If you're indoors, you need adequate ceiling height to jump rope.

- **Quick.** The regimen can be compressed into a tidy five minutes if you're starting out and extended to a 10-, 20- or 30-minute workout when you're ready to up your game.

Perfecting Your Technique

To get the maximum benefits and reduce your risk for injuries, it's important to do both of these exercises properly...

- **Burpees.** Unless this exercise is already part of your workout, start slowly to make sure you've got the right technique. Ready?
- **Stand straight with your arms at your sides.**
- **Squat down until you can put your hands on the ground in front of your feet.**
- **Kick your legs back into the plank position, straight behind you.**
- **Do a push-up on your toes or on your knees.**
- **Pull your legs back into the squat position.**
- **Jump up as high as you can with your arms overhead.**

The Workout Work-Around

Do you find it difficult to keep up with the standard exercise recommendation of 150 minutes per week?

Recent study: When the activity levels of 6,000 women ages 63 to 99 were tracked for seven days, just 30 minutes of light housework per day (such as sweeping or doing the laundry) was linked to a 12% lower risk for death over the next three years. Those who added another half-hour of daily exercise slashed their risk by 39%.

Takeaway: As you age, don't get hung up on "working out"—just keep moving!

Michael LaMonte, PhD, research associate professor of epidemiology, University at Buffalo, New York.

For a somewhat easier version: Do the same exercise without the push-up and jump. If the plank position is too difficult, modify it by kicking your legs back only halfway.

• **Jumping rope.** Maybe you haven't jumped rope since you were a kid, but it will come back to you. Keep the jump low to minimize the impact on your ankles and knees. When you feel ready, try using a weighted jump rope (which incorporates 1-, 3- or 5-pound weights) to rev up your heart rate and build upper-body strength. Skip the added weight if you have existing shoulder, arm or wrist problems. Use a jump rope that feels right to you—whether it has anti-slip handles or plastic beads strung on a nylon cord.

Warming Up

Jumping jacks and running in place are great ways to warm up. These exercises are also good substitutes for burpees and jumping rope if you haven't been physically active in a while and/or want a gentler way to ease into your routine.

If jumping jacks and running in place don't appeal to you or you are concerned about your risk for falling or joint pain, there are other ways to modify the burpee–jump rope regimen while you increase your fitness.

Instead of burpees, try: Knee bends (also known as "squats"). If you're worried about your knees, skip the knee bends and simply stand with your back against a wall and lift up one leg with your knee bent as high as you feel comfortable. Repeat with the other leg.

Or try push-ups, either on the floor or against a counter.

Instead of jumping rope, try: Brisk walking—set a pace that puts you at the edge of being short of breath.

The Workout

To begin a burpee–jump rope regimen, do five burpees alternating with 30 seconds of jumping rope. Do each set three to five times (for a total of 15 burpees and a minute and a half of jumping rope…or 25 burpees and two and a half minutes of jumping rope). Then work up to sets of 10 burpees alternating with one minute of jumping rope. As your stamina builds, continue to alternate exercises until you work up to longer sets of up to two minutes of each. Try to do the burpee–jump rope workout two to three days a week with brisk walking or cycling on the other days.

Important: If you have any chronic medical conditions, consult your doctor before trying this workout. Stop immediately if either activity causes pain. It will take time to build up your stamina. Scale up according to your age and ability.

These Exercises Keep You Fit for Daily Living

Debra J. Rose, PhD, FNAK (Fellow of the National Academy of Kinesiology), director of the Center for Successful Aging and a professor in the department of kinesiology at California State University, Fullerton (HDCS.Fullerton.edu).

You're unloading groceries from your car trunk when—ouch!—there goes your back.

You're pulling on a sweater and—snap!—you tweak your shoulder.

Want to help protect yourself from these annoying—and often painful—everyday injuries? *Functional fitness training can help you…*

In the Top 10

Functional fitness training is the official name for exercise that improves strength, balance and flexibility in ways that allow you to safely and effectively perform your real-life activities. It's not a new concept. It's been used for more than a decade to help patients get back to their normal daily activities after heart attacks, stroke, surgeries and other medical setbacks.

Latest development: Functional fitness training is increasingly being used preventively to stave off injury and maintain independence. In fact, it has reclaimed a spot on the top 10 list of fitness trends in the US and around the world for 2018, according to a survey of more than 4,000 exercise physiologists and other fitness professionals.

What's different about this form of exercise? Unlike traditional fitness moves that work just one or two muscle groups at a time (for example, up-and-down bicep curls or the cyclical motion of an elliptical machine), functional fitness training focuses on whole-body movements that mimic the twisting, bending, turning, crouching and reaching you do all day long.

Scientific evidence: When researchers published a review in *European Review of Aging and Physical Activity* of 13 trials looking at functional fitness training, this form of exercise beat out strength training alone (such as weight lifting) when assessing one's ability to perform daily activities.

New and Improved

Most signature exercises of functional training haven't gone away—they are just being supplemented by recent (and some would say improved) ideas such as introducing unstable surfaces (using Bosu balls, for example) or equipment that elevates the exercise challenge (for instance, suspension exercises, described in the next column).

Traditional functional fitness exercises include…

- **Chair Sit to Stand,** which engages your abdominal, back and leg muscles. This exercise, which involves rising from a seated position, helps you get out of a chair, car or bathtub.
- **Medicine Ball Low-to-High Chop** involves squatting down, picking up a weighted ball positioned next to one of your ankles, and standing up while hoisting the ball overhead and then swinging it to the opposite side. This helps prepare you for unloading groceries, stashing items on high shelves and picking up an item from the floor. It also can help your golf swing!

Among the newer additions to functional fitness workouts…*

*Consult an exercise professional for advice on the frequency and appropriate number of repetitions for you.

- **TRX Suspension Training.** If you've seen these black-and-yellow straps dangling from an overhead anchor point at your gym and felt intimidated, fear not. With this type of suspension exercise (TRX is short for total-body resistance exercise), the strap's handles can be gripped with your hands or looped around your feet, letting you leverage your body weight and gravity for a full-body workout. It can be a smart option for active older adults—it offers the opportunity to perform hundreds of moves that can be made increasingly more challenging as strength improves.

Sample TRX move #1: **Squats.** Let's say you want to do squats, which strengthen the muscles needed to climb stairs or lower yourself into the bathtub. With this form of suspension exercise, you can shorten the straps to increase stability as you lower your body and rise back up. When the straps are lengthened, however, more strength and body control are required throughout the exercise.

Sample TRX move #2: **Assisted Row.** Beginning with shortened straps, hold one handle in each hand. Your hands should be chest height with your palms facing in and your elbows fully bent. Slowly lean your upper body back and away from your hands, keeping your back straight. Once your arms are fully extended, pull back up to the starting position. Increase the number of repetitions and sets as strength improves.

Note: The TRX Suspension Training System is available at more than 25,000 gyms worldwide. If you're interested in a home system, TRX Home2 System is available for $159.95. TRXtraining.com.

Important: For beginners with very poor balance or poor body awareness and control, the TRX may not offer sufficient support. To avoid injury, good body form and movement technique should be maintained throughout the exercises performed on the TRX. If you're concerned about your balance, ask your doctor if suspension exercises are right for you.

- **Resistance Bands.** These stretchy bands have been around for a while, but are now being used in fresh, new ways. With resistance band–walking, for example, a long band is tied around the user's hips while a trainer holds the other end. As the user walks far enough away to create tension in the band, the trainer then gently tugs or releases the band, forcing the user to quickly adjust to the instability.

You also can perform a number of different solo exercises by attaching your band to a post or door handle. For example, you can lower your body into a semi (partial) squat or staggered stance position and perform an alternating push-and-pull exercise with or without trunk rotation.

Getting Started

One-on-one training is the safest way for beginners to start a functional fitness training program. For those who are more experienced exercisers, group classes are a more affordable option. Check with your local Y or community center.

For personal guidance, look for an exercise professional with a degree in kinesiology or sports science and/or a Senior Fitness Specialist certificate from the National Academy of Sports Medicine or American Council on Exercise.

Another option: You also can use a DVD for a functional fitness workout at home. Search "functional fitness workout DVD" online.

Weekend Warriors Live Longer

Bob Barnett, editor, *Bottom Line Personal,* with I-Min Lee, MD, ScD, professor of medicine at Harvard Medical School.

My wife swims three times a week, works out at the gym on other days…fits in yoga at home frequently…and walks our Labradoodle most mornings.

Me, I plan to exercise about twice as often as I do. I squeeze in workouts on weekdays, yes, but to be honest, there are weeks that I say hi to the gym only on Saturday.

So I was happy to learn the good news—I might not die young!

Fitness guidelines traditionally stress exercising at least three to five times per week. The goal is to accumulate 150 minutes of "moderate" intensity exercise such as brisk walking or 75 minutes of "intense" exercise such as running.

But it turns out that procrastinators, even fitness underachievers, live longer, too. In a recent study published in *JAMA Internal Medicine*, researchers tracked activity habits and longevity of more than 63,000 people, age 40 and older, over a period of nearly 20 years.

Findings: "Weekend warriors" who exercised only once or twice per week enjoyed virtually the same longevity advantages as several-times-a-week go-getters—even when they didn't quite make the 75/150 goal. They were 30% less likely to die over that period than inactive folks who almost never exercised.

Is a daily exercise habit good? Of course it is. But the point is, any regular exercise is a lot healthier than none. "We need to dispel the myth that you have to run marathons or do triathlons for health benefits," says study coauthor I-Min Lee, MD, ScD, professor of medicine at Harvard Medical School. "We don't even say 'exercise'—it's just 'physical activity.'"

Skipping the Gym, Ladies? Try the Stairs

JoAnn Pinkerton, MD, professor of obstetrics and gynecology, University of Virginia Health System, Charlottesville, and executive director, North American Menopause Society, Pepper Pike, Ohio.
North American Menopause Society, news release.

Older women don't have to hit the gym to stay healthy, because a stair-climbing workout appears to do the trick, researchers report.

Finding the right type of exercise can be difficult for postmenopausal women, according to the North American Menopause Society. For example, high-intensity resistance training reduces age-related muscle loss, but can increase blood pressure.

Combining aerobic and resistance training can minimize this problem. But many women say they don't have the time, the money, access to a gym or decent weather for getting out.

Study Findings

"This study demonstrates how simple lifestyle interventions such as stair climbing can be effective in preventing or reducing the negative effects of menopause and age on the vascular system and leg muscles of postmenopausal women with hypertension," said JoAnn Pinkerton, MD, the Menopause Society's executive director.

This doesn't mean climbing just one or two flights of stairs a day, however. The study included postmenopausal women in Korea who climbed 192 steps, two to five times a day, four days a week.

A typical house in the United States has 13 steps per story. So you'd need to climb more than 14 flights of stairs several times a day to gain the reported benefits.

According to the study, this exercise program improved artery health, lowered blood pressure and increased leg strength.

Additional benefits included fat loss, improved cholesterol profiles and reduced risk of the bone-thinning disease osteoporosis, the researchers said.

The results were published in the journal *Menopause*.

The National Institute on Aging has more about exercise and physical activity at NIA.NIH.gov. Search "exercise."

Are You Hurting Your Knees?

Wayne L. Westcott, PhD, professor of exercise science, Quincy College, Massachusetts.

If jogging up a flight of stairs is part of your workout, are you hurting your knees?

Maybe, but you can modify your routine to reduce your chance of knee (and hip, lower back and muscular) injuries.

Your best bet is to jog up the stairs, then walk back down.

Here's why: When you're running, the fraction of time your feet are in contact with the ground and supporting your weight decreases. Add the impact of bouncing, and the average "landing force" absorbed by your ankles, knees and hips is about three times your body weight. (Walking reduces the landing force absorption by about half.) Jogging up those stairs reduces this force because your foot does not drop as far as it would on level ground. Jogging down the stairs increases the landing force because your foot has to fall farther. Walking, of course, is a lower-impact exercise and less risky.

The New, Sleeker Electric Bikes

Michael Yozell, senior test editor of *Bicycling* magazine. Bicycling.com

E-bikes—bicycles that you can pedal but that also have electric motors to deliver a boost any time you want—used to be heavy and ungainly, but thanks to updated technology, they now are sleek and surprisingly light. You can rely on the electric power for up to 100 miles per charge, and you can go 20 miles per hour (mph) or faster with electric assist. You probably have at least one neighbor with an e-bike—US sales doubled last year.

These bikes are not for exercise slackers, either—most models provide electric assist only when you are pedaling, and research shows that they encourage exercise. They charge in about four or five hours from any standard household outlet. The price, though, is closer to that of mopeds than most regular bicycles. To get a reliable ride, you'll want to spend $2,800 to $3,000...and if your goal is high speed or carrying a lot of cargo, expect to spend $4,000 or more.

Before buying any electric bike, consider whether you'll primarily use it as a general-purpose recreational ride...or to commute, go on long tours, carry cargo or children or even to go off-roading. Also, think about whether you would like a model that gives you power without pedaling. Here are five excellent e-bikes for different needs...

Best affordable, dependable electric bike: Cannondale Quick NEO. This is the Honda Accord of electric bikes—reliable and not too expensive.

Maximum electric-assist speed/range: 20 mph/50 miles. $2,799.99.* Cannondale.com

Best for speed: Specialized Turbo Vado 6.0. The Porsche of e-bikes, the Turbo Vado 6.0 can attain speeds up to 28 mph with electric assist.

Electric-assist range: 25 miles in "turbo" (high speed) mode, 50 miles in "eco" (battery-saving) mode. $5,000. Specialized.com

Best for carrying cargo or kids: Tern GSD. You can carry multiple shopping bags and/or up to two young children in child seats—totaling 400 pounds, rider included. Unlike other cargo-carrying e-bikes, the Tern GSD's center of gravity is low, making it easier to pilot when loaded.

Maximum electric-assist speed/range: 20 mph/150 miles. $3,999. TernBicycles.com

Best for comfort: Riese ller Swing. Riese ller includes suspension on both wheels of most models for an impressively smooth ride, but its Swing model adds suspension under the seat as well.

Maximum electric-assist speed/range: 20 mph/100 miles. $4,209. R-M.De/en-us

Best if you don't always want to pedal: Elby S1 9-Speed. With this e-bike, you can get an assist while you're pedaling and can stop pedaling and let the motor do all the work or use the active-regeneration mode to charge the battery while you ride.

Maximum electric-assist speed/range: 20 mph/90 miles. $2,999. ElbyBike.com

*Prices are manufacturer's suggested retail prices. Maximum electric-assist ranges are estimates.

Group Workouts are Better for Stress Reduction

People who worked out in a group had 26% less stress than those who worked out on their own—and reported better quality of life. While people who did individual fitness routines worked out twice as long as group participants, they reported only an 11% increase in mental health, compared with 12.6% for those in a group. The group members also reported 24.8% better physical health and 26% improved emotional health by the end of the study.

Dayna Yorks, DO, University of New England College of Osteopathic Medicine, and coauthor of a study of 69 medical students participating in a 12-week exercise program, published in *The Journal of the American Osteopathic Association.*

Chapter 13

HEAL NATURALLY

Powerful Plants for a Smooth Menopause

Medicinal plants have very powerful properties and have been used for centuries to help heal conditions ranging from migraines to high blood pressure. For a smooth transition into menopause and beyond, here are a few of my favorites...

Black Cohosh (Cimicifuga racemosa)

Black cohosh, the most widely used and most thoroughly studied natural supplement for menopausal symptoms, has been clinically proven to reduce hot flashes and night sweats. While black cohosh's exact mechanism of action is unknown, compounds in the herb appear to bind to estrogen receptors without changing hormone levels in the body. Because black cohosh does not have estrogenic action, it is safe for use in patients with a history of breast cancer. My usual recommendation is 40 mg of black cohosh, standardized to 2.5% triterpene glycosides, daily. Please note, while some women experience a decrease in hot flashes almost immediately, maximum benefit may not be apparent for as long as 12 weeks.

Panax Ginseng

Often, women going through the menopausal transition experience a lack of energy due to fluctuations or depletions in reproductive hormone levels. Panax ginseng to the rescue! In fact, a double-blind, placebo-controlled study of postmenopausal women showed overall symptom relief and improvement in mood and well-being after ginseng supplementation. I've found great success using a product called Ginseng Phytosome—ginseng formulated with a patented process that results in superior absorption. It contains one part Panax ginseng extract standardized to contain 37.5% ginsenosides, bound to two parts phosphatidylcholine—a source of the nutrient choline that serves as a precursor to the neurotransmitter acetylcholine, which is important for nerve and muscle function.

Holly Lucille, ND, RN, a naturopathic doctor whose private practice, Healing from Within Healthcare, in West Hollywood, California, focuses on comprehensive naturopathic medicine and individualized care. She is author of *Creating and Maintaining Balance: A Woman's Guide to Safe, Natural Hormone Health.* DrHollyLucille.com

Green Tea (Camellia Sinensis)

Green tea is a rich source of flavonoids and polyphenols that have been studied for their support of immune system health. Green tea also contains small amounts of caffeine, which supports stamina and reduces fatigue. There is some evidence that green tea supports daily energy expenditure and may be beneficial in weight management. An effective dose for women is 250 mg of green tea leaf extract standardized to contain 35 mg of caffeine.

Rhodiola (Rhodiola Rosea)

While somewhat new to American practitioners, rhodiola has been used to support healthy energy levels for centuries in Russia, Scandinavia and Iceland.

Animal research demonstrates that rhodiola reduces levels of the stress hormone cortisol, and boosts *adenosine triphosphate* (ATP) synthesis, a coenzyme important for energy production. For women struggling with energy drain related to menopause, rhodiola may support mental concentration and alertness and support healthy endurance levels.

Chaste Tree (Vitex agnus-castus)

Vitex has been widely used for the management of menstrual disorders, premenstrual syndrome (PMS) and hot flashes in menopause. The key actives in chaste tree fruit seem to support the pituitary gland's regulation of ovarian hormone production, directing menstruation, fertility and other processes.

Women have used Vitex preparations for menstrual difficulties for at least 2,500 years. In a double-blind, multi-center study, 175 female patients were randomized to receive either chaste tree extract or pyridoxine (vitamin B-6) for relief of PMS. Using self-report and physician assessment to determine results, the women in the Vitex group had significantly reduced breast tenderness, edema (swelling), tension, headache, constipation and depression.

Natural Ways to Beat Constipation

Christopher Vasey, ND, a naturopathic physician who specializes in detoxification and rejuvenation in Chamby-Montreux, Switzerland. He lectures regularly about natural health in Europe, Canada and the US, and is the author of *Freedom from Constipation: Natural Remedies for Digestive Health*. ChristopherVasey.ch/anglais/home.html

Constipation is a topic that many people are too embarrassed to discuss with their doctors. But there's no need to suffer in silence.

It's widely known that infrequent and/or painful bowel movements often have relatively simple explanations—you're not getting enough water...you're skimping on fiber... and/or you're too sedentary. If you drink more fluids, add fiber to your diet and get some exercise, you're usually good to go, right? Unfortunately, that is not the case for everyone.

What you may not know: For approximately 15% of Americans, constipation is a chronic problem. This can occur if you're taking a certain medication, such as an antacid, antidepressant or narcotic painkiller...or have a medical problem, such as low thyroid (hypothyroidism), Parkinson's disease or multiple sclerosis, that can cause constipation.

Is a pharmaceutical laxative (pill or liquid) the next best bet? Not always. These products can cause side effects, such as bloating, cramping or gas, and may even interfere with the absorption of some medications and nutrients.

A better way: Most people can beat constipation without using a pharmaceutical. *Here's how...*

Start with These Strategies

If you are troubled by constipation, make sure you give the strategies below a try...

- **Drink up!** A healthy bowel movement is about 75% water. Constipation can occur when the stool water content falls below 70%—this can cause the stool to become too hard for the body to evacuate easily.

To avoid constipation, most people need 2 to 2.5 quarts of fluids a day. You don't need that much if you eat a lot of vegetables, fruit and other plant foods—they have a high water content that counts toward the daily total.

But: If you exercise or sweat a lot, you will need more than the recommended 2 to 2.5 quarts of fluids a day.

My advice: Drink a big glass of water (or a mug of herbal tea) all at once, several times a day. Like many naturopaths, I advise against drinking fluids with meals to avoid diluting digestive juices.

- **Get your roughage.** Plant fibers take up space in the large intestine and cause the intestinal walls to stretch—the process that triggers intestinal peristalsis (contractions) and bowel movements.

Important: All plant fibers are good for constipation, but the water-soluble type—found, for example, in vegetables, fruits (raspberries, figs, dates and passion fruit are especially beneficial), flaxseed and beans—is particularly good because it absorbs water and can double or even quadruple in size in the intestine, which helps move things along.

My advice: Be sure to get enough fiber each day. For people over age 50, that's about 30 g daily for men and 21 g daily for women. Those who are constipated may need even more fiber.

- **Avoid constipating foods and beverages.** These include bananas, blueberries, fresh apricots, white rice and red wine. Generally, you would need to have these foods/drinks on a regular basis to have a problem, but sometimes having the food/drink just once causes an issue.

- **Walk the right amount.** Walking is very effective for constipation because it stimulates nerves that trigger peristaltic activity.

My advice: To work for constipation, you need to walk for at least 40 minutes a day. If it's more convenient, you can break it up into two, 20-minute sessions.

Note: Other types of exercise can also help constipation, but walking is the easiest and most convenient for most people.

For More Help

If the advice above does not give you relief within 15 days, then it's time to step up your game. *The following tips can help—you can try all of them...*

- **Heat the liver.** According to the principles of Eastern medicine, a loss of heat from the liver—often triggered by fatigue or stress—causes blood capillaries to shrink...reduces circulation...and lowers production of bile, which you need for healthy digestion.

What to do: Place an old-fashioned rubber hot-water bottle over the liver—halfway down the right side of the abdomen, on the ribs under the right breast. The heat will increase circulation and cause the liver to expand, which has a stimulating effect on bowel movements.

Keep the bottle in place for about 15 to 30 minutes. Repeat the treatment up to three times a day, preferably after meals. People who do this for a month in addition to the steps above often find that constipation is no longer a problem. Or you can use the hot-water bottle indefinitely if you feel that it is continuing to help.

- **Self-massage.** To stimulate the peristaltic muscles that push stools out of the intestine, it helps to stretch, knead and compress the intestines with self-massage.

What to do: Using your fist or fingertips, firmly rub your abdomen (the area surrounding the navel) in a clockwise direction. This mimics the clockwise direction of intestinal peristalsis and stimulates different parts of the intestine. Once a day, rub the area for five to 10 minutes, at least two hours after a meal. You will most likely start to notice an improvement in bowel movements within three or four days.

- **Improve your bacterial balance.** There's an ideal ratio of bacteria in the gut—about 85% of the organisms should be "good" bacteria involved in fermentation (the dividing of food particles)...and the rest of the organisms should be "bad" bacteria that cause putrefaction (the decomposition of the particles). People who eat a lot of animal foods tend to have an excess of the second type and not enough of the first.

To restore a healthier balance, cut back on animal foods and eat more high-fiber plant foods such as fruits, vegetables and whole grains. These foods have probiotic effects—they increase levels of the fermenting organisms.

Another option: A daily probiotic supplement that provides high doses (numbering in the billions) of beneficial bacteria, such as bifidus and/or acidophilus strains. Follow label instructions.*

• **Strengthen the "push" muscles.** Because of their sedentary lifestyles, many Americans don't have the strength in the abdominal and/or intestinal muscles to readily generate the pressure needed for a bowel movement. This exercise can help.

What to do: Sit on the floor with your knees bent. Recline backward and rest your weight on your forearms. Extend one leg straight out in front of you...slowly bend it to bring it back to the starting position...then do the same with the other leg. Alternating legs, extend-and-bend each leg five times, then rest and repeat the cycle two more times. Do this daily. As you get stronger, increase the number of leg extensions to 10 or 20. You can extend-and-bend both legs at the same time, but it's more challenging.

• **A better position.** Our early ancestors squatted on their heels to evacuate. This position strongly facilitates evacuation of the bowels because it relaxes the muscles of the anal sphincter, encouraging it to open, and puts the colon in a vertical position. To achieve these benefits on a toilet, raise your feet four to eight inches with a stool.

What Is Normal?

Depending on what's being eaten, it can take about 30 to 40 hours for food to be transformed into stools and evacuated from the body. But sometimes the body doesn't work as intended.

Doctors define constipation as having fewer than three bowel movements a week... straining or having hard stools more than 25% of the time...and/or feeling that your bowel movements are often "incomplete."

*Although probiotics are generally considered safe, anyone with a weakened immune system, including those who take corticosteroids, as well as pregnant women, should check with their doctors before taking them.

Surprising Benefits of Acupuncture

Stephen Chee, MD, MPH, MA, MTOM, LAc. He is dual-trained and dual-licensed as a medical doctor and acupuncturist. He is board-certified in family medicine, integrative medicine, medical acupuncture and acupuncture, and Traditional Chinese medicine. Dr. Chee has a private practice in Beverly Hills, California. DrSteveChee.com

A recent *Vanity Fair* cover story about actress Angelina Jolie revealed that she had suffered from Bell's palsy (temporary weakness or paralysis and drooping of one side of the face). But Jolie said she no longer had the disorder—and credited acupuncture for her full recovery.

It took acupuncture a very long time to move from its roots as an ancient Chinese therapy to being accepted as "real medicine" in the West—and even today, most people, including most doctors, think of acupuncture mainly as a treatment for pain such as low-back pain, headaches and pain from arthritis. And acupuncture does treat pain effectively, probably because its placement of very fine needles into the skin in particular spots blocks the transmission of pain signals to the brain and also releases the body's natural endorphins.

What most people don't know: Acupuncture also is an excellent treatment for a wide variety of other illnesses and conditions.

Research shows that acupuncture reduces inflammation...improves circulation...regulates the autonomic nervous system (which controls heart rate, breathing, digestion and other body functions)...and balances the production of neurotransmitters, brain chemicals that control mood—all therapeutic keys to treating many health problems.

Here are surprising conditions that acupuncture can treat…

Overactive Bladder Syndrome (OAB)

This problem afflicts one in six Americans and becomes more common with age. You feel a sudden, uncontrollable urge to urinate (which can lead to incontinence), and you may have to urinate many times a day and even several times overnight.

How acupuncture helps: When medications can't control the problem, electroacupuncture—in which the needles conduct a very mild, nonpainful electric current—often can. The proven approach is using electroacupuncture to stimulate a point in the ankle along what Traditional Chinese medicine practitioners call the "kidney meridian." This also happens to be the location of the posterior tibial nerve, which controls the bladder.

Recent finding: A team of researchers from several major institutions—including Johns Hopkins School of Medicine, Columbia University Medical Center and Brown University—reviewed studies on nondrug treatments for OAB, publishing the results in *American Journal of Obstetrics Gynecology*. The researchers found that electroacupuncture was effective for the problem and improved quality of life.

What works best: Weekly electroacupuncture for 12 weeks. Discontinue the treatment if it isn't improving the condition after four or five weeks. Patients who respond to the treatment may require additional therapy at individually defined treatment intervals (for example, every three weeks) for sustained relief of symptoms.

Acupuncture may help for incontinence as well: Stress urinary incontinence—passing urine inadvertently when you cough, sneeze, laugh, exercise or lift a heavy object—afflicts an estimated 35% of women, most of them older. A recent study of about 500 women with this condition, published in *JAMA,* showed that electroacupuncture decreased urine leakage after six weeks. (Using electroacupuncture to treat stress urinary incontinence is still being researched.)

Diabetic Peripheral Neuropathy

An estimated 50% of older people with diabetes develop this nerve disorder, which can cause numbness, burning, tingling and pain in the feet, legs, hands and/or arms—and also increases the risk for infected diabetic foot ulcers and the need for amputation.

Recent finding: A study published in *Journal of Acupuncture and Meridian Studies* showed that 10 weekly sessions of acupuncture improved the symptoms of diabetic peripheral neuropathy in three out of four patients.

Another new finding: Acupuncture also may help control high blood sugar itself. In a study published in *Nutrition & Diabetes,* treatment with a diabetes medication (*metformin*) and acupuncture controlled high blood sugar more effectively than the medication alone.

What works best: Electroacupuncture and scalp acupuncture weekly for 10 weeks. (Scalp acupuncture utilizes advanced acupuncture needling techniques and points on the scalp that have been identified not by Traditional Chinese medicine but by neuroanatomy. In my clinical experience, it often is the most effective type of acupuncture for treating neurological problems such as neuropathy, stroke and mental decline and usually requires additional training by the acupuncturist.)

Asthma

I have used acupuncture to treat a number of patients with asthma, helping them decrease the frequency and severity of asthma attacks—and reduce the dosage of their asthma medication. (As with all the medical problems discussed here, I almost always use acupuncture in combination with other medical and nondrug treatments—in the case of asthma, those nondrug treatments include certain supplements, conscious breathing, meditation and eliminating environmental and potential food triggers.)

Recent finding: In a study published in *The Journal of Alternative and Complementary Medicine*, German and Swiss researchers added acupuncture (15 sessions over three months) to standard asthma treatment in 184 patients, comparing them with people who had asthma but did not receive acupuncture. Compared with those not getting acupuncture, those receiving it had a 70% greater improvement in asthma symptoms and in limits to their daily activity. They also had two to four times greater improvement in perceived physical and mental health.

What works best: Any style of acupuncture can be effective for asthma, with treatments once a week for 10 to 15 weeks. Patients who respond to the treatment may require additional therapy at regular intervals (for example, every three to four weeks) for sustained relief of symptoms.

Post-Stroke Rehabilitation

Research shows that acupuncture can treat a variety of post-stroke symptoms including pain, depression and insomnia—and can help restore the basic nerve and muscle function that strokes rob from patients.

Recent finding: Researchers from Australia and China analyzed the results from 22 studies on 1,425 stroke patients, publishing their results in *Archives of Physical Medicine and Rehabilitation*. They found that electroacupuncture reduced spasticity (in which muscles involuntarily shorten or flex, causing stiffness and tightness) by more than 40% and improved everyday functioning.

What works best: Scalp acupuncture combined with either electroacupuncture or standard acupuncture.

Finding an Acupuncturist

Word-of-mouth is the most effective way to find a competent acupuncturist. Ask your doctors, family members and friends for recommendations. You also can use the "Find a Practitioner" feature at the website of the National Certification Commission for Acupuncture and Oriental Medicine (NCCAOM.org).

Talk to the acupuncturist before your treatment to see whether you feel comfortable with him/her, which, I think, is a key element of healing. (Avoid treatment from any acupuncturist who is not willing to talk to you or answer your questions before charging you or starting treatment.)

---

6 Natural Fixes for Neuropathy

Janice F. Wiesman, MD, FAAN, associate clinical professor of neurology at New York University School of Medicine in New York City and adjunct assistant professor of neurology at Boston University School of Medicine. She is author of *Peripheral Neuropathy: What It Is and What You Can Do to Feel Better.*

Nerve damage can be both mysterious and maddening. It's mysterious because about one-third of those with neuropathy never discover what's causing the pain, tingling and numbness. It's maddening because damaged nerves recover slowly—if they recover at all. Even when an underlying cause of neuropathy is identified (diabetes, for example, is a big one) and corrected, the symptoms may persist for months, years or a lifetime.

More Than Pain

About one in every 15 American adults has experienced some form of neuropathy, also known as peripheral neuropathy. The symptoms vary widely—from sharp, shooting pains that feel like jolts of electricity...to burning sensations...tingling...numbness...muscle fatigue...and/or a lack of muscle strength in the feet. Symptoms typically start first in both feet, then slowly move up the legs and to the hands. Nerves that control functions such as sweat, blood pressure, digestion and bladder control can be affected as well.

There are hundreds of different causes of neuropathy. Diabetes, mentioned above, accounts for about one-third of all cases. Elevated blood sugar damages nerve cells and blood vessels and can cause numbness and other symptoms.

Other common causes of neuropathy: Heavy alcohol use, rheumatoid arthritis, vitamin deficiencies (including vitamin B-12) and certain medications, especially some chemotherapy drugs.

Important finding: One-third to one-half of patients with neuropathies of unknown origin have inherited neuropathies—that is, they're genetically susceptible to nerve damage, even in the absence of a specific disease/injury, according to research conducted at Mayo Clinic.

A few medications are FDA-approved for neuropathy, but the side effects may be more uncomfortable than the condition itself. Fortunately, there are some surprisingly effective nondrug therapies.

Natural Treatments

It can be a challenge for doctors (usually neurologists) to identify what is responsible for neuropathies. But it's worth making the effort because treating the cause early can stop ongoing damage and potentially allow injured nerves to regenerate. When nerves repair there may be some increased sensitivity, but this is usually temporary.

When the cause of neuropathy can't be identified, the symptoms can still be treated. If your symptoms make you very uncomfortable, there are medications that can help. The drugs that have been FDA-approved for neuropathic pain include *pregabalin* (Lyrica), also often used for seizures...and *duloxetine* (Cymbalta), also used for depression. Lyrica can cause drowsiness and weight gain...and Cymbalta can cause drowsiness as well as sweating in a small number of people. *Gabapentin* (Neurontin) and tricyclic antidepressants, such as *amitriptyline* (Elavil) and *nortriptyline* (Pamelor), are used off-label for neuropathy. Neurontin is similar to Lyrica with the same side effects...and the antidepressants can cause sedation, dry mouth and, in high doses, arrhythmias.

My advice: If you'd describe your symptoms as uncomfortable and annoying—but not debilitating—you might want to start with nondrug treatments. They probably won't eliminate the discomfort altogether, but they can make it easier to tolerate. Plus, if you do decide to use medication, these treatments may enable you to take it for a shorter time and/or at a lower dose. *Try one or more of the following at a time...*

- **Natural fix #1: Vibrating foot-bath.** Most patients will first notice tingling, numbness or other symptoms in the feet. Soaking your feet in a warm-water vibrating footbath (available in department stores, pharmacies and online) for 15 to 20 minutes dilates blood vessels and increases circulation in the affected area. More important, the vibrations are detected and transmitted by large-diameter sensory nerve fibers. Because of their large size, these fibers transmit signals very quickly. The sensations of vibration reach the spinal cord before the pain signals from damaged nerves, which blunts the discomfort.

The pain relief is temporary but reliable. You can soak your feet as often as you wish throughout the day.

Helpful: Soak your feet just before bed—the pain relief you get will help you fall asleep more easily.

For discomfort in other parts of the body, you can get similar relief from a whirlpool bath or a pulsating showerhead.

Important: Some people with neuropathy are unable to sense temperatures and can burn their feet in too-hot water. Test the temperature with your hand first (or have someone else test it).

- **Natural fix #2. Menthol cream.** The smooth muscles in arterial walls are lined with receptors that react to menthol. When you rub an affected area with menthol cream (such as Bengay), the blood vessels dilate, create warmth and reduce discomfort. Creams labeled "menthol" or "methyl salicylate" have the same effects. These creams can be used long-term as needed.

• **Natural fix #3. Transcutaneous electrical nerve stimulation (TENS).** This therapy delivers low levels of electric current to the surface of the skin. It's thought that the current stimulates nerves and sends signals to the brain that block the discomfort from damaged nerves.

How well do the devices work? The research is mixed. In 2010, a meta-analysis of TENS in patients with diabetic neuropathies found that the treatment led to a decrease in pain scores. Other studies, however, have shown little or no benefit.

Battery-powered TENS units cost about $30 for low-end models. The treatment is largely without side effects, and some people have good results. Treatments are typically done for 30 minutes at a time and can be repeated as needed throughout the day. Treatments should not be done on skin that is irritated.

My advice: If you want to try TENS at home, start using it under the direction of a physical therapist so that he/she can suggest the appropriate settings and amount of time for treatment.

• **Natural fix #4. Percutaneous electrical nerve stimulation (PENS).** Percutaneous means that the electric current is delivered under the skin, using short needles. Studies have shown that the treatments, done in rehabilitation/physical therapy offices, decrease pain, improve sleep and may allow patients to use smaller doses of painkilling medication. After each treatment, the pain relief can potentially last for weeks or longer. The treatments take about 30 minutes per session and are generally repeated three times a week, until the patient achieves the desired amount and duration of pain relief. The risks are minimal, although you might have mild bruising or a little bleeding. Infection is possible but unlikely. Most patients have little or no pain during the treatments. PENS is not advised for those with pacemakers and should not be done on areas of irritated skin. The treatments might or might not be covered by insurance—be sure to ask.

• **Natural fix #5. Self-massage.** Firmly rubbing and/or kneading the uncomfortable area is another way to block pain signals. You don't need to learn sophisticated massage techniques—but you (or a loved one) must use enough pressure to stimulate the big nerves that carry the pressure sensations. A too-light touch won't be helpful.

Caution: If you have a history of deep vein thrombosis, ask your doctor before massaging your legs.

• **Natural fix #6. Relaxation techniques.** Stress and anxiety do not cause neuropathy, but patients who are tense may feel pain more intensely. A multiyear study found that patients with chronic pain who completed a mindfulness/stress-reduction program reported significantly less pain—and the improvement lasted for up to three years.

Helpful: Meditation, yoga and other relaxation techniques. Most large medical centers offer programs in anxiety/stress management. Excellent guided meditations are also available on YouTube.

Medicinal Mushrooms

Mark Stengler, ND, a naturopathic doctor in private practice at Stengler Center for Integrative Medicine in Encinitas, California. He is author of more than 30 books, including *The Health Benefits of Medicinal Mushrooms* and *The Natural Physician's Healing Therapies*. He is coauthor of *Bottom Line's Prescription for Drug Alternatives*. MarkStengler.com

---

Mushrooms may not seem like a big health deal—most people think of them simply as earthy additions to meals and salads.

What most people don't realize: Dozens of varieties of mushrooms are medicinal. Rich in unique carbohydrates (polysaccharides) called beta glucans, they can energize the body's disease-fighting immune cells.

Here's what you need to know about three effective medicinal mushrooms…

Note: Mushroom supplements generally are safe, but because they activate the immune system, they should not be taken by organ-transplant recipients on immunosuppressive drugs. Also, look for a hot-water (or hot-water/ethanol) extract. This may be stated on the supplement label—if not, check the company's website. I typically recommend that patients take one mushroom supplement at a time, rather than two or three.

Maitake

I consider the maitake mushroom (*Grifola frondosa*)—native to northern Japan and called the "King of Mushrooms" throughout Asia—to be one of the most powerful allies in the battle against cancer. It can be used for immune enhancement in addition to conventional cancer treatment.

Compelling research: Chinese doctors studied more than 300 people with bladder cancer after they had surgery for the disease, tracking the effectiveness of five standard and natural therapies, including supplements of a maitake mushroom extract. After an average of seven years, those taking maitake had the lowest rate of cancer recurrence (35%). And in a study of 36 cancer patients published in *Alternative Medicine Review*, maitake supplements improved symptoms and decreased the size of tumors in 69% of breast cancer patients, 63% of lung cancer patients and 58% of liver cancer patients. The supplements also boosted the cancer-killing power of chemotherapy by up to 40%—doses ranged between 50 milligrams (mg) to 150 mg daily (some patients received chemotherapy and some did not).

Decades of research from Japan show that one "fraction" or extract of maitake—the D-fraction—is most effective in boosting the immune system and fighting cancer. Specifically, D-fraction boosts the number and power of natural killer cells, immune cells that can "recognize" and kill cancer cells and viruses.

Best product and dose: For my patients with cancer, I often prescribe the over-the-counter product MaitakeGold 404, used in many studies on cancer. I prescribe a daily dose of 0.5 mg to 1 mg per kilogram (2.2 pounds) of body weight. For everyday immune-strengthening, I often recommend 5 mg to 15 mg daily taken 20 minutes before meals or on an empty stomach.

You can find maitake mushrooms in your supermarket, farmers' market or gourmet market—and add them to your diet to help prevent cancer. The mature mushroom—also called "Hen of the Woods"—has large, fleshy grayish-brown caps. Cut off the tough white base, then slice and sauté the caps for 10 to 15 minutes with salt, pepper and garlic. They're great in pasta, risotto, eggs and other dishes. I recommend two to three servings of maitake mushrooms weekly.

Turkey Tail

The turkey tail mushroom (*Trametes versicolor*) grows around the world and has a fan-shaped, brown-and-tan cap that resembles turkey feathers. Used for centuries in folk and traditional medicines in China and Japan, this mushroom can treat lung infections, hepatitis (liver infection) and cancer. Modern medicine has focused on cancer.

Compelling research: More than 400 studies show that turkey tail can fight cancer. Nearly all the studies on people have been with PSK (krestin), a proprietary extract that has been used as a supportive therapy by thousands of cancer patients in Japan. In one study published in *Anticancer Research*, Stage 1 and 2 lung cancer patients taking the extract had a five-year survival rate of 39%, compared with 16% for patients taking a placebo. Other studies show higher survival rates in people taking PSK for colorectal, esophageal and stomach cancers.

Best product and dose: For those with cancer, I often recommend 1,000 mg to 1,500 mg, twice daily, taken in the morning and evening on an empty stomach. Look for a product that has 20% beta glucans. As for your diet—turkey tail is not an appetizing mushroom.

Reishi

Reishi (*Ganoderma lucidum*)—a shiny fan-shaped mushroom with colors ranging from reddish brown to black—has been used for thousands of years by traditional healers in

Japan and China. (Chinese healers call this the "Mushroom of Immortality.") Among mushrooms, it's your best choice for an everyday tonic to boost the strength of your immune system. And it also strengthens the rest of the body. *Proven benefits include...*

• **Reversing fatty liver disease.** Fatty liver afflicts an estimated 25% of Americans and can lead to liver disease and liver cancer. In a new study published in *Pharmaceutical Biology*, the livers of people with fatty liver completely normalized after they took reishi for six months. And their levels of cell-damaging oxidants fell by 42%. The participants made no other changes in diet, exercise or anything else.

• **Improvement in fibromyalgia.** In a recent study by Spanish researchers published in *Nutrición Hospitalaria*, people with the pain, stiffness and poor fitness typical of fibromyalgia saw improvements in flexibility, strength and endurance after taking reishi for six weeks.

• **Eliminating oral HPV virus.** Oral infection with some strains of human papillomavirus (HPV) can cause throat cancer. In a study of 61 people with cancer-causing oral HPV, published in *International Journal of Medicinal Mushrooms*, 88% of people who took reishi for two months had complete clearance of the virus.

• **Easing rheumatoid arthritis pain.** In a study of people with rheumatoid arthritis published in *Arthritis & Rheumatism,* people who took reishi had less inflammation and pain compared with those taking a placebo.

• **Raising HDL "good" cholesterol in people with diabetes.** In a study published in *British Journal of Nutrition*, people with diabetes who took reishi had an increase in "good" HDL cholesterol.

• **Preventing altitude sickness.** Reishi is a favorite natural remedy of travelers and trekkers to prevent altitude sickness. Start taking the supplement 10 to 14 days before you travel to a higher altitude.

Best product and dose: Look for an extract product containing a minimum of 10% polysaccharides (beta glucans) and 4% triterpene (another active ingredient). Take 800 mg two to three times daily.

Reishi is bitter and woody-tasting and not ideal for culinary use.

---

3 Weeds That Really Heal!

Jamison Starbuck, ND, a naturopathic physician in family practice and a guest lecturer at the University of Montana, both in Missoula. She is a past president of the American Association of Naturopathic Physicians and a contributing editor to *The Alternative Advisor: The Complete Guide to Natural Therapies and Alternative Treatments.* DrJamisonStarbuck.com.

Every spring, when the dandelions poke their yellow heads out of the soil, I smile with gratitude. This hardy, and often maligned, weed has several under-recognized but well-established health benefits. In fact, it's one of a trio of herbs that I used years ago to clear up a stubborn case of eczema before I had become a naturopathic physician. This "herb tonic" did the job in a matter of weeks and convinced me that natural medicine really does work! My favorite medicinal weeds (available in natural-food and herb stores)...*

• **Dandelion.** This weed, which contains vitamins such as vitamin C, is a member of the daisy family. With roots and leaves that are rich in medicinal properties, dandelion supports liver and gallbladder health...promotes digestion...acts as a diuretic to reduce edema (water retention) in the ankles and hands...and lowers blood pressure.

Note: Check with your doctor before trying dandelion—especially if you take a blood thinner, diabetes medication, a blood pressure drug (such as a diuretic) or other prescription medication.

To consume dandelion, you can eat the leaves in salads or on sandwiches or add to soup as a raw garnish.

*Before trying any herbal therapy, consult your doctor if you have a chronic medical condition or take prescription medication.

Important: Don't cook dandelion leaves in soup or you will lose many of the medicinal benefits—simply add them to the top of your soup for steaming before you serve.

You can also enjoy medicinal dandelion tea. Just put two teaspoons of dried dandelion root in one cup of boiling water. Reduce heat, and simmer for 15 minutes. Drink one cup two times a day, at least 15 minutes before or after eating. Doing this will aid your digestion and help ease one or more of the conditions described above. For example, edema will typically improve in a few days, while it can take three to four weeks to lower blood pressure. If you like dandelion tea, you can drink it indefinitely. If you opt for dandelion tincture, a typical daily dose is one-quarter teaspoon, in two ounces of water, twice a day, 15 minutes before a meal.

- **Burdock.** Like dandelion, burdock is ubiquitous in the US, popping up around the edges of sidewalks and in abandoned areas. Burdock is also in the daisy family and has what herbalists call "bitter properties"—that is, constituents that help improve digestion. I also use burdock in formulas for skin problems such as psoriasis, eczema and dandruff. Burdock root is mild tasting and can be used in soups and stews as you would carrots. Consult your doctor before using it if you take a blood thinner, diabetes drug or diuretic.

- **Yellow dock.** Because yellow dock is a mild laxative, it relieves constipation in a few days. It's also a good plant source of iron. Like burdock, yellow dock can help with scaly, itchy skin conditions. It is a member of the buckwheat family and tastes very bitter, so it's best taken in tincture (see above for dosage, under "Dandelion") once daily...or mixed in small amounts with other milder plants in a tea.

Caution: Do not use yellow dock if you take *digoxin* (Lanoxin), a diuretic or *warfarin* (Coumadin).

Because these herbs are generally safe for long-term use, I often combine all three in my treatment plans for liver, gallbladder or skin conditions. Many of my patients become fans of these herbs—just as I did—when they experience firsthand the plants' healing powers.

Hypnosis Works! How to Make It Work for You

Roberta Temes, PhD, a psychotherapist, hypnotist, former faculty member, SUNY Downstate Medical Center, Brooklyn. She is author of *The Complete Idiot's Guide to Hypnosis.* DrRoberta.com

Hypnosis is a powerfully effective mind-body medicine. But it's underutilized—partly because of confusion about what hypnosis can and can't do...and because it's too often misused and abused.

Hundreds of scientific studies show that hypnosis can help with a wide range of physical and emotional issues, including pain, depression, phobias, unwanted habits, performance enhancement and much more. But not everything called "hypnosis" is helpful.

A hypnotic trance is nothing extraordinary. In fact, when you've been so intensely focused—maybe in a book, a TV program or a craft project—that you're unaware of your surroundings, you've been in a hypnotic trance. If someone asked you for a dollar bill, you would probably hand it over—because the power of suggestion is uniquely effective during a hypnotic trance.

However, since anyone can call himself/herself a hypnotist, you need to know what to look for and what to avoid. *Pitfalls to watch for...*

- **The "hypnotist" is unqualified.** There are no state or national certifications nor any formal licensing required to call yourself a hypnotist. "Training" can be a YouTube video or a three-hour course. Instead, look for training from the American Society of Clinical Hypnotists or the Society for Clinical and Experimental Hypnosis. Both offer programs and workshops that are open only to health professionals.

Better: In my opinion, word of mouth is the only way to find a competent hypnotist.

If a friend has used hypnosis and it worked, ask if he would recommend his hypnotist. A good endorsement might be, "I was afraid of flying, and now I can get on a plane with no problem" or "I smoked two packs of cigarettes every day, and now I cannot stand the thought of cigarettes." If none of your friends have tried hypnosis (or would recommend theirs), ask your doctor or dentist for a recommendation.

• **Hypnosis masks an underlying health problem that requires medical care.** Many people (and unqualified "hypnotists") believe hypnosis can fix any problem, but it's important to know when hypnosis should not be the first thing you try.

Example: I can easily hypnotize someone with a headache to relieve the pain. But if the cause of the headache is an undiagnosed brain tumor, what the person needs most is a neurologist.

Better: A doctor visit—not hypnosis—should be the first response to a new symptom. Make sure that any underlying medical condition is appropriately addressed first.

• **The hypnotic suggestions are inappropriate.** Many years ago, asthmatic patients in a hospital in North Wales in the UK were hypnotized to not panic, remain calm and slowly and carefully seek help when having asthma attacks. These turned out to be terrible suggestions. Some of the asthmatics were so calm and deliberate when they had a life-threatening asthma attack that they almost died!

Better: Both hypnotist and client should evaluate the safety of the suggestions that are going to be used and write them down so that there is no ambiguity—before the client is brought to a hypnotic state.

• **The hypnotist recommends long-term treatment.** Some psychotherapists offer "hypnotherapy" as an adjunct to standard treatment—sometimes for a year or longer—usually as a way to uncover "repressed" material to help achieve psychological health. I don't endorse this approach.

I believe hypnosis works rapidly and should be used for changing habits and attitudes, not for delving into the unconscious. For instance, a patient undergoing psychotherapy might benefit from one session of hypnosis to deal with a particular issue—such as unhealthy eating habits, fear of public speaking or reluctance to meet a certain person—that is preventing him from moving forward with therapy.

Better: A good hypnotist should need to see you only one or two times.

Helpful: Hypnotic suggestions can "wear off." Ask if you can record the session on your phone to replay later if you need it. Some of my clients play their recording once a week…others never, but like to keep it as a "security blanket."

• **The hypnotist helps you to "recover" a repressed memory.** A memory "recovered" during hypnosis, especially a new memory about a past supposedly traumatic event, is almost always a false memory. In fact, there's a name for this common phenomenon—false memory syndrome.

Problem: Such memories are usually "recovered" by a therapist with an agenda, such as proving that you're a victim of childhood sexual abuse, something that's too easy for a hypnotist to create and reinforce.

Better: If you don't remember an event when you're not in a hypnotic trance, it probably didn't happen.

• **You're hypnotized on stage—and feel anxious afterward.** I love stage hypnosis! But I never volunteer to be hypnotized, and I don't think you should either. A stage hypnotist rapidly induces a hypnotic state and rapidly ends it. If your mental state is at all fragile—if you're stressed or didn't sleep well the night before—such rapid transition into and out of a hypnotic state could create a few days of mental imbalance and anxiety.

Better: Enjoy the show, but don't participate!

How I Do Hypnosis with My Clients…

I start a session by informally chatting with a client to establish a comfortable rapport.

We then decide together on verbal suggestions—the words I will say, slowly and deliberately, while he/she is in a hypnotic state.

Example: For a claustrophobic client scheduled for an MRI, we agreed that I would suggest that the cramped quarters of the MRI machine were a protective womb...and that the loud noise was a lullaby that would put her to sleep.

Finally, I help the client enter a hypnotic state. A typical session takes about one hour, although the actual hypnosis portion is usually about 20 minutes. I suggest that my clients record their sessions, but some of my clients prefer instead to return to my office for another session when or if they feel they need reinforcement.

Having Trouble Meditating?

Amy Zabin, DA, MT-BC, founder and director of The Music Therapy Center of Greenwich and a music therapy consultant at Greenwich Hospital and Stamford Hospital, all in Connecticut. She previously served as an adjunct professor in New York University's music therapy graduate program for 20 years. AmyZabin.com

Despite the incentive of its amazing health benefits (meditation has been shown to reduce blood pressure, improve sleep, relieve pain, minimize anxiety, ease depression and more), many people have a lot of difficulty meditating. Some people even feel anxious when they meditate—they wonder if they're doing it properly...get upset when the mind wanders...or feel like they're wasting time by sitting around and doing "nothing."

Good news: If you have tried to meditate without success, listening to music while you meditate may be the secret. And if you already meditate regularly, adding music can enhance the experience.

How Music Helps

For traditional meditation, you find a quiet place, remove as many distractions as possible—bright lights, cell phones, etc.—and focus on your breath or a mantra. When music is added to meditation, it offers a new and enjoyable focal point. Instead of feeling pressured to concentrate solely on your breath or mantra, you can focus on the music.

Choosing Meditative Tunes

Pick a genre of soothing music that you truly enjoy, but try to stick with instrumental pieces, since lyrics can be distracting. Music with a slow beat can create brain wave activity similar to that of meditation. Avoid aggressive music with a fast tempo—it can work against you by speeding up your heart and breathing rates. *Some good options...*

- **Classical music**—This type of music has been proven to slow heart rate, boost memory and more. Choose slow pieces that are captivating but not bombastic, such as Pachelbel's Canon in D, Bach's Air on the G String from Orchestral Suite No. 3 in D Major and Mozart's Piano Concerto No. 23, 2nd Movement, Adagio. There are many selections available for purchase online or streaming for free on YouTube or other websites.

- **New Age music**—There are lots of choices in this genre as well. An album I like is *In a Silent Place* by Eric Roberts.

- **Irish music**—Good choices include relaxing Irish and Celtic music and, my favorite, *Watermark* by Enya.

- **Guitar and flute combinations**—Various selections by Peder Helland feature guitar, violin, flute, cello and harp music. And on Music and Meditation (available at AmyZabin.com), I lead listeners into a deep meditation using guitar and flute music as well as crystal singing bowls.

Note: In my opinion, meditating to music might not be ideal at night—while the process feels relaxing, music activates so many parts of your brain that the overall effect is invigorating...you'll feel focused and alert afterward. Music meditation is best done in the morning or as an alternative to a midafternoon cup of coffee.

How to Meditate with Music

To start, sit or recline in a peaceful spot, free from distractions—your bed, a couch or even in your car parked on a quiet street.

Close your eyes and take a few breaths in through the nose and out through the mouth. Some people like to breathe in to a count of four and exhale to a count of eight, while others prefer to simply breathe in and out as deeply as possible.

Tune into your body and how it feels—do you notice any areas of tension or tightness? Take notice of these sensations, then release them. You can try shrugging your shoulders and releasing them and rolling your head a few times to let go of tension.

Next, turn on the music…you can play it out loud or use headphones or earbuds. Continue slowly breathing in and out as you turn your full attention to the music. Allow the music to lead the experience—to wash over, around and through you. Notice the tempo and the various instruments. Maybe you find yourself tuning into the cello in an orchestral piece or the ping of a triangle in a New Age song. Ask yourself—"How does this music make me feel?" Maybe it's relaxing you all over, or you notice your chest opening up, or you find yourself smiling.

If your mind wanders, that's fine. Think of these thoughts as clouds passing through the sky—simply notice them without judgment and gently return your focus to the music.

Interesting: Some experts believe the power of meditation lies in shifting and returning to focus. The more you practice it in the soothing, controlled environment of meditation, the easier it will be for you to calm yourself during stressful times.

Remarkable: I've found that just three to five minutes, three times a week, is all you need to reap the rewards of meditating with music.

The Sleep-Better Yoga Plan

Carol Krucoff, a yoga therapist at Duke Integrative Medicine in Durham, North Carolina. She is cofounder and codirector of the Yoga for Seniors trainings and network, Yoga4Seniors.com. Ms. Krucoff is also author of several books, including *Yoga Sparks: 108 Easy Practices for Stress Relief in a Minute or Less* and *Healing Yoga for Neck and Shoulder Pain.* HealingMoves.com

The day is waning, your warm bed beckons…and yet your mind continues to race, making peaceful slumber a far-off dream. What's the best way to bring on the z's?

Many Americans opt for a powerful sleeping pill or even a nightcap to help drift off at bedtime. Even though these so-called sleep "aids" may help you doze off, they leave you vulnerable to wee-hour awakenings…or pose dangerous side effects such as dizziness that make you prone to falls.

An under-recognized solution: Yoga is a safe approach that can easily be added to your sleep-hygiene toolbox. *Here's how…*

The Yoga Solution

Yoga is a perfect sleep inducer because it is designed to quiet the mind—targeting the racing thoughts that can keep us from drifting off. Yoga is also a proven pain-fighter, easing backaches, arthritis and other common sleep saboteurs.

When adults over age 60 who had insomnia took three months of twice-weekly classes incorporating yoga poses, meditation and daily home practice, they reported significant improvements in their sleep, according to a 2014 study in *Alternative Therapies in Health and Medicine*.

How to Breathe Right

When we are drifting off to sleep, the pace of our breathing naturally slows. But when our racing mind keeps us awake, turning our attention to our breath and deliberately slowing and deepening the breath can trigger a cascade of relaxing physiological changes—the heart rate slows, blood pressure decreases, muscles relax, anxiety eases and the mind calms.

Surprisingly, many people do not know the basics of correct deep breathing.

What to do: Put yourself in a comfortable position—lying on your back, for example—and place one of your palms on your belly. Relax your abdomen, and invite your breath to completely fill your lungs. You might notice that when you inhale fully this way, your belly rounds and your hand rises. With the exhale, your belly gently drops inward and your hand falls.

To get the most from abdominal breathing: Go a step further by making the exhale a bit longer. This type of breathing sends a clear signal to your central nervous system that everything is fine...just let go.

The Sleep-Inducing Poses

Once you have become comfortable with the relaxed breathing described above, here are some sleep-better yoga poses to do right before bed. For each pose below, start by lying on the floor (on a yoga mat or carpet for comfort) or on your bed with your knees bent and your arms at your sides. If your chin juts up, place a small pillow or folded towel under your head so that your chin is at the same level or slightly lower than your forehead.

- **Knees to chest.** *What to do:* Do the relaxed abdominal breathing described above for several minutes.

Once you're feeling relaxed, bring both knees toward your chest, holding onto your thighs or using a yoga strap (or a bathrobe tie) to catch your thighs and bring them toward your chest. Notice where you feel the sensation of stretch, and use your breath to help relax any tension. On the exhalation, draw your thighs in toward your body...on the inhalation, allow your thighs to drift away from your body. If it's uncomfortable to hug both legs, hug one leg at a time. Continue for six to 10 cycles of breath—each inhalation and exhalation is one breath cycle.

- **Neck release.** *What to do:* Take an easy, full breath in, then as you exhale, rotate your head to the right. Your eyes can be open or closed, whichever feels better.

Inhale as you bring your head back to center, then exhale as you turn your head to the left. Continue for six to 10 breaths, moving with your breath. Next, turn your head as far as it will comfortably go to the right and relax your left shoulder toward the ground. Linger here for three to five easy breaths, then bring your head back to the center and repeat to the left.

- **Arms overhead.** *What to do:* With your arms alongside your body and your palms facing down, tune in to your breath. As you inhale, extend your arms up and back so that the backs of your hands move toward the surface behind you. If your hands don't reach the surface behind you, that's fine. As you exhale, return your arms to their starting position along your sides. Repeat six to 10 times, moving with your breath—inhale your arms up and over...exhale them back down to your sides. Sleep tight...

Natural Fixes for 3 Foot Problems

Jamison Starbuck, ND, a naturopathic physician in family practice and producer of Dr. Starbuck's Health Tips for Kids, a weekly program on Montana Public Radio, MTPR.org, both in Missoula. She is a contributing editor to *The Alternative Advisor: The Complete Guide to Natural Therapies and Alternative Treatments.* DrJamisonStarbuck.com.

Foot problems are hard to ignore. When your tootsies are unwell, something as simple as shopping for groceries becomes a chore. *Fortunately, some well-chosen natural remedies can really help these common foot problems...*

- **Toenail fungus.** This is a stubborn problem, particularly for people with poor circulation or diabetes. You'll know you have a fungal infection if your nail is yellowed and/or raised or if there's white, flaky debris under the nail. Keeping your nails clipped, clean and dry can reduce the chances that the problem will spread to other toes. In mild cases, which usually involve just the top of the nail and/or skin around the nail, applying full-strength white vinegar two times daily to the site of the infection can reduce fungus. In more severe cases, an effective prescription topical drug regimen is *ketoconazole* (an antifungal) mixed with DMSO, a liquid substance made from wood pulp. DMSO enables the penetration of other liquids—such as ketoconazole—through skin and nails. This regimen is usually prepared by a compounding pharmacist and must be prescribed by a physician. (To find a compounding pharmacist, search online or ask your drugstore pharmacist.) Apply this mixture twice daily to nails and the surrounding skin for several months.

• **Cracked heels and soles.** If you have deep cracks in those thick, unsightly calluses on your feet, lotions, herbal salves and petroleum jelly offer little benefit because the problem is caused more from the inside than the outside. Deep cracks on the bottoms of your feet can indicate a deficiency in vitamin A. Vitamin A is not abundant in food (except in liver). Instead, the body makes vitamin A from beta-carotene, a nutrient that is plentiful in beets, carrots, cantaloupe, sweet potatoes and squash. You can also take a beta-carotene supplement. A typical dose for callus cracks is 50,000 international units (IU) daily, taken with food. You may need to do this for several months for lasting results. After your feet improve, consider taking 25,000 IU of beta-carotene daily as a maintenance dose.

Caution: If you have lung, liver or heart disease, are a smoker or heavy drinker or take prescription medication, check with your doctor before using a beta-carotene supplement. Do not use if you take a multivitamin that contains vitamin A.

• **Swollen feet.** Edema, a term used to mean puffy and swollen, can be caused by circulatory problems, heart and kidney disease, standing for long hours, pregnancy and air travel. Done properly, hydrotherapy can relieve edema by improving your circulation so that your blood vessels and lymph system move excess fluid out of your feet.

Do-it-yourself hydrotherapy: Put hot water (enough to cover your ankles) and one cup of Epsom salts into a basin. Place another basin filled with cold water next to the hot water basin. Soak your feet in the hot water for three minutes, then in the cold for one minute. Alternate between the basins three times, always beginning with hot and ending with cold. Thoroughly dry your feet, and then elevate them above your navel for five minutes. You can do this once or twice daily for as long as needed.

Important: If you have neuropathy and cannot feel hot or cold sensations in your feet, be sure to test the water temperature with your hand first.

Also helpful: Walk for at least 10 minutes twice daily...and elevate your feet while sitting.

Chapter 14

OPTIMUM AGING

The End of "Old Age": Change Your View... Live Longer...

"Old age" has long gotten a bad rap. The conventional thinking has been that it's a time for rocking chairs, fading memory, illness and decrepitude.

Now: As an increasing number of Americans are living—and thriving—into their 80s and beyond, it's more important than ever to cast aside those outdated and harmful attitudes.

What the new thinking can mean for you: Older adults who see aging as a positive stage of life have fewer cardiovascular problems and actually outlive those with gloomier self-perceptions by more than seven years, according to landmark research conducted at Yale University.

So what are you waiting for? There are simple steps you can take to make sure that you aren't missing out on the richness of aging—and this uniquely positive life stage.

The Gifts of Age

As a geriatric psychiatrist, I have worked with hundreds of older adults who have developed life skills and perspectives that, in many ways, enable them to live more successfully than younger adults.

Of course, we can't kid ourselves. Old age does bring some challenges. We become more susceptible to disease. Our brains and bodies slow down. Daily life gets harder in many ways. The flip side is that some of the traits that come with age make us more adept at dealing with adversity and finding purpose in our lives.

Don't believe the myth that older adults get stuck in the past and can't handle new challenges. For example, research has shown that many older adults excel at divergent thinking, the ability to generate different solutions to particular problems. A lifetime of experiences helps them sort through complexities and explore novel ideas.

Other significant benefits that come with growing older—and what you can do to cultivate them in your own life...

• **A reserve of wisdom.** You can be smart and capable at any age, but wisdom is some-

Marc E. Agronin, MD, vice president, behavioral health and clinical research, Miami Jewish Health Systems, and an adult and geriatric psychiatrist and affiliate associate professor of psychiatry and neurology at University of Miami Miller School of Medicine. He writes about senior health for *The Wall Street Journal* and is author of *The End of Old Age*. MarcAgronin.com

thing different. It's an amalgam of all the knowledge, skill and attitudes that you've gained over time.

Wisdom is a trait that we often attribute to the world's great thinkers, but it also has a smaller, day-to-day scope.

Example: Mary, a woman in her 90s, had no earth-shattering life experiences. She wasn't known by anyone outside her small circle of family and friends. But within that circle, she had tremendous influence.

She had two Sunday rituals that gave her a sense of purpose—Catholic Mass in the morning and a family dinner in the afternoon. Her son-in-law would take her to church. After that, she would spend hours with her daughter and other family members preparing a multicourse Italian meal. She was the glue that held the family together—the one who shared recipes...passed along family stories...and overflowed with love. These are powerful forms of wisdom.

My advice: People sometimes ask, "How do I achieve wisdom?"

The answer: You already have it. Think of wisdom as your life's résumé. It might consist of knowledge from previous careers...military experience...being a good listener...a tolerance for different ideas, etc.

• **Resilience.** Hurricane Katrina, which devastated the Gulf Coast, was one of the deadliest hurricanes in history. Older adults were among the most vulnerable and suffered disproportionately. Thousands lost their homes, support networks and even their lives.

Yet subsequent research found that many of them coped just as well with the chaos as younger adults—and, in many cases, even better. Decades of experience increased their stores of resilience, the ability to manage life's obstacles without feeling helpless.

Examples: They didn't sweat the storm-related loss of cell-phone service or the Internet because they tended to view these things as luxuries, not necessities. Shortages of food and water? People who have lived through tough times know how to be resourceful when things are scarce. They could see beyond the chaos and find glimmers of acceptance and hope.

Resilience has physical benefits, as well. Not getting overwrought about difficulties allows the body to quickly recover from stress-related changes—muscle tension, increased heart rate, elevated stress hormones, etc.

Remarkable finding: A study of hundreds of older victims after the storm found that they often had the emotional and psychological strength to deal with the widespread loss of electricity and other basic services. In a way, it's not surprising—these were the same people who went through the Great Depression and World War II. Unlike younger victims, they already knew how to be resourceful in these types of situations.

My advice: Even resilient adults will eventually hit what I call an "age point," in which their resources and coping skills are temporarily overwhelmed. It's important to get help—from a therapist and/or friends and family members—when you suffer such a potentially serious setback. The ultimate resolution can bring growth and greater resilience.

For example, one of my elderly patients had a blood test that indicated abnormal liver enzymes. She was convinced that she had a terminal disease and would be unable to care for her husband who had Alzheimer's disease. Her emotional state started to rapidly deteriorate.

Along with therapy, I treated her with a short-acting tranquilizer, which allowed her to get out of bed, leave the house and function more normally overall. She eventually recovered and was able to go off the medication—and, in some ways, grew stronger.

After further tests showed that she was fine, she recognized that she'd had a turning point that clarified what she wanted from life. She felt that she had been given a second chance to do what really mattered—to care for her husband, be a guide for her son, be active in the community and form a close network of friends.

• **Reinvention.** Older adults can do some of their best work late in life. After a serious illness, the French painter Henri Matisse turned his attention, in his 70s and 80s, to the paper cutouts that appeared in the influential book *Jazz* and eventually revolutionized the world of art. He brought a lifetime of experience to the new medium, along with a sense of freedom that's often missing in the young.

Gene Cohen, MD, a well-known psychiatrist, describes an encore phase that starts in the late 70s and continues until the end of life. People often take up new activities during this phase. It can be artistic endeavors...more reading...landscape design...or even real estate investing!

Important: You can reinvent yourself even if you're dealing with physical/cognitive issues. In fact, these issues mean that you should reinvent. You can shape your interests to circumvent otherwise detrimental changes.

My advice: Start small. Manage your expectations to match your current reality.

For example, one of my clients, a retired professor, suffered from memory loss that made it difficult to keep up with the high-powered, distinguished people she had always spent a lot of time with. She was deeply depressed.

We decided that she should find new intellectual opportunities that didn't require her to be on stage or to "compete." She started taking art and adult-education classes. Family members helped her get used to a computer and an iPad. She was able to pursue her intellectual interests in new (and more comfortable) ways. The opportunities are endless!

Unexpected Health Risks of Menopause... and Beyond

JoAnn V. Pinkerton, MD, NCMP, executive director of the North American Menopause Society, Pepper Pike, Ohio, and professor of obstetrics and gynecology and division director of Midlife Health at the University of Virginia Health Center, Charlottesville.

If you're approaching menopause or are postmenopausal, you already know about bothersome symptoms such as hot flashes and night sweats. And you're likely aware that your risk for serious health conditions, including osteoporosis and heart disease, is now higher.

What you may not know is that the shift in hormone levels that occurs during menopause and continues into postmenopause may be behind other physical and emotional changes—everything from achy joints to dry skin.

We asked Dr. JoAnn V. Pinkerton, executive director of the North American Menopause Society, about some of the less obvious effects menopause and postmenopause may be having on your life and your health...and what you can do.

• **Changes in your skin.** Your biggest organ, the skin, takes a hit from menopause-related hormonal changes in several ways...

You lose collagen, a protein that gives skin its elasticity. Women lose up to 30% of skin collagen in the first five years after menopause, although the exact link to menopausal estrogen loss isn't clear. The less collagen you have, the looser, drier and flakier your skin looks and feels.

Acne, which probably has not been a problem since you were a teen, may rear its head again. Blame a shift in the balance between estrogen and androgen. This hormone-related acne usually develops on your lower face or around your chin, jawline, neck and even upper back.

A more rare, yet disturbing, skin issue that can be related to menopause is formication—an itching, tingling sensation that feels like ants crawling on your skin! It usually develops during early postmenopause. Short-term hormone therapy—two to 12 weeks—may relieve symptoms. It also can have nonhormonal causes, such as allergens or side effects from medications.

What you can do: Follow basic rules of good skin care—drink plenty of water, exercise, eat well, get a good amount of sleep and avoid sun exposure. If you take estrogen in the first five years after menopause (the safest time to do so), it may help you maintain collagen and avoid some of the issues of aging skin...but not all studies agree that it helps.

Advice: Don't take hormone therapy for the sole purpose of skin care. But it might be an added bonus.

• **Achy bones and joints.** Waking up with more than your usual aches and pains? It's a normal part of aging, but women after menopause have it worse than men. Compared with men their age, twice as many postmenopausal women develop osteoarthritis—a "wear and tear" degenerative joint condition. Although how estrogen affects women's joints is not well understood, it is known that there are estrogen receptors in muscles, tendons and cartilage, which all support and protect joints. So it stands to reason that there would be some effect when estrogen levels dip.

Observational studies reveal clues. In the Women's Health Initiative study, the largest US study of postmenopausal women, women on estrogen therapy had fewer hip replacements than women who didn't take estrogen. Those who were taking both estrogen and progestin had less joint stiffness and pain. Finally, women who take aromatase inhibitor drugs to block estrogen (usually to treat estrogen-fueled cancers) commonly do have joint pain.

What you can do: As with skin issues, while hormone therapy may help ward off arthritis, it is not a good reason to start taking it. Instead, whether you take hormone therapy or not, remain as active as you can, since moving your muscles and joints is key to preventing arthritis. Look for low-impact activities that don't stress joints, such as brisk walking, swimming or tai chi. If you're overweight, losing even a small amount of weight can relieve stress on joints. A healthy Mediterranean-style, anti-inflammatory diet may help even if you don't lose weight.

• **Sleep apnea.** Sleep problems are common in menopause, especially if hot flashes and night sweats interrupt sound sleep. And after menopause your risk of developing sleep apnea, a sleep disorder characterized by repeated pauses in breathing during sleep, also rises. Sleep apnea makes you more vulnerable to heart disease and stroke, among other problems.

Postmenopausal women are twice as likely to develop sleep apnea as premenopausal women. In one large study, researchers found that postmenopausal women had different apnea symptoms than men. Men's apnea symptoms were primarily snoring or interrupted breathing at night, while women were more likely to suffer from insomnia, morning headaches, tiredness, depression or anxiety—or even bed-wetting. The increased risk after menopause is believed to be related to hormonal decreases, which may be associated with weight gain. But it can happen even if you don't gain weight.

What you can do: Lifestyle approaches, such as losing weight, not smoking and sleeping on your side, may help. An oral appliance that shifts your jaw position may help, too. But if these approaches don't work, you may need to use a continuous positive airway pressure (CPAP) machine to keep your airway open so that you can breathe normally all night long. If you even think that you might have sleep apnea, talk to your doctor to get diagnosed. In small trials, hormone therapy improved sleep-disordered breathing and sleep disruption.

• **Changes in your senses.** Some women report that their sense of taste, specifically for salty, peppery or sour foods, shifts after menopause. And some women report a strange burning mouth sensation.

There is also evidence that declining estrogen may hasten hearing loss. Your eyes undergo changes, too—they may become dry and itchy after menopause.

What helps: In the case of sensory changes and complaints, research isn't clear about the role of estrogen—or hormone therapy. But understanding that they may be related to the normal menopause process can ease your mind.

Note: Just because some of these health issues are more likely after menopause doesn't mean they'll happen to you! But if you are concerned, talk to your doctor.

And although declining estrogen levels can trigger these conditions and symptoms, the best treatment may not be hormone therapy. Always weigh the benefits against your individual risks.

Is Hormone Therapy for Menopause Back?

JoAnn Manson, MD, DrPH, chief, division of preventive medicine, Brigham and Women's Hospital, Professor, Harvard Medical School, Boston, Massachusetts, and lead author of the study, "Menopausal Hormone Therapy and Long-term All-Cause and Cause-Specific Mortality: The Women's Health Initiative Randomized Trials," published in *JAMA*.

Women who take hormones to ease menopausal symptoms are at no greater risk for early mortality than women who skip them, according to new long-term findings. The findings have just been announced by researchers with the Women's Health Initiative (WHI), and they come from the largest, longest-term study conducted to date on hormone therapy—either estrogen by itself or, more commonly, an estrogen/progestin combination.

In the hormone wars, you might call it a draw. On the one hand, the new data confirm that earlier dire warnings about increased health risks for all women who take these drugs don't translate into shorter lives. On the other hand, this study provides the strongest evidence to date that hormone therapy, while it helps with symptoms, won't provide protection for all women against heart disease and stroke.

The devil, of course, is in the details. Health risks are different depending on how old a woman is when she begins hormone therapy. Younger women (those in their 50s when they enrolled) turned out to have a 30% lower risk for premature death with hormone therapy than without it, but there was no reduction in risk for premature death for women who began the therapy when they were in their 60s and 70s. And the new study leaves unanswered many questions that some women and their doctors are still struggling with. For starters, many "hormone therapy" options are different now than in the 1990s, when they were almost always moderate-to-high doses of conjugated equine estrogens (Premarin)—a complex of estrogenic compounds that are not exactly the same chemically as human estrogen—and *medroxyprogesterone* (Provera), a synthetic form of the hormone progesterone.

In the years since the study began, the way ob-gyns and other physicians prescribe hormone therapy to menopausal women has been transformed. Today, lower doses of the above drugs are more common. Plus, besides the pills that used to be the only way to take hormone therapy, there are now FDA-approved patches that deliver hormones directly into the blood, vaginal inserts that deliver hormones locally to vaginal tissue, bioidentical hormones that are (as the name implies) identical in structure to what a woman produces herself, hormone precursors such as vaginal DHEA and many other options for women experiencing menopausal symptoms.

Help for Hot Flashes

A modest exercise program can help you to navigate the sometimes-turbulent waters of menopause. A recent study followed 166 postmenopausal sedentary women (none were using hormone therapy). Half of the women participated in a cardio/strength fitness program three hours per week for 20 weeks. They also received psychological counseling to help them set goals and deal with setbacks.

Results: Compared with the sedentary women, the active women had fewer hot flashes and better moods, lost weight, reduced blood pressure and increased flexibility.

JoAnn Pinkerton, MD, executive director, The North American Menopause Society and professor, University of Virginia Health System, Charlottesville.

To clarify how the new research affects a woman's decision about hormone therapy, we interviewed menopause expert JoAnn Manson, MD, DrPH, a professor at Harvard Medical School and Brigham and Women's Hospital and lead author of the new research.

Background: When a now-famous large WHI study of estrogen plus progestin that started in 1993 was abruptly halted in 2002—because it seemed so clear that the risks of the hormone therapy outweighed any benefits—many women panicked. For years, women going through menopause had been taking hormones because it not only treated hot flashes but also might protect them from osteoporotic fractures and heart attacks. It did help to reduce bone fractures and type 2 diabetes but also appeared to increase the risk for heart attack and stroke in some women. Estrogen plus progestin increased breast cancer risk, while estrogen alone reduced this risk. Use of hormone therapy plummeted after the 2002 WHI report.

Then in 2013, new data from the same study revealed that the risks were mostly among the women who had begun hormone therapy 10 years or more after menopause. For women who had begun hormone therapy around the time of menopause, there were fewer risks than for older women and even some long-term health benefits. But we still didn't know whether hormone treatment affected lifespan, including the long-term effects on overall death (all-cause mortality) or death from any specific disease (cause-specific mortality). Now, the latest analysis sheds more light on this question.

Latest study: Researchers picked up where the earlier studies stopped and followed the women for another dozen years—for an average follow-up of 18 years. Overall, 7,489 of the WHI participants have died since the study began.

Results: On average—meaning not accounting for the age at which each woman started hormone therapy—there was no statistically different rate of all-cause, cardiovascular or cancer mortality between women who took hormones and those who took placebos. But age made a difference. For all-cause mortality over 18 years, the data suggested a 21% reduced risk with estrogen alone, and minimal reduction for estrogen plus progestin, for women who started hormones before age 60, compared to placebo.

Surprising finding: Deaths from Alzheimer's disease and other forms of dementia were 26% lower among women who used estrogen alone compared with placebo. The finding was intriguing because some earlier studies had suggested that using hormones may actually increase risk for dementia. The researchers point out the possibility that the beneficial effects of hormone therapy on insulin resistance and diabetes, both major determinants of cognitive decline, may have contributed to this surprising finding. Estrogen-only therapy is an option only for women who have had a hysterectomy, however.

The Hormone Decision: What to Do Now

This latest, longer-term study provides reassuring evidence that the hormone treatment used in the WHI didn't lead to excess mortality and remains a reasonable option for management of menopausal symptoms, especially for women in early menopause. However, the treatment should not be used to try to prevent cardiovascular disease or other chronic diseases of aging. Although the same medications used in the study dating back to the 1990s still are available, women have more treatment options now. These include lower doses, different formulations, non-oral routes of hormone delivery, and nonhormonal choices. The North American Menopause Society (NAMS) has a free mobile app (MenoPro, for iOS and Android devices) that helps women work together with their clinicians to individualize decision making about treatment options. What's right for you depends on your menopausal symptoms and how much they are bothering you, your personal medical history and risk factors and, just as important, your personal preferences. The more you know, the better your conversation with your doctor can be—and the more likely that your decision will be right for you.

Menopause Age and Your Risk for Diabetes

Study titled "Age at natural menopause and risk of type 2 diabetes: a prospective cohort study" by researchers at Erasmus University Medical Center in Rotterdam, the Netherlands, published in *Diabetologia*.

The average age at which a women hits menopause is 51. In the years that follow, her risk for diabetes goes up dramatically. You can't blame menopause—entirely. Risk increases with age for everyone—men and women—especially over age 45.

But the hormonal changes that happen with menopause play a role. Starting in the perimenopausal years and accelerating through postmenopause, declining levels of estrogen can lead to rising blood sugar levels and higher insulin levels. Low estrogen also increases a woman's chances of developing abdominal obesity (e.g., becoming more "apple" shaped), which in turn increases diabetes risk. And women who use hormone therapy, which increases their estrogen levels, have a statistically reduced risk of developing diabetes.

Now researchers have found a new twist. It's not just going through menopause that increases diabetes risk. It's how old you are when menopause hits. In this case, being relatively older when you have your last period appears to be a distinct advantage.

Background: Technically, menopause begins one year after a woman's final menstrual period. For most women, this is between the ages of 45 and 55—the average age is 51. Some women reach menopause earlier due to surgery (such as a hysterectomy in which both ovaries are removed). But some women go through natural menopause between 40 and 44 (early menopause), and some even experience it before age 40 (premature menopause). Other women don't reach menopause until after age 55 (late menopause).

It's known that early menopause is associated with increased heart disease risk. But how menopause age affects diabetes risk in women hasn't been well-researched.

Study: Researchers from the Netherlands examined medical histories, lifestyle information and many other health factors related to about 3,600 women. None of the women had diabetes at the start of the study. All of the women provided the age when they entered menopause. Over an average of 9.2 years of follow-up, 348 of the women developed diabetes.

Finding: After adjusting for known risk factors such as obesity, menopause age still made a big difference...

- **Premature menopause.** Women who reached natural menopause before age 40 were nearly four times more likely to develop diabetes than women who reached it after age 55 (late menopause).
- **Early menopause.** Women who reached menopause between the ages of 40 and 44 were more than twice as likely to develop diabetes as those who reached it after 55.
- **Normal menopause.** Even women who reached menopause at so-called normal age (45 to 55 years) had 60% increased risk of developing diabetes compared with women who experienced late menopause.

Overall, for each year of delay reaching menopause, diabetes risk was reduced by 4%.

What about surgical menopause? When the researchers added those numbers in, they found the same statistical phenomenon—the earlier the menopause, the greater the diabetes risk.

Bottom line: While this study can't identify how menopause age affects diabetes risk, the researchers suggest that it may be a signal of early aging. Whatever the reason, the new research suggests that the age at which you hit menopause is a clue to your future risk of diabetes. According to the National Institutes of Health, every American adult age 45 or older should get tested for diabetes.

(The same tests are used to diagnose prediabetes, too.) Yet millions of Americans go undiagnosed. If you hit menopause on the early side, you have a new incentive to get tested as soon as possible.

Underweight Women and Early Menopause

Underweight women risk early menopause. Compared with women who had a body mass index (BMI) of 18.5 to 22.4—considered the normal range—those with BMI less than 18.5 had a 30% higher risk for early menopause, defined as reaching menopause before age 45.

Kathleen L. Szegda, PhD, MPH, postdoctoral researcher, University of Massachusetts, Amherst, and leader of a study of 78,759 women, published in *Human Reproduction.*

FDA-Approved Bioidentical Hormones for Menopause

Mache Seibel, MD, member of the faculty at Beth Israel Deaconess Medical Center and Harvard Medical School, both in Boston, and an expert in women's health and menopause. He is the author of *The Estrogen Fix: The Breakthrough Guide to Being Healthy, Energized, and Hormonally Balanced.* DrMache.com

There are two ways to get bioidentical hormone therapy (BHRT)—through FDA-approved prescriptions or through a compounding pharmacy. The first choice is much safer.

First, though, let's explain what bioidentical hormones are. They are hormones that are manufactured to have the same chemical structure as the ones that are produced by women's bodies. The primary form of estrogen that women make in their ovaries is estradiol. FDA-approved Premarin, the most common prescription hormone treatment in the US, is not bioidentical—it is 17% estradiol but also contains dozens of other compounds. In contrast, bioidentical hormones can be produced that contain nearly 100% estradiol. Some are derived from plant sources, such as a special kind of yam. Some studies suggest that they are better for women's health—for example, by not raising the risk for breast cancer, cardiovascular disease or cognitive issues as much as Premarin does—but the research is not conclusive. I believe they are comparable in risk.

The good news for women who make this choice is that there are many FDA-approved bioidentical hormone products that supply estradiol that you can buy...with a prescription, of course...at any neighborhood pharmacy. They have names such as Estrace, Alora, Climara, Estring and Vagifem. A woman who still has her uterus and who goes on hormone therapy for menopause symptoms should also take progesterone to reduce her risk for uterine cancer. FDA-approved bioidentical progesterone products, such as Prometrium, are available as well. (At present, there are no combined estrogen/progesterone prescriptions that are bioidentical, except for pharmacy-compounded ones, but they are in development.)

The other type of place where you could get bioidentical hormones is a compounding pharmacy. This type of pharmacy makes medication to order based on health-care providers' specific instructions. You might assume that custom-compounded drugs would be ideal, since they're made to order, but in fact they aren't approved by the FDA...and experience has shown that their quality varies widely. In fact, you might not get what your doctor ordered. Research in the last years has found this can lead to serious health problems.

Example: In one study, researchers had 12 different compounding pharmacies fill the same prescription, then had each filled prescription analyzed at a chemical lab. It turned out that estrogen was provided by these pharmacies at doses of as much as 173% more than what had been prescribed, and progesterone was provided at doses of up to 40% less than what had been prescribed. Because of the incorrect estrogen/progesterone ratios, taking such incorrectly filled prescriptions could lead to a condition called hyperplasia, an increase in cell production that can lead to uterine cancer—and that is just one of the potentially serious outcomes that could possibly result from incorrectly compounded hormones.

I would encourage you to choose FDA-approved hormones. If you're set on the path of compounded hormones, though, I'd recommend that you have your uterine lining checked once a year for abnormality. Most health-care providers who prescribe these compounds will do this with a biopsy or ultrasound—and if the ultrasound reveals that the thickness of the uterine lining is more than four millimeters, you'll need a biopsy anyway, regardless of whether you are using hormone therapy. It's also a good idea to seek out a compounding pharmacy that is accredited by the Accreditation Commission for American Health Care. That's helpful, although it's no guarantee.

Bottom line: If you want bioidentical hormones, stick with the FDA-approved drugstore preparations. You can get patches, gels, creams, sprays and pills in a wide variety of doses. Talk to your doctor about which one is best for relief of the menopause-related symptoms that bother you the most. These products are regulated, so you and your doctor will know exactly what you're getting.

Are You Afraid of Hormones?

Holly Lucille, ND, RN, a naturopathic doctor whose private practice, Healing from Within Healthcare, in West Hollywood, California, focuses on comprehensive naturopathic medicine and individualized care. She is author of *Creating and Maintaining Balance: A Woman's Guide to Safe, Natural Hormone Health.* DrHollyLucille.com.

I can't tell you how many women come in to my practice seeking help for symptoms associated with perimenopause and menopause and exclaim, *I am miserable but I don't want hormones—they're dangerous.* While it is true I will always seek to find the least invasive way to diagnose and treat any symptom or condition in the spirit of doing no harm, let me tell you—I have prescribed plenty of hormones. I do so when I detect an imbalance in the body's highly sophisticated hormone system that I believe is contributing to the woman's symptoms and clinical issues.

Let me explain.

We're bombarded with information from TV, radio, brochures, blogs, tweets, posts, newspapers, webinars, you name it...on a daily basis. For most people, these sources have become their main source of information on hormone therapies. As is the case with most health matters these days, some of this information can indeed be helpful. But it may be only part of the story—or, at times, completely biased and misleading.

Part of the problem when discussing hormones is that many highlights, headlines and media statements discuss them in general terms and do not distinguish between bioidentical and other, nonbioidentical forms. In fact, the studies conducted to actually test the safety and benefits of hormone therapies

Safer Hormone Therapy

The latest research on vaginal estrogen for menopausal symptoms shows that these creams, inserts or rings are safer than oral estrogen, which may increase stroke and breast cancer risk. A study of 45,663 women, followed for more than six years, found that those who used vaginal estrogen, compared with women who didn't use any hormonal product, had no greater risk for breast cancer, stroke, heart disease or hip fracture. Vaginal estrogen relieves symptoms including vaginal dryness, itching and urinary urgency.

Carolyn J. Crandall, MD, MS, professor of medicine, David Geffen School of Medicine at the University of California at Los Angeles.

are directly responsible for confusion and misinformation. For example, the landmark study known as the Women's Health Initiative (WHI), that was constructed to demonstrate the long-term effects of non-biodentical estrogens and progestin hormone therapies and to assess the risk for heart disease, fractures and breast cancer, suffered from a major limitation. The hormone products used were Premarin, which comes from pregnant horse urine, and Prempro, which contains Premarin and a synthetic progestin called *medroxyprogesterone*.

The Prempro arm of this study was initially halted due to an increased risk for breast cancer, heart disease, stroke and blood clots. Then, the Premarin portion of the study was also stopped, due to an increased risk for stroke. These results and the attention they received terrified not only women but also their practitioners, leaving many questions regarding hormone therapies.

Then in 2013 a different story emerged from the same study. For women who began Prempro hormone therapy around the time of menopause, there actually was no increased cardiovascular risk—and even some benefit.

Worse yet, the results were broadly attributed to bioidentical hormones as well. You see, the agents used in this study and bioidentical hormones do not have the same effects on the body. They are very different compounds.

Bioidentical hormones are chemically indistinguishable from the hormones in our bodies. They produce the same physiologic response as our own naturally occurring hormones, and they are the only hormone therapies that I use in my practice. As research is finally starting to include bioidentical hormone preparations, current evidence demonstrates that the bioidentical hormones are associated with lower risks than their nonbioidentical counterparts.

To be sure, bioidentical hormones that are prepared in compounded pharmacies have been controversial. There have been some cases of inaccurate doses, so it's important that you work with a health-care provider who has a good relationship with a compounding pharmacy that can be trusted. Also, there are now FDA-approved bioidentical formations.

Part of my job, as well as a tenet that I practice by, is to be a "doctor as teacher." Because of their history and "word on the street" surrounding hormone therapy, I do understand the fear and reservation many women have around their use. However, I have seen compounded bioidentical hormones provide so much relief for so many when symptoms become overwhelming and nothing else is working. If I feel hormones are an option that could help improve the life of my patient, I carefully explain about bioidentical hormones and together we assess the risk for her.

Awareness, education and individualized treatment are the key to healthy and safe hormone balance. Don't let fear and misinformation stop you from getting the best care. There are plenty of educated and astute practitioners who specialize in these therapies that you can partner with. Consider finding one at Naturopathic.org.

Anxiety After Menopause

JoAnn V. Pinkerton, MD, executive director of The North American Menopause Society and professor of obstetrics and gynecology and division director of midlife health, The University of Virginia Health System, Charlottesville.

Anxiety is common in perimenopause. But new research finds that it's common in postmenopause, too—and is linked to severe symptoms that can interfere with your quality of life.

According to a recent study of 3,503 postmenopausal women ages 40 to 59, published in *Menopause*, the likelihood of having severe menopausal symptoms—especially hot flashes, sleep problems, a racing heart, and muscle and joint pain—was five times higher in those who reported that they felt anxious. One possible explanation is that anxiety boosts the stress-related neurotransmitter norepinephrine, which can trigger symptoms such as hot flashes.

What to do: Find ways to reduce menopausal symptoms and anxiety. A number of approaches could help, including regular exercise, breathing exercises, relaxation techniques such as mindfulness meditation and reducing caffeine. Using the supplement hops and aromatherapy with neroli oil may also offer relief.* If anxiety symptoms persist, be sure to seek professional help.

*Hops can cause drowsiness—do not combine with alcohol or sedatives. If you have allergies or asthma, check with your doctor before trying aromatherapy.

Menopause Can Make Your Breasts Hurt

Mache Seibel, MD, member of the faculty at Beth Israel Deaconess Medical Center and Harvard Medical School, both in Boston, and an expert in women's health and menopause. He is the author of *The Estrogen Fix: The Breakthrough Guide to Being Healthy, Energized, and Hormonally Balanced.* DrMache.com

Discomfort, even pain, is fairly common for menopausal women in one or both breasts. Most of the reasons are not dangerous but, of course, it's important to find out the cause, and when something is hurting, you'll want to find a solution as soon as you can.

The breasts are extremely sensitive to the hormones estrogen and progesterone. In the months leading up to menopause and in the year or two after, hormones are still being produced, though at lower levels, and levels are quite unbalanced. These suboptimal fluctuations of estrogen and occasionally progesterone can influence the breasts and cause them to feel tender or swollen or feel as if the skin is stretched tightly. You may even feel sharp, stabbing pain.

If you are on hormone therapy, the reintroduction of higher hormone levels can cause one or both breasts to feel quite sensitive and to enlarge—and the increased size can lead to discomfort. As your body gets used to the steady dosage of hormones, your breast pain symptoms should subside.

Sleuthing Out Breast Pain

The first step to dealing with breast discomfort is to make sure there isn't something else going on besides normal hormonal fluctuations.

There could be a physical cause. You may have stretched a ligament (the fibrous connective tissue that supports your breast), and that would definitely cause discomfort. Similarly, if you've recently bruised a rib, it may feel like your breast hurts when in fact it's the bone underneath. It's also possible to have strained the muscles that cover the ribs and lie beneath and surrounding the breasts, which often happens to women who lift heavy objects, rake, shovel or do weight training. Breasts can also become inflamed, a condition called mastitis. Often there is warmth associated with this. There could also be a cyst in the breast causing pain. Caffeine can also bring on breast pain in some women.

Is It Cancer?

Breast pain can be a symptom of cancer, though typically pain isn't an early symptom. But because breast pain is so frightening for most women and because of the potential serious nature of breast pain, if you have any kind of breast pain, make an appointment to see your health-care provider soon. A simple exam will provide answers in many instances. Some testing, such as a breast ultrasound, a mammogram or other testing, may be ordered to confirm a diagnosis. The good news is that more times than not, the answer to, *What is causing my breast pain?* is going to be something other than cancer.

In the short term, wear a well-fitted and supportive bra...wear a sports bra during exercise...limit caffeine...try an anti-inflammatory such as *ibuprofen*...and apply cold packs.

The 6 Best Foods for Your Skin

Torey Armul, MS, RD, CSSD, LD, a registered dietitian, nutritionist and national media spokesperson for the Academy of Nutrition and Dietetics. She is author of *Bun Appétit: A Simple Guide to Eating Right During Pregnancy.* Armul provides private counseling and consulting services in Columbus, Ohio.

Want healthier skin and fewer wrinkles? Men and women can look younger and lower their risk for skin cancer, psoriasis, eczema and more by eating certain foods. *The following foods have been scientifically proven to boost the health, strength and appearance of your skin...*

Yellow Bell Peppers

Yellow bell peppers are one of the most abundant sources of vitamin C. The body depends on vitamin C to form collagen, a protein that provides strength, support and elasticity to skin, hair, muscles and other tissues. Collagen also assists with cell regrowth and repair. As we age, our bodies produce less collagen, which can lead to reduced elasticity of the skin and more wrinkles.

The relationship between vitamin C and skin appearance was studied in more than 4,000 women in a report published in *The American Journal of Clinical Nutrition.* Researchers found that higher dietary intake of vitamin C was associated with lower likelihood of skin dryness and fewer wrinkles, as assessed by dermatologists. These results were independent of age, race, sun exposure, body mass index and physical activity.

Why not eat oranges, famous for their vitamin C, instead? A typical large orange contains 163% of the recommended daily value (DV) of vitamin C. That's good—but just half a yellow bell pepper contains nearly 300% of the DV of vitamin C. (Red and green peppers have less vitamin C than yellow ones but still are excellent sources.)

Eat yellow peppers raw to maximize the nutrient content. Vitamin C is sensitive to cooking and, as a water-soluble vitamin, leaches into cooking water. If you prefer to cook yellow peppers, keep the heat as low as possible for your recipe. Use the cooking juices, too (whenever possible), so that the vitamin C in the water is not wasted.

Sweet Potatoes

Sweet potatoes are an excellent source of carotenoids, the antioxidant pigments that give many foods their bright red, orange, yellow and green colors—and help keep skin cells healthy.

In a study published in *British Journal of Nutrition*, participants who ate more carotenoid-rich vegetables had significantly fewer facial wrinkles.

Eating carotenoids also can make you look healthier overall and more attractive to others. Carotenoid levels in skin contribute to healthy skin coloration. In fact, researchers from University of St. Andrews, Scotland, found that people whose faces were rated as healthy by others had consumed an average of 2.9 fruit and vegetable portions each day... and whose faces were rated separately as attractive had consumed 3.3 daily portions.

Carotenoids are fat-soluble, which means that they're better absorbed when paired with a fat-containing food—so sprinkle nuts or drizzle olive oil over your sweet potatoes for a delicious skin boost.

Salmon

Although protein in your food does not directly affect protein in your body's collagen, some research shows that amino acids (the building blocks of protein) are related to collagen synthesis in the skin.

Some amino acids are "essential," meaning that they're necessary for life but are not made in the body. They must be provided by food or supplements. Salmon contains all the essential amino acids—and essential amino acids play a unique role in skin health. In a study published in *Amino Acids,* researchers found that consuming a combination of essential amino acids significantly increased the rate of collagen synthesis in mice with UV-damaged skin.

Salmon also is a good source of monounsaturated fat, which was found to be positively associated with skin elasticity in older women in a study published in *British Journal of Nutrition*.

Don't love fish? Essential amino acids also are found in poultry, eggs, beans and whole grains.

Walnuts

Walnuts are rich in omega-3 polyunsaturated fatty acids, which help the body make the collagen needed for healthy skin. Omega-3s help reduce inflammation and have been shown to reduce symptoms in inflammatory skin diseases such as psoriasis and acne.

The European Journal of Cancer published research comparing omega-3 fat intake to the development of malignant melanoma in more than 20,000 women. Data showed that higher intakes of omega-3s were associated with an 80% lower risk for skin cancer, leading researchers to conclude that these fats "have a substantial protective association" against melanoma.

Like essential amino acids, omega-3 fats are vitally important but are not made in the body. You must get them from your diet or supplements. Aside from walnuts (and salmon, discussed above), other excellent sources of omega-3s include flaxseed oil, ground flaxseed, chia seeds, canola oil and tofu.

Raspberries and Pomegranates

There is exciting research on collagen and how it is affected by ellagic acid, an antioxidant found in certain fruits and vegetables.

A study published in *Experimental Dermatology* found that mice who received ellagic acid had significantly reduced collagen breakdown from UV light, compared with mice who did not receive ellagic acid. The treatment group also developed fewer wrinkles. While most research focuses on the treatment of skin damage, this study was unique in its ability to show the role of nutrition in the prevention of collagen breakdown, wrinkles and skin damage.

Foods that are high in ellagic acid include raspberries and pomegranates (as well as blackberries, strawberries and cranberries).

Chickpeas

Zinc is an important ingredient for skin health because it supports the regeneration of new skin cells. The benefits are most apparent with skin repair and wound healing, but zinc also may be able to help with other skin problems such as rashes, eczema and acne.

A study published in *BioMed Research International* found a correlation between participants' zinc levels and the severity of their acne symptoms. Researchers believe that this is partly due to zinc's ability to inhibit the overgrowth of *Propionibacterium acnes,* a bacterium that contributes to acne.

Legumes were the focus of another study in *The Journal of the American College of Nutrition*. Researchers found that higher intakes of legumes, such as chickpeas, appeared to protect against sun-induced wrinkles in people with a variety of ethnic and geographic backgrounds.

Chickpeas are a good source of zinc, as are other beans, oysters, poultry, tofu, oatmeal and zinc-fortified cereals.

Got Age Spots?

Valori Treloar, MD, CNS, a board-certified dermatologist in private practice at Integrative Dermatology in Newton, Massachusetts. A fellow of the American Academy of Dermatology, she is coauthor of *The Clear Skin Diet*. Dr. Treloar is also a Certified Nutrition Specialist, a credential awarded by the American College of Nutrition.

Soaking in the sun can leave you with more than just wrinkles. Age spots—those flat, roundish marks that appear on sun-exposed areas such as the face, chest and backs of hands—also result from exposure to ultraviolet (UV) light, which stimulates the production of pigment known as melanin. Sometimes called liver spots, these brown, tan or black marks actually have nothing to do with the liver...or with age, for that matter. Age spots are more common among fair-skinned and light-haired individuals, and they affect men and women about equally.

Harmless or Not?

True age spots, also called solar lentigines, are harmless. If you find them unsightly, you can significantly lighten them or, in some cases, render them almost invisible with the therapies described below.

Important: Some skin cancers can masquerade as age spots. That's why it's crucial that you show any new or changing growths or spots to a dermatologist. Be aware of the ABCDE signs of skin cancer—Asymmetry, Border irregularity, Color that is not uniform, Diameter greater than 6 mm (size of a pencil eraser) and Evolving size, shape or color.

A Natural Approach

Over-the-counter (OTC) topical products cost significantly less than prescription treatments...but they don't work quite as well. Even with consistent use and rigorous sun protection, it can take a month or so to see some improvement. *For an OTC product, consider one that contains one of these ingredients...**

- **Niacinamide (vitamin B-3).** Topical niacinamide lightens age spots without irritation. Hundreds of skin creams contain this ingredient. Look for one with a 2% to 5% concentration for best results. This cream can be used on your face, chest, arms, hands, etc.
- **Glycolic acid.** Originally sourced from sugarcane, glycolic acid is used in varying concentrations in facial peels, cleansers, moisturizers and serums. Also called a fruit peel, it exfoliates the outer layer of dead skin cells. When purchasing a product, make sure glycolic acid is listed as an active ingredient...or look for a product with 5% to 10% glycolic acid. It can be used all over the body if it's tolerated—glycolic acid can be irritating for some people.

Niacinamide works better for some, but for others glycolic acid is more effective.

Eat to Beat Age Spots

A plant-based diet, filled with antioxidant-rich produce, may help combat sun-induced skin damage by fighting harmful free radicals. Eat plenty of berries, dark leafy greens and tomatoes. Foods rich in beta-carotene may be particularly helpful—the carotenoids that give sweet potatoes and other orange produce their color get converted to vitamin A in the body, speeding cell turnover and perhaps helping the top layer of skin to shed more quickly.

These foods alone won't prevent age spots, but they may slow their growth and help prevent new spots from forming.

My advice: Eat nine fist-size servings of vegetables that have a variety of colors each day.

Prescription Creams

The following products, which can be prescribed by your doctor, are considered the most effective topical treatments for age spots. *Note:* Insurance companies generally will not cover age spot treatments as they are considered cosmetic.

- **Hydroquinone.** This bleaching cream interrupts pigment production. With a prescription-strength cream containing 3% or 4% hydroquinone, you may notice lightening within a few weeks...maximum effect occurs after a few months. Apply it twice daily to the spots only, not the surrounding skin. This cream can be used all over the body if it's tolerated.

Note: Do not use if you are pregnant or breastfeeding or are using peroxide products.

- **Tretinoin.** This vitamin A–based product slows melanin production and increases skin cell turnover. Sunlight causes tretinoin to break down, so you should apply it only at night. I recommend applying it to your face or other affected area one to two times

**Caution*: Products made outside the US may contain mercury. Use caution if buying online.

a week to begin. Then when any redness or irritation has subsided, use it nightly. For initial treatment of the face, dilute the tretinoin with a mild face cream. Tretinoin can take up to 40 weeks for noticeable results.

I like a combination hydroquinone/tretinoin product that includes a topical steroid, which helps calm possible irritation.

Topical treatments cost an average of $50 to $200 per tube. A course of treatment may require one or more tubes.

Want a Healthy Glow? Feed Your Flora!

Ginger Hodulik Downey holds a BS in foods and nutrition, an MS degree in nutrition and a CNS (Certified Nutrition Specialist). She is currently the co-owner and vice president of R&D for DermaMed Solutions.

Did you know that your skin is crawling with bugs? This may sound scary, but it's true! But don't worry, the good bacteria feeds our flora (and our flora makes us beautiful)!

Our skin supports a delicate ecosystem of microorganisms, including yeast and bacteria. We can't see them, but they are there and they serve an important function. When most of us think of microorganisms we think of bad things. The bacteria living on our skin offer immunity and support skin health... these are good bugs! When we over-strip our skin by using harsh cleansers and chemical peeling agents, we can kill our good flora and allow bad bugs to move in. Over the past several years, research has begun to show that the application of topical probiotics can help keep the bad microbes in check and improve skin condition.

Probiotics do this in three ways…

- **Act as a protective shield** (protecting skin from redness and inflammation)
- **Have antimicrobial properties** (specific strains poke holes in bad bacteria and kill it)
- **Offer calming of irritations** (preventing threat reaction and signals that flare acne and rosacea).

Many progressive skin care lines are incorporating topical probiotic strains, like *lactobacillus* into their products in response to this compelling research. For those who want to harness the power of live bacteria to improve skin health with items found in their own homes, you can make a yogurt mask and apply it to the skin for 15 or 20 minutes. (Another home mask idea is to break open a probiotic dietary supplement capsule, mix with water, olive oil or your favorite lotion, and apply it to the face for 15 minutes.)

There's an inside-out/outside-in story to be told here as well. Your gut is also lined with beneficial flora. These bacteria help to digest food, metabolize vitamins and provide immune support. Many nutritionists believe that your gut health is reflected in the condition of your skin. When gut flora are out of balance many people experience rashes, allergies and overall skin inflammation.

Antibiotic use, stress, travel, and poor diet can disrupt the balance of the skin and gut bacteria and cause red, puffy skin, rashes, inflammation, and even acne and psoriasis. A proper diet, rich in prebiotics and probiotics can help maintain your healthy bacterial balance and in turn give you healthy skin. To clarify, the probiotic foods are the ones which contain the live bacteria. Prebiotics are foods rich in a certain type of fiber called FOS (Fructooligosaccharides) and these feed the bacteria.

Good food choices to include in your regular diet are…

- **Yogurt** (check label for live active cultures)
- **Keifer**
- **Sauerkraut**
- **Miso, tempeh and natto** (fermented soy foods)
- **Kimchi**
- **Buttermilk**
- **Fortified foods** like cottage cheese and/or other foods fortified with probiotics

• **Probiotic supplements**

• **Prebiotic rich foods** like asparagus, leeks, garlic and onions

Our understanding of the role of the bacteria that resides on and in our bodies is limited, but growing every day as scientists make new and exciting discoveries. It's becoming more and more clear that we need to pay attention to—and nourish—these bugs both internally and externally as a tool for improving our skin health.

Why not add a probiotic-enhanced skin care product in your daily skin-care regimen to improve the texture and integrity of your skin? That, combined with a diet rich in probiotic and probiotic laden foods will help you to achieve a healthy glow!

The Best Anti-Aging Exercise for Your Muscles

Study titled "Enhanced Protein Translation Underlies Improved Metabolic and Physical Adaptations to Different Exercise Training Modes in Young and Old Humans" by researchers at Mayo Clinic, Rochester, Minnesota, published in *Cell Metabolism*.

Exercise benefits the body at any age, but a certain kind of exercise, new research finds, is particularly effective at counteracting the effects of aging on your muscles. It stimulates literally hundreds of genes that enhance the ability of muscle cells to convert nutrients into energy—an essential function that tends to decline with age. For younger people, this form of exercise is a good way to get fitter and healthier.

If you're older, it's a great way.

Background: There's no question that exercise is key to aging gracefully—being fit and strong fights age-related risks for disease and disability. As we age, our muscle mass decreases—and our muscles become less efficient at turning oxygen and nutrients into energy. Exercise counters both trends. But little has been known about what kind of exercise is most effective at keeping older muscles younger.

Study: Researchers from Mayo Clinic in Rochester, Minnesota, enrolled healthy men and women in a study that looked at the effects of three different types of exercise. The first was resistance (strength) training. The second was high-intensity aerobic interval training (HIIT), during which the exerciser pushes all-out for a brief spurt and then recovers while exercising at a reduced pace, and then repeats the process. The third was a combination of moderate-intensity aerobic exercise plus less intense resistance training. The researchers evaluated various markers of health.

Unlike similar studies, however, this one was conducted on two groups of people in very different stages of life. The younger group was 18 to 30 years old…the older group, 65 to 80. Baseline laboratory tests and muscle biopsies were conducted at the beginning of the study and after it ended 12 weeks later.

Results: All three exercise types improved insulin sensitivity, a key way that exercise helps prevent diabetes. Both HIIT and combined aerobic/resistance training led to improvements in aerobic capacity. Resistance training increased muscle mass. None of these results was surprising—and the effects were similar in both age groups.

But HIIT was really a hit for the older set in the way it increased the activity of genes that are thought to improve mitochondrial function. Mitochondria are tiny power plants inside every cell. As we age, the mitochondria in our cells diminish in both quantity and quality…and that leads to reduced ability to convert oxygen and nutrients into energy.

In the older study group, muscle biopsies showed that nearly 400 genes that affect mitochondria became more active with HIIT. In the younger group, 274 such genes became more active. In the older exercisers, HIIT was particularly effective at reversing low activity levels of 11 genes that are known decline with age.

Bottom line: HIIT is a great approach to fitness, especially if you're older. Here's the program that was used in the study…

Three days a week, exercisers pedaled stationary bikes—fast and hard for four minutes, followed by a three-minute interval of slow pedaling. They repeated that cycle for a total of four times.

Twice a week, on other days, they ran on a treadmill at 70% of capacity for 45 minutes. That's not interval training, but it rounded out the weekly aerobic program.

If this program seems intense, that is because it is! Although the study didn't look at less intense intervals, do what you are comfortable doing and work your way up. You may not reap the same benefit of the study participants right off the bat, but you will be on the right track.

How to Protect Your Eyesight!

Mrinali Patel Gupta, MD, a retina specialist and assistant professor of ophthalmology at Weill Cornell Medicine in New York City. Her research has been published in many professional journals, and she was a recipient of the Howard Hughes Medical Institute-National Institutes of Health Research Fellowship for her work on AMD at the National Eye Institute.

How would you feel if you lost your eyesight? When asked this question, nearly half of Americans recently surveyed by researchers at Johns Hopkins University said that it would be the worst possible thing that could happen to their health. Ironically, half of the respondents in the same survey were completely unaware of age-related macular degeneration (AMD), a leading cause of blindness in the US.

The Basics of AMD

The word "age" in AMD doesn't mean that the condition affects only the elderly. Rather, it means that the incidence of AMD rises with age. The exact causes of AMD are unknown, but some risk factors are well established—such as age, gender (women get it more often than men) and race (whites face a higher risk than other races).

Other risk factors: Having blue eyes... obesity...and high blood pressure. A healthy lifestyle that includes not smoking and a nutritious diet are the best ways to help reduce the risk for AMD.

Dry and Wet AMD

AMD affects and damages the macula of the retina—the region of the retina responsible for central vision (seeing what's right in front of us) and fine acuity vision (seeing fine details).

There are two forms of AMD—dry and wet. The dry form accounts for 90% of people with AMD. In the early stages, dry AMD may cause no visual symptoms, which is why routine eye exams are important for diagnosis. As dry AMD progresses, patients may start to notice subtle changes or distortions in central vision such as straight lines that appear wavy or written words that seem to be missing letters. In the late stages of dry AMD, patients may have severe vision loss. In general, however, the progression of dry AMD is slow and occurs over many years, and some patients may never have vision loss.

Wet AMD is characterized by abnormal blood vessels that grow under and into the retina. The blood vessels can leak blood and fluid that reduce vision and damage the retina. Wet AMD causes the majority of cases of AMD-related blindness and can progress rapidly.

The dry form of AMD can progress to the wet form—risk of conversion from dry to wet AMD is approximately 14% to 20% over five years. There may be no symptoms early in the conversion of dry to wet AMD. Subsequently, patients may notice subtle vision changes such as those described above. Severe vision loss, such as dramatic reduction in overall vision or a large dark area in central vision, can develop, especially if wet AMD goes untreated.

Diagnosis of AMD

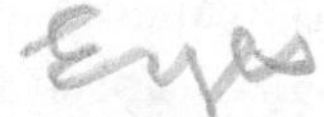

Because most people with dry AMD may have no symptoms, regular eye exams are important to identify the early signs of the disease. AMD can be diagnosed during a routine dilated eye exam done by an oph-

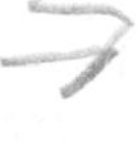

thalmologist or optometrist. The American Academy of Ophthalmology advises a baseline eye exam at age 40 (earlier if you have eye disease or are at risk for developing eye disease) and an exam every year or two at age 65 and older. However, your doctor may advise more frequent exams based on your specific situation.

If you experience any slowly progressive (over weeks or months) vision changes, get promptly evaluated by an ophthalmologist. And if you have severe and sudden vision loss, see an eye doctor immediately, preferably on the same day, for an evaluation to determine if you need emergency treatment.

Treatment for Dry AMD

If you have dry AMD, there are currently no medical treatments, but it can be effectively managed to prevent progression. *What to do...*

• **Maintain a healthy lifestyle**—don't smoke and eat a nutritious diet.

• **Get an eye exam once or twice yearly,** including an optical coherence tomography scan to check for progression from dry to wet AMD. This noninvasive imaging test allows doctors to examine the retina to detect the abnormal blood vessels of wet AMD at very early stages. Your doctor may repeat the test at every visit. The test is also used to monitor wet AMD.

• **Self-monitor.** Use the Amsler grid—with horizontal and vertical lines—at least a few times a week to check for subtle vision changes in each eye. If there's any change in the grid when looking at it, such as straight lines that appear crooked/wavy or parts of the grid are missing, you should contact your eye doctor. A downloadable Amsler grid is available at AmslerGrid.org, and grids are also available as a smartphone app.

Also: For some patients, getting the right nutrients may prevent dry AMD from worsening. An eye doctor can tell you if your situation warrants vitamins for your eyes.

What the research shows: A large clinical trial led by the National Institutes of Health found that patients with intermediate or advanced AMD in only one eye who took an antioxidant mix—500 mg of vitamin C...400 international units (IU) of vitamin E...15 mg of beta-carotene...80 mg of zinc...and 2 mg of copper (known as the AREDS formula)—were less likely to have progression of AMD.

Note: Current or former smokers should use the newer AREDS2 formula, which has lutein and zeaxanthin instead of beta-carotene—beta-carotene is associated with increased risk for lung cancer in smokers.

These mixes are available over-the-counter in pharmacies.

Breakthrough Injections

Previously, the average patient with wet AMD quickly lost significant vision (two to three lines on the vision chart in the first two years alone). But with the advent of anti-vascular endothelial growth factor (VEGF) therapy, vision can be stabilized or improved in roughly half of patients.

Multiple large clinical trials have demonstrated that intravitreal injection (into the eye) of medications that block VEGF, such as *bevacizumab* (Avastin) and *aflibercept* (Eylea), dramatically reduce vision loss in wet AMD.

The procedure is done with local anesthesia in the ophthalmologist's office. It's quick and usually painless. The injections are often given monthly...or on a less frequent basis, depending on how the patient is doing. Some people need long-term therapy, while others can over time reduce or discontinue it but are monitored closely as many patients subsequently need additional treatments (when the wet AMD becomes active again). The treatment controls wet AMD but is not a cure. The risk associated with injections is very low but includes cataracts, retinal detachment, bleeding or infection/inflammation in the eye.

eyes

The Cataract Fix

David F. Chang, MD, clinical professor of ophthalmology at University of California, San Francisco. He is coauthor of *Cataracts: A Patient's Guide to Treatment.*

No one wants to have surgery—any surgery. But once you have had cataract surgery, you'll probably wonder why you waited so long.

Recent developments: Cataract surgery now takes about 20 minutes for most people. You'll go home soon after the procedure...serious, vision-threatening complications, such as infection, are extremely rare...and it's successful in about 99% of cases, making it one of the most effective of all surgeries.

The benefits are undeniable. Within days, you'll see better—with sharper vision, better nighttime eyesight and fewer bright-light "halos." But that's not all.

The procedure, which usually is done on one eye at a time, is performed while you're awake and while your eye is numbed with eye-drop anesthesia, so it's not even painful. Most health insurance plans pick up the tab.

But is it for you?

Is It Your Time?

Most people are familiar with the telltale signs of cataracts—the normally clear lens within your eye becomes cloudy and/or discolored. Because the lens focuses incoming visual images and transmits them to the retina, these changes, though generally gradual (occurring over a period of years), can cause significant vision loss if untreated.

Important: The lens sits behind the iris and pupil, so you can't self-diagnose cataracts by looking in a mirror. Only an eye doctor using a special microscope can actually see cataracts.

That's why it's important to see an eye doctor (in addition to having routine eye exams) if you're experiencing vision problems, including blurred vision, difficulty seeing details (such as small print or road signs) and glare or poor night-driving vision.

Age is the main risk factor for cataracts. When you're young, the proteins that form the lenses of your eyes are arranged in a way that makes the structures crystal-clear. Over time, these proteins eventually start to clump together and reduce the amount of light that passes through.

By your 60s and 70s, these changes will have gradually begun to occur. Most people, if they live long enough, will develop cataracts that are advanced enough for them to consider surgery.

Earlier-onset of cataracts has been associated with such risk factors as smoking, diabetes, prior retinal surgery, severe nearsightedness, excessive sun exposure and prolonged use of certain medications such as steroids.

What Are You Waiting For?

Cataracts can affect one or both eyes, either simultaneously or at different times. In the past, doctors advised patients to delay surgery until a cataract was "ripe"—meaning that it was so advanced that the benefits justified the lengthy recovery and the potential for complications due to the large incision that was used at that time. Unfortunately, many people are still operating under this misconception.

Newer thinking: You don't need to wait so long. If the cataract is impairing your daily activities, such as reading and/or driving, it makes sense to have cataract surgery sooner rather than later because of the procedure's exceptionally high success rate.

Now the lens is broken up into many small pieces using ultrasonic vibrations within the eye, then suctioned out. The incisions are so small that stitches aren't required—and cataracts can be safely removed at an earlier stage. The replacement artificial lens lasts a lifetime and is folded so that it can pass through the tiny (about one-eighth inch) incision.

The timing is important because cataracts can get so bad that they increase a person's risk for falls and auto/pedestrian accidents, as well as contribute to depression.

These factors may have something to do with the recent research regarding cataract surgery that was published online in the journal *JAMA Ophthalmology*.

Key findings: This study of more than 74,000 women ages 65 and older found that those who had undergone cataract surgery had a 60% lower risk of dying over the 20-year study period than those who did not get treated.

Better Vision Without Glasses

You'll obviously see better once a cataract is removed. What some people don't realize is that they might see better than they ever did.

The surgeon will remove the cloudy lens and replace it with a clear, artificial lens that comes in more than 50 different powers.

Suppose that you have always worn glasses to see well in the distance. When you have cataract surgery, a replacement lens can be chosen to correct your particular type/degree of optical error. For example, some lenses correct for astigmatism (blurred vision that is caused by incorrect corneal curvature). Certain artificial lenses function like bifocals and reduce how frequently people must rely on reading glasses.

In most cases, cataract surgery won't completely eliminate the need for glasses. Most people will have excellent distance vision without glasses following cataract surgery. However, most will need reading glasses—but can perhaps use them less often and/or get by with a lower-power prescription.

What Else Can You Do?

Surgery is the only treatment for cataracts, and it is a permanent solution—the new lens will remain transparent forever. Unfortunately, there is no medication that can halt or reverse cataract formation. What can one do to prevent cataracts?

- **Wear sunglasses outdoors.** The UV radiation in sunlight damages eye proteins and can lead to cloudiness. A large study that reviewed data from more than a half million people found a strong association between cataracts and skin cancer—more evidence that UV exposure is a major risk factor.

What to do: Wear sunglasses with UV protection whenever you plan to spend prolonged periods of time outdoors. Virtually all sunglasses today are UV-protected.

- **Wear a broad-brimmed hat to block UV radiation.** It will reduce your risk for eyelid skin cancer as well as cataracts.

- **Eat a nutritious diet.** Many studies have found an association between a healthy diet and fewer cataracts—but that's not the same as proof.

For example, several studies have suggested that particular nutrients—alone or in combination—can help prevent cataracts. The large Age-Related Eye Disease Study (AREDS) reported that people with cataracts who got the most lutein and zeaxanthin (antioxidants that are found in leafy greens and other fruits/vegetables) were 32% less likely to need cataract surgery.

Other research has looked at the effects of fish oil supplements (or regular meals including fatty fish)...vitamin C...vitamin E...and other nutrients.

It's common sense to eat a nutritious diet. If you want to take one of the AREDS formulations, check with your doctor first if you are a current or former smoker. Certain versions of these supplements (with lutein and zeaxanthin) also contain beta-carotene, which has been linked to increased risk for lung cancer in current and former smokers.

Could a Hot Cup of Tea Preserve Your Vision?

Anne Coleman, MD, PhD, professor, ophthalmology, University of California, Los Angeles.

Davinder Grover, MD, MPH, clinical spokesperson, American Academy of Ophthalmology, and ophthalmologist, Glaucoma Associates of Texas, Dallas.

British Journal of Ophthalmology.

A spot of hot tea in the afternoon might help you save your sight, new research suggests.

The study of US adults found that people who drank hot tea on a daily basis were 74%

less likely to have glaucoma, compared to those who were not tea fans.

Experts were quick to stress that it may not be tea, itself, that wards off the eye disease. There could be something else about tea lovers that lowers their risk, said senior researcher Anne Coleman, MD, PhD.

But the findings do raise a question that should be studied further, according to Dr. Coleman, a professor of ophthalmology at the University of California, Los Angeles.

"Interestingly," she said, "it was only hot, caffeinated tea that was associated with a lower glaucoma risk."

Decaf tea and iced tea showed no relationship to the disease. Neither did coffee, caffeinated or not.

It's hard to say why, according to Dr. Coleman. "Is there something about the lifestyle of people who drink hot tea?" she said. "Do they exercise more, for example? We don't know."

About Glaucoma

Glaucoma refers to a group of diseases where fluid builds up in the eye, creating pressure that damages the optic nerve. It's a leading cause of blindness in older adults, according to the American Academy of Ophthalmology (AAO).

Some people face a higher risk than others, the AAO says: They include blacks, people with a family history of glaucoma, and people with high blood pressure, diabetes or other conditions that affect blood circulation.

Some studies have suggested that people who drink a lot of coffee have a heightened glaucoma risk. Others have hinted that caffeine can temporarily boost pressure within the eye.

On the other hand, some studies have failed to find a coffee-glaucoma link, Dr. Coleman said.

Study Details

Her team decided to see whether there is any connection between glaucoma and not only coffee, but also tea or soda—caffeinated or not. So the researchers turned to data from a nationally representative government study where US adults underwent eye exams and filled out nutrition surveys.

Of nearly 1,700 survey participants, 5% had glaucoma.

Overall, Dr. Coleman's team found, the odds of having glaucoma were 74% lower among people who said they drank hot tea more than six times a week, versus nondrinkers.

That was with a number of other factors taken into account—including age, weight, diabetes and smoking habits.

The findings were published in the *British Journal of Ophthalmology*.

Possible Explanation

Still, it's impossible to conclude that tea, itself, deserves the credit, Dr. Coleman said.

Other lifestyle factors might be at work, she explained. And with diet, Dr. Coleman noted, it's always hard to disentangle any effects of a single food or nutrient from the rest of a person's eating habits.

That said, she pointed to some theoretical reasons why tea could be beneficial. It contains a range of plant chemicals that may fight inflammation and protect body cells from accruing damage.

Recommendations

For now, Dr. Coleman recommends focusing on some proven steps.

"The important first step is to not take your eyes for granted," she said. "Go in for that comprehensive eye exam."

Davinder Grover, MD, MPH, a clinical spokesperson for the AAO, agreed.

He said people should get a "baseline" eye exam with an ophthalmologist at the age of 40—a time when early signs of eye disease may start to emerge.

Some people may need to start earlier, Dr. Grover noted—such as those with relatives who developed glaucoma early, in their 40s or 50s.

As for prevention, there is no surefire way to ward off glaucoma. But people may curb

the risk by minding their overall health—their cardiovascular health, in particular, he said.

"So if you have diabetes or high blood pressure, try to get that under control," Dr. Grover said.

Dr. Coleman stressed another point: Even when glaucoma is already present, it can be treated—with eye-drop medications or laser surgery, for example. That can prevent damage to the optic nerve and vision loss.

Damage to the optic nerve is not, however, reversible, Dr. Grover said. So early detection and treatment are vital.

"The name of the game is prevention," Dr. Grover said. "If we catch glaucoma early and treat it appropriately, the vast majority of the time, we win."

For more information about glaucoma, visit the website of the AAO, AAO.org, and search "What is glaucoma?"

Stop Neglecting Your Eyesight

Jeffrey D. Henderer, MD, professor of ophthalmology and the Dr. Edward Hagop Bedrossian Chair of Ophthalmology at the Lewis Katz School of Medicine at Temple University in Philadelphia. Dr. Henderer is the Secretary for Knowledge Base Development for the American Academy of Ophthalmology and has authored numerous articles and text-book chapters on glaucoma and genetics.

When it comes to staying on top of our health, far too many people take their eyesight for granted. It's obvious that we should get regular eye exams (see next page), but there are other steps that often slip under the radar. *Here are the strategies that ensure you're doing all you can to protect your vision…*

Eye-health secret #1: **Use the right eyedrops.** Older adults and those of any age who are heavy users of computers and/or electronics know that they're more likely to suffer from dry eye. Lubricating drops, sometimes called artificial tears, are effective for this condition. But when you're in the store, it's easy to mistakenly pick up redness-reducing eyedrops, which temporarily constrict the blood vessels. These drops do not help with dry eye.

In fact, daily use of redness-reducing drops can cause rebound redness and set off an unhealthy cycle of using more eyedrops. For this reason, redness-reducing drops should be used only occasionally—and if the redness persists, see your eye doctor to find out why.

Best for dry eye are lubricating drops such as Refresh, Systane, GenTeal, Bion Tears and even pharmacy brands.

Caution: If the preservatives they contain irritate your eyes, look for preservative-free brands.

Lubricating drops come in three viscosities—liquid, thicker gel-like formulas and ointments. The thicker drops and ointments last longer but can temporarily blur vision.

Eye-health secret #2: **Watch your medication.** Steroids—taken orally, inhaled or in eyedrop form—can cause cataracts and glaucoma. Cataracts can start to develop within months of regular steroid use, while glaucoma is slower and subtler. If you must take a steroid, ask your doctor for the lowest dose possible, schedule an eye exam one to two months after starting any form of the drug, then return every six to 12 months for monitoring. *Other drugs that can affect the eyes…*

Tamoxifen (Nolvadex), used to treat and prevent recurrences of breast cancer, can cause eye irritation and dryness…lead to cataracts (usually after five years of use)…and accumulate in the retina, weakening color vision and central vision. Fortunately, as oncologists have started prescribing lower doses of tamoxifen, these side effects happen less often.

Self-defense: Have an annual dilated eye exam with a retina specialist while you are taking tamoxifen and have him/her examine your retinas to be sure there is no accumulation in the retina.

Eye-health secret #3: **Keep diabetes well-controlled.** People with diabetes tend to develop cataracts at an earlier age than people without diabetes. They also have an elevated risk for visual impairment and

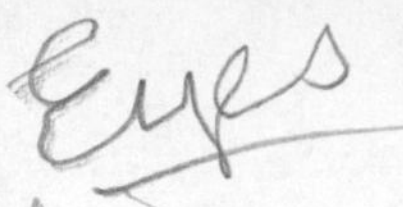

blindness due to diabetic retinopathy, when high blood sugar levels damage blood vessels in the retina.

What to do: Get a dilated eye exam annually or more often if recommended by your doctor, particularly if you struggle to keep your sugar under control. Early treatment can prevent an astonishing 95% of diabetes-related vision loss!

Also important: The better you are able to control your blood sugar with diet, lifestyle changes and medication, the better your chances of delaying the onset of cataracts and diabetic retinopathy.

Eye-health secret #4: **Take this eye supplement.** If you're at high risk for advanced age-related macular degeneration (AMD)—that is, you have intermediate AMD or advanced AMD in one eye only—taking high levels of certain antioxidants plus zinc can reduce the risk of developing an advanced form of AMD by about 25%, according to a major National Eye Institute clinical trial called the Age-Related Eye Disease Study (AREDS). A leading cause of blindness among Americans age 50 and older, AMD causes damage to the retina that may lead to central vision loss.

What to do: Look for a supplement labeled "AREDS formula" (such as Bausch & Lomb PreserVision AREDS 2 Formula). It's not an AMD cure, but it may help preserve vision in susceptible individuals. Ask your ophthalmologist if it's right for you.

When Was Your Last Eye Exam?

Adults between the ages of 55 and 64 who are risk-free and have no eye symptoms should have eye exams every one to three years, but nearly half of those recently surveyed have not.

People who are over age 65 or of any age with a risk factor, such as high blood pressure, diabetes or a family history of eye disease, should have an eye exam at least every one or two years, according to the American Academy of Ophthalmology.

Because your eyes offer an unobstructed view of your blood vessels, nerves and connecting tissue, any abnormalities that show up in an eye exam may indicate similar changes elsewhere in the body. This means your optometrist or ophthalmologist can give you crucial information about your risk for serious conditions such as stroke, high blood pressure, diabetes and autoimmune disease, such as Graves' disease, a thyroid disorder. Insurance should cover these exams.

Keep Your Voice Young

Murray Grossan, MD, otolaryngologist, Tower Ear, Nose and Throat Clinic, Cedars-Sinai Medical Towers, Los Angeles. His most recent book is *The Whole-Body Approach to Allergy and Sinus Relief.* DrGrossanTinnitus.com

Is your voice making you sound old—maybe older than you are or feel? If you've been having concerns about the quality of your voice, your answers to the following four questions might give some clues about what's going on…

1. Do you have trouble speaking loudly or being heard in noisy situations?

- Never
- Sometimes
- Often

2. Do you run out of air and need to take frequent breaths when talking?

- Never
- Sometimes
- Often

3. Do you feel like you don't know what sound will come out when you begin speaking?

- Never
- Sometimes
- Often

4. Do you have to repeat yourself to be understood?

- Never
- Sometimes
- Often

A weak, quavering "old person" voice is not an automatic accompaniment to accruing years. Many people still sound strong and vigorous in their 80s and 90s. *If you answered sometimes or often to any of the above questions, here's what might be happening to your vocal cords and what you can do about it...*

What happens: Your voice is produced when folds in your vocal cords come together while air from your lungs passes through the folds, causing them to vibrate and create sound waves. As you age, your muscle mass shrinks and your mucous membranes become thinner and drier as a normal process throughout your whole body. These changes include your vocal cords and cause the tissues in your throat to become less elastic and lose volume—so your vocal cords no longer come together as tightly or they may even gap. The condition, vocal cord atrophy and bowing, is technically called *presbylaryngis* or *presbyphonia.* The result—a weak or breathy voice.

The good news is that most voice disorders are treatable, especially if you see an ear, nose and throat specialist for help. You can find a more detailed voice-related quality of life quiz and an ENT locator on the American Academy of Otolaryngology-Head and Neck Surgery site. You can also try an easy daily "workout" that will keep your vocal-cord muscles fit and your voice strong. (It will benefit your lungs, too!) The only "equipment" you need is a straw...and all you do is hum into the straw in a certain way.

What to do: Start with a wide drinking straw, and make a simple "hmmmm" or "oommm." Do this daily for about 10 minutes, but stop if your voice begins to feel tired. As you build stamina, try a smaller-diameter straw, even working your way down to a hollow coffee stirrer—the narrower the straw, the greater the resistance to your airflow and the more robust the workout. Also vary the pitch of your humming—for example, imitate the two-tone sound of a siren or hum a tune.

In fact, there's no need for voice strengthening to be a drudge—have some fun! Singing in the shower, crooning in the car, reading aloud, doing tongue trills—even making the motorboat sound that kids make with their lips—all help. But do avoid yelling, as that puts wear and tear on your vocal cords.

The Health Risks of Iron After Menopause

Study titled "Serum ferritin level is positively associated with insulin resistance and metabolic syndrome in postmenopausal women: A nationwide population-based study" by researchers at Yonsei University College of Medicine in Seoul, Republic of Korea, published in *Maturitas.*

After menopause, a woman's risk for diabetes and heart disease goes up. One likely culprit is the loss of estrogen because of menopause. But another factor also may play an important role—excess iron.

Background: After menopause, women are at higher risk for metabolic syndrome, a cluster of symptoms including abdominal obesity and high blood sugar, often due to insulin resistance. The syndrome increases the risk of developing diabetes and heart disease.

Why does the risk go up after menopause? It's true that the loss of estrogen is known to negatively affect the lining of blood vessels in ways that increase many of these risk factors. But another line of evidence points to excess iron as an additional risk factor. Because iron in blood is no longer lost with each menstrual cycle, iron levels generally increase after menopause. Korean researchers set out to determine whether there was a statistical link between high iron levels, insulin resistance and metabolic syndrome.

Study: 2,734 postmenopausal women in a large health database all had extensive exams that included blood samples, so the researchers could sort them into four groups based on blood levels of ferritin, a protein that's a marker for body levels of iron. They then analyzed ferritin levels against rates of insulin resistance and metabolic syndrome.

Results: After the researchers adjusted for other known factors (age, smoking, drinking and amount of exercise), it was evident that women with the highest levels of ferritin, compared to women with the lowest levels, were…

- **More than twice as likely to have insulin resistance**
- **Almost twice as likely to have metabolic syndrome.**

What's so bad about excess iron? It promotes oxidation (think: rust), which can lead to body-wide inflammation—and that in turns increases all the above risk factors. Plus, there is evidence that too much iron may interfere with normal glucose and insulin activity in muscles. Because this is an observational study, however, it can't determine whether high ferritin levels cause insulin resistance/metabolic syndrome—or are simply a marker for these risk factors.

Bottom line: The authors advise that getting your iron level checked—it's part of a regular checkup anyway—could be an early tip-off to these risk factors. Then you can take lifestyle steps, including weight loss if needed, that can independently reduce your risks.

You may also want to talk with a nutritionist about your diet. After menopause, a woman's daily iron requirement goes from 18 mg to 8 mg. However, recent research has found that some postmenopausal women may still be at risk for iron deficiency anemia—an issue best dealt with by eating more iron-rich foods.

In particular, be cautious about your vitamin/mineral supplement(s). According to the National Institutes of Health, postmenopausal women should not take a supplement that includes iron unless they have been diagnosed with iron deficiency. If you are concerned about anemia, get tested and discuss with your doctor whether supplementing with iron is appropriate for you.

The Menopause Lesson Whales Can Teach Us

Study titled "Reproductive Conflict and the Evolution of Menopause in Killer Whales," by Darren P. Croft, PhD, professor of animal behavior, director of research (psychology), University of Exeter, England, and colleagues, published in *Current Biology*.

Why does human menopause even exist? After all, it's pretty rare in nature. Even female elephants, who can live to a ripe old age of 70 in the wild, continue to be able to reproduce throughout their life spans.

Women are different. So are orca (aka killer) whales, it turns out. Now pioneering animal biology research has uncovered the most likely reason that killer whales stop reproducing in their 30s or 40s yet live for many decades afterward.

The findings shed new light on the role that menopause may play in the lives of humans, too.

Hint: It's about sharing wisdom.

Background: One somewhat downbeat hypothesis holds that when humans first evolved, we didn't live past reproductive age…but now we do. That makes menopause a kind of accident. Scientists who study killer whales, however, hypothesized that living well beyond reproductive age has benefits. There was already evidence for the "grandmother hypothesis"—the idea that by helping find scarce food supplies, based on their age-earned knowledge, older females help the species survive. But that's true for animals such as elephants that continue to reproduce. A newer hypothesis holds that menopausal whales compete less with their daughters in having offspring—and that's good for the entire species, too.

Study: Using an extraordinary database tracking killer whales over 43 years, English researchers analyzed how likely offspring were to survive if both older and younger whales had babies in the same season.

Results: When both younger and older whales bred at the same time, the offspring of the older whales were 70% more likely to die than those of the younger whales. It wasn't age—the increased mortality didn't occur for older whale offspring when the younger generation wasn't simultaneously having babies. It was competition, especially for food supplies. For the sake of the survival of the species, it would be better if older whales didn't breed—and instead used their food-finding skills to help the entire pod find food supplies during scarcity. Hence, menopause evolved. That benefitted everyone—including their adult sons, who stay with their mothers' pods and do particularly well when mom showed them where to find salmon. In short, by not having more offspring, grandma killer whales helped the entire species.

Bottom line: Humans aren't whales, so you can't draw one-to-one conclusions. But the evidence that menopause has an evolutionary benefit in killer whales adds support to the idea that human menopause isn't some deficiency or aging problem—it's a new phase of life in which women can use their hard-earned knowledge to benefit their children…and everyone else. As British writer Christa D'Sousa, author of *The Hot Topic: A Life-Changing Look at the Change of Life*, put it to the British Broadcasting Service, "The idea of women passing on information; the idea of wisdom with age—there's a beauty in that that is about something other than being able to reproduce."

Feet Getting Bigger???

Neil A. Campbell, DPM, FACFAS, DABFAS, staff podiatrist, Cuero Regional Hospital, Texas.

You may have had a recent panic when shopping for shoes. It might seem as if suddenly your usual shoe size is too small.

Here's the good news: Your feet are not growing.

Now the bad: As we age, we lose some of the elasticity in the ligaments and connective tissues in our bodies. This is the reason why various body parts start to "sag." In the foot, that means the supporting tendons and ligaments become lax and can't hold the bones and joints in the same position as when we were younger, causing the arch to flatten and the feet to expand. Pregnancy and weight gain also can cause your feet to spread, due both to hormones and the added pressure on the feet, and this change is generally permanent. An injury to the bones or tendons that causes a rupture or dislocation is another reason feet can change shape.

For all these reasons, it's normal for feet to become longer and wider, perhaps gaining a half size or more every decade or so. However, if change in size is also accompanied by pain, see a podiatrist to rule out a more serious foot problem such as arthritis, tendon dysfunction or nerve damage. And always try on shoes before purchasing them—you may also find you need a wider size.

Chapter 15

YOU AND YOUR DOCTOR

8 Mistakes to Avoid If You Get Bad News

Sooner or later, it happens to most of us: We find ourselves sitting in a doctor's office hearing some very bad news. The diagnosis is heart disease, breast cancer, dementia, kidney failure, Parkinson's disease or some other serious (and possibly terminal) illness. At that moment, we are scared and vulnerable. It's easy to make mistakes when we're in a frantic quest to beat back illness. *Here's how to avoid or overcome these common mistakes...*

MISTAKE #1: **Making rash decisions.** Even when a diagnosis is dire, jumping right into treatment can be a mistake. So slow down, and make sure you have all the information you need. That means asking how your illness and the treatments you are considering will affect your day-to-day life...how likely it is that treatments will work...and what "working" means. To truly understand the answers, you need to also (politely) insist that doctors cut the jargon—so you won't end up thinking, for example, that a "response rate" is the same as a "cure rate."

Cancer patients often are surprised to learn that they can wait a bit before starting chemotherapy or other treatments—it is almost always safe to wait two to three weeks, but the doctor can tell you if it's not. These days, this short pause will often include waiting for a genetic analysis of the tumor, which might point to a more effective, targeted treatment. Getting extra information like that can make a wait worthwhile.

MISTAKE #2: **Believing everything you read online.** By now, everyone knows that all online information is not created equal. But many people cannot resist reading everything they find—and, in the process, they stumble across a lot of information that is scary, wrong or not relevant to their personal situation.

Best approach: Ask your doctor for reputable information sources, and discuss what you find with him/her.

MISTAKE #3: **Not focusing on what you really want.** Let's say you might benefit from a cutting-edge treatment, but you learn that getting it will mean frequent trips or a long stay in another city.

Steven Z. Pantilat, MD, a palliative-care physician and the Kates-Burnard and Hellman Distinguished Professor in Palliative Care, University of California, San Francisco School of Medicine. He is author of *Life After the Diagnosis: Expert Advice on Living Well with Serious Illness for Patients and Caregivers.*

Those trips might be worth the hassle if your goal is to explore every avenue for treating the illness and taking any chance, no matter how small, to find a cure or at least manage an illness—but not if your primary goal is to enjoy the comforts of home and family in what might be precious remaining weeks or months.

The right question to ask is: Will this procedure or medicine help me to get back to my home and family? If it won't, what will?

MISTAKE #4: **Focusing on death instead of living.** It's important to think and talk about the end of life, but not at the expense of planning for the weeks, months or years that might still lie ahead. What will you need to do to keep up cherished hobbies and habits for as long as possible? Can you take a long-delayed trip, reconnect with long-lost friends or reach other personal goals?

To do that planning, you need to know the truth, so do not be afraid to ask your doctor how much time you have left, even if he has to estimate. You might have a lot more (or less) time than you assume.

Helpful: Regardless of your prognosis, ask about "palliative care"—care aimed at helping you function better, with less pain and stress and more emotional and spiritual support.

MISTAKE #5: **Keeping your illness a secret.** It might come as a surprise in this age of online over-sharing, but many people still keep serious illness a secret from family members, friends and others. That's a mistake. At the very least, you want a support person to go with you to important medical appointments to act as a second set of ears.

But you also may find a wider network of people eager to help with everything from meals to rides to lawn-mowing. Let them help. Share your hopes and fears with people you love and trust to help keep your stress levels in check.

Helpful: If you are wondering whether to tell someone close to you, try turning the table. What if you learned that this person had a serious illness and had not shared it so that you could help him? If you wish this person had told you, then you should think about sharing your news with this person.

MISTAKE #6: **Assuming that the most aggressive or newest treatments are best.** Even if your main goal is to live as long as possible, the most aggressive treatments are not always the best choices. You might sacrifice both quality and quantity of life by going ahead with a treatment that has little chance of helping you and a high probability of harming you.

For example, for some people with heart failure, a left ventricular assist device (LVAD), a pump surgically implanted into your heart to help pump the blood, might seem like a great idea. But there are serious complications, such as bleeding and stroke. Many people who have an LVAD implanted feel better, but some never get over the operation or have complications early and may feel that they are worse off with the LVAD than without it.

Helpful: Ask your doctor what is the best case, worst case and likely case with a particular treatment...and ask for the same assessments if you don't get that treatment.

MISTAKE #7: **Limiting your care to alternative treatments.** Complementary therapies—especially yoga, meditation, acupuncture and others that have been shown in research to have benefits—can be helpful when combined with standard treatments or when the benefits of standard treatments are exhausted. But patients who rely only on unproven approaches, including those pitched by pricey foreign clinics and online hucksters, sometimes wait too long to get evidence-based treatments that could have made a difference in how well and long they live.

MISTAKE #8: **Beating yourself up.** Many people blame themselves for getting sick—a woman may have forgotten to get a mammogram, for example, and developed breast cancer. Give yourself a break. It's true that there are risk factors for serious diseases. But generally speaking, the development of illness is more complex than that.

Also, don't beat yourself up for not staying positive enough. While cultivating joy, hope, gratitude and love will help you face your illness, blocking off all sadness, worry and grief will not help. Find a balance.

Helpful: Talk about things that are real, meaningful and personal with those who care about you.

Don't Let a Diagnosis Ruin Your Dreams

VJ Periyakoil, MD, director, Stanford Palliative Care Education and Training, and associate professor of medicine, Stanford University.

When you're facing a medical decision, it's easy to feel rushed and get lost in the details. What are my options? What are the side effects? Will it work? But there's an equally important question to ask—how will this treatment affect the things I really want to do in my life?

You may get started on a treatment plan without realizing how much it will affect your plans and dreams—whether that means going to your annual family reunion or seeing Paris. That's why Stanford University's VJ Periyakoil, MD, director of the university's palliative-care training program, asks her patients not only about their health but also about their life goals.

Dr. Periyakoil's advice: If your doctor tells you that you have a serious or long-term health condition—or recommends that you begin a new treatment—bring up your short- and long-term goals and desires.

Why? Because sometimes, treatment can wait. One of Dr. Periyakoil's patients, for example, had advanced gallbladder cancer. He had always wanted to go to Hawaii but figured it would have to wait until next year because he needed radiation therapy. She gently told him that the treatments would likely leave him terribly debilitated and his survival chances wouldn't be good.

Result: He took his family to Maui for two weeks and came back "beaming like a jack-o'-lantern."

It's not always about life or death. If you're living with a chronic condition, talk to your doctor about more than your medications and prognosis—talk about your dreams. And if you're healthy and aren't yet planning to do something that you always wanted to do, what are you waiting for?

Can't Remember What Your Doctor Said?

Glyn Elwyn, MD, PhD, professor, physician and researcher at The Dartmouth Institute for Health Policy and Clinical Practice in Lebanon, New Hampshire, and at the Scientific Institute for Quality of Healthcare, Radboud University Nijmegen Medical Centre, in the Netherlands. He leads an international team examining shared decision-making among patients and providers. GlynElwyn.com

So how did your doctor visit go? We've all heard that question from family and friends, but it can quickly lead to a frustrating exercise in trying to remember exactly what did happen during those precious minutes you spent with your doctor.

Perhaps you recall something about needing to return for some tests...but you're not quite sure what the tests are for. Or maybe your doctor suggested a better way to monitor your symptoms...but you don't remember what it was.

Luckily, most of us have a cure for this common ailment right in our pockets or purses—our smartphones. Pull it out and press a recording app the next time you sit down with your doctor, and you never have to wonder again about what happened at your appointment. It's easier to make a recording than to take notes. Plus, you can relisten to what was discussed during the appointment...and share it with others electronically.

Sounds easy, right? It is—but there are some important points to consider before you hit "record."

A Commonsense Solution

Very few people are blessed with perfect recall, and our memories tend to become less efficient as we age. Add on the possibility of hearing loss—a common problem for adults over age 50—and you've got a recipe for miscommunication.

Throw in the overall stress of a medical encounter—especially one where you may be receiving new or distressing information—along with the high probability that your doctor may have lapsed into medicalese while explaining a complex concept, and it's no wonder that so many of us struggle to remember and understand what we hear under those conditions.

Among patients who have access to recordings of their doctor visits, studies suggest that there are benefits. One review, published in *Patient Education & Counseling,* found that about 72% of patients took the time to listen to the recording after the appointment...and 60% shared it with caregivers, including family and friends. Just knowing that a conversation is being recorded may also encourage patients and doctors to express themselves more clearly.

Important Considerations

Before you whip out your smartphone at your next doctor visit, keep these key points in mind...

POINT #1: **Know the law.** In 38 states and the District of Columbia, you can legally record a conversation with another person—even a medical provider—with or without the other person's consent. In the following 12 states, you do need consent from both the patient and the physician (verbal consent is acceptable)—California, Connecticut, Florida, Illinois, Maryland, Massachusetts, Michigan, Montana, New Hampshire, Oregon, Pennsylvania and Washington.

So if you ask a doctor for permission to record your visit in one of these 12 states, he/she could refuse. If you went ahead and made a recording without permission and the doctor finds out, you could be reported to legal authorities. You could also get into legal trouble for sharing the recording.

As mentioned above, in the 38 states and District of Columbia that don't require permission, you could record and share the doctor visit secretly, but there are good reasons not to do that (more on that shortly).

Important: If you use a recording to damage the reputation of a doctor—by posting a damning conversation on Facebook, for example—you could face legal consequences. If you sue a doctor for medical malpractice, a recording may or may not be admissible as evidence. An attorney would need to advise you.

POINT #2: **Don't jeopardize your relationship with your doctor.** Even if you are in a state where it's legal to secretly record a doctor visit, it's a bad idea.

Here's why: Good patient/doctor relationships are built on trust. If your doctor finds out that you are secretly recording him, that's going to undermine trust. And even if your doctor doesn't find out, many patients will find themselves feeling anxious about the deception.

Better idea: Let the doctor know that you would like to record the visit, emphasizing the potential benefits to you.

You might say: "You know, sometimes I have real trouble recalling everything. Would you mind if I recorded this conversation so I can review it later and perhaps share it with my relatives?"

We don't have much data on how doctors respond to such requests. In some states, as noted earlier, they can legally say "no." But as more patients ask, it will be interesting to see what happens.

Ideally, groups representing medical providers and patients will get together to develop guidelines for recording doctor visits so that eventually it will become common practice. Until then, doctors might be reassured by preliminary evidence suggesting that patients rarely set out to use a recording against a doctor—as evidence in a malpractice case, for instance.

***POINT #3:* Know the technical details.** Don't own a smartphone? A simple digital recorder will work fine, and it costs a lot less (prices start at about $20). If you still own an old-fashioned cassette tape recorder, that will work, too.

But if you do have a smartphone, making a recording is easy.

On an iPhone: You can just tap the Voice Memos icon and then press the red button to record. You can download other recording apps, for both iPhone and Android phones, and many are free. Some come with bells and whistles—like the ability to type in notes as you tape or convert audio to text.

To make the process even more user-friendly, some providers are experimenting with secure online systems that are specially designed to record and store audio from medical visits and make key exchanges easier to find and play back.

What About Privacy?

One law that patients do not need to worry about if they are recording and sharing a doctor visit is the Health Insurance Portability and Accountability Act (HIPAA). This health-privacy law limits what health providers, insurers and other professionals can do with your medical information, but it doesn't stop you from making or using your own audio medical recordings.

Is Your Doctor a Bully?

Rebecca Shannonhouse, editor of *Bottom Line/ Health*

You might excuse rudeness from your doctor, especially if he/she is very highly regarded or tops in the field. But boorish behavior can be dangerous when it involves your health.

Interesting finding: Patients of surgeons who don't show respect for their medical staff have much higher rates of adverse effects—including more infections, delayed wound healing and excessive post-operative bleeding—than patients of their more congenial colleagues, according to a new study.

"As a patient, you're also a member of the health-care team," explains Gerald B. Hickson, MD, of Vanderbilt University Medical Center. If your doctor is condescending or dismisses your concerns, you're getting poor care. *Dr. Hickson's advice...*

• **Give your doctor a chance.** If he doesn't explain an issue clearly, you might say, "I didn't understand. Would you repeat that, please?" If he won't return phone calls, ask if there's a better way to communicate, such as by e-mail. If your doctor still can't extend basic courtesies, find another doctor. *But first...*

Say something! Most hospitals and health-care groups have patient-relations representatives who want to know if a doctor is rude. Only one in 70 to 90 dissatisfied patients bothers to complain. Most simply leave the practice.

But hospitals and group practices know that a patient who has been treated rudely is more likely to sue than one who is treated with respect. In any health-care group, just 5% of doctors account for 40% of malpractice claims.

Fortunately, once a doctor's bad behavior is called to his attention, he is likely to do better—and so will his patients.

Don't Let Your Doctor Become Your "Drug Dealer"

Anna Lembke, MD, a psychiatrist, assistant professor and chief of addiction medicine at Stanford University School of Medicine in California, where she is also chief of the Stanford Addiction Medicine Dual Diagnosis Clinic. She is the author of *Drug Dealer, MD: How Doctors Were Duped, Patients Got Hooked, and Why It's So Hard to Stop.*

With all the alarming headlines warning us against the full-blown opioid epidemic that is gripping the US, you'd think that patients and doctors would be on high alert for possible misuse of these drugs. *Yet the problem continues...*

Shocking statistics: More than 91 Americans die every day from an opioid overdose, according to the Centers for Disease Control and Prevention (CDC).

Surprisingly, only 7% of people who misuse or are addicted to these powerful painkillers get them from strangers or dealers—the vast majority are obtained with legitimate prescriptions or from friends or relatives who presumably obtained them from their doctors.

Why do doctors continue to prescribe drugs that are known to cause addiction—and why do so many patients demand drugs that are not effective for long-term pain?

To learn more, we spoke with Anna Lembke, MD, a psychiatrist and addiction specialist who has extensively studied the misuse of prescription drugs.

Which drugs are most likely to cause addiction?

The opioid painkillers—*morphine*, *hydrocodone* (Vicodin), *oxycodone* (OxyContin, Percocet), *fentanyl* (Sublimaze, Duragesic), etc.—are the main offenders. They're classified by the FDA as Schedule II drugs, meaning they carry a high risk for addiction.

Some stimulant drugs, including methylphenidate (Ritalin) and other medications used to treat attention deficit hyperactivity disorder, can also be addictive, particularly when they're used by patients who are also taking opioid painkillers or other mood-altering drugs.

Are prescription medications more addictive than street drugs?

They may not be inherently more addictive (this would depend on the different chemical properties), but they're more readily available—and that's a big part of addiction. In the 1960s, 80% of heroin (an illicit opioid) users started out with heroin. Today, most heroin users begin with prescription opioid painkillers before moving on to heroin.

Opioids are routinely prescribed by pain specialists, surgeons and family doctors. Patients acquire the drugs from emergency rooms, walk-in clinics and online pharmacies. They're everywhere.

Who is most likely to get addicted?

Patients with a previous history of addiction—to alcohol and/or drugs—have the highest risk. Addiction is also common in those with a family history of addiction or a personal history of depression or other psychiatric disorders. Before prescribing opioids, doctors should ask if a patient has any history of addiction or mental illness as well as if there is any family history of addiction. If a doctor does not ask about this (many don't), a patient should be sure to alert his/her doctor regarding these issues.

However, we've also found that patients with no history of addiction/drug use are also at risk. Studies have shown that about 25% of patients who use these drugs for legitimate medical reasons for three months or more will begin to misuse these medications—meaning they take more than prescribed or don't take the medication as prescribed (for example, they binge or hoard medication). This is a first step on the road to addiction.

Why do doctors keep prescribing opioids?

Many believe, mistakenly, that patients who take these drugs for pain—as opposed to using them recreationally—are unlikely to become addicted. There's an old (and flawed) statistic that pain patients have less than a 1% chance of becoming addicted. We now know that this is not true.

Other factors: Doctors want to ease pain...pleasing patients is part of their DNA. Prescribing a powerful painkiller can feel like a better alternative than possibly letting someone suffer.

How do patients get more medication than they need?

Many of them "doctor shop"—they exaggerate their symptoms while collecting prescriptions from many different doctors. Some patients claim to have lost or misplaced their prescriptions before the refill date. Others create so much disruption in doctors' offices—begging for drugs, threatening lawsuits, intimidating the staff, etc.—that they're given prescriptions just to be rid of them.

Note: Some insurance companies are now closely monitoring claims and alerting prescribers about suspicious activity, so some patients pay out of pocket to avoid getting caught.

Don't patients know that they're becoming addicted?

Surprisingly, they don't. Addictive drugs work on the brain's reward pathways. Patients feel so good when they take the drugs that they lose insight into all the negative consequences—lost jobs, damaged relationships, etc.

Who should take these drugs?

Opioids are very effective painkillers. Anyone who's suffered a severe, acute injury—a broken leg, for example—will clearly benefit in the short term. Those who have had major surgery almost always need them. They're also a good choice for those with acute pain related to cancer, such as metastatic cancer lesions on the bone. And opioids are an essential tool in the last few hours of life to help ease the passage to death.

But for chronic pain, opioids should be the very last choice. Nonmedication alternatives, such as psychotherapy, physical therapy, acupuncture, massage, meditation, etc., should be tried first, followed by nonopioid medications, such as *ibuprofen* (Motrin) or *acetaminophen* (Tylenol). These approaches can also be tried in combination.

For people who don't respond to the approaches above, opioids may be required, but doctors need to proceed with caution. I advise intermittent dosing—say, using the drugs three days a week, without using them in between. This will still reduce pain but with less risk for addiction. Patients don't take the drug regularly enough to build up a tolerance and dependence, so they shouldn't have withdrawal symptoms.

Can anything else be done to help?

Doctors who prescribe these drugs should take advantage of prescription drug monitoring programs. These state-by-state databases (available in every state except Missouri) allow doctors to see every prescription (for opioids and other scheduled drugs) that a patient has received within a certain time. They'll know how many prescriptions a patient has received...how many doctors they're getting them from...the doses they're taking, etc. This information goes into the database when a patient picks up the prescription at the pharmacy.

Drugs That Can Turn Deadly

Jack E. Fincham, PhD, RPh, professor of pharmaceutical and administrative sciences, Presbyterian College School of Pharmacy, Clinton, South Carolina.

Americans use a lot of medications, filling prescriptions and buying over-the-counter (OTC) drugs several billion times each year. All these medications come with potential benefits and risks. But in the ubiquitous TV and print ads targeted to consumers, the benefits get much more attention than the risks.

Surprising danger you should know about: A medication that you take to feel better might twist your thoughts, suddenly and powerfully, so that you feel bad enough to consider ending your life.

My analysis: When I recently completed a search of Clinical Pharmacology powered by ClinicalKey, a trusted database of drug information, suicide as a potential side effect is listed for 188 different drugs, including both prescription and OTC medications that are taken by several million Americans. Use of certain drugs with this possible side effect has also been linked to increased risk for suicide attempts and completed suicides.

To be fair, just because this possible side effect is listed does not mean that a drug always causes suicidal thinking...nor that the drug is to blame if this frightening problem does occur. But it does mean that cases have shown up—either in clinical trials conducted before the drug was approved or in reports sent to FDA regulators after it hit the market.

Unfortunately, it is impossible to say with any certainty how often people experience this (or any other) side effect in real-world use. That's because not everyone having a problem reports it, nor do regulators hear from people who have no problems with the drug.

Still, if suicidal thinking is a possible side effect of a drug you're taking for, say, depression, asthma, allergies or acne, it's something you want to know so that you, your doctor and the people close to you can be on the alert—and fully consider all the risks and benefits of that medication or alternatives.

Important: Do not stop taking a medication your doctor has prescribed without checking with the doctor or pharmacist. Some drugs may have additional side effects if stopped abruptly.

Drugs on the Danger List

Among the medications that have been linked to suicidal thinking...

• ***Montelukast*** **(Singulair).** Singulair is the best known of a group of medicines known as leukotriene inhibitors. Usually taken in pill form, it is used to treat asthma and, in some cases, nasal allergies. Other drugs in this class include *zafirlukast* (Accolate) and *zileuton* (Zyflo).

Since 2009, the FDA has required these drugs to carry labels saying that suicidal thinking and actions (and mental health problems such as anxiety and depression) have been reported in some patients.

My advice: Assuming you've talked with your doctor about the risks and potential benefits and have decided to use a leukotriene inhibitor, stay alert for any changes in your typical feelings and thoughts. If any occur, it may be that you could safely use another drug, such as a beta-agonist, or switch to something else entirely, such as an inhaled corticosteroid. These medications have not been linked to suicidal thinking.

• **Antidepressants.** While studies in older adults have not found a definitive link between antidepressant use and suicidal thinking, studies in children, teens and adults under age 25 have been concerning enough to lead the FDA to put so-called black-box warnings (the strongest kind) about the possible risks for young people on all antidepressants.

It's unclear why young people might be especially vulnerable to such a drug side effect. Perhaps medical providers and parents are more vigilant and more likely to report known suicidal thoughts or attempts when the patient is young. Or perhaps young brains react differently to the drugs. Whatever the reason, the FDA says the risk appears greatest in the early weeks of treatment or right after a dose is increased or decreased.

My advice: When anyone you know—but particularly a young person—is taking an antidepressant, be alert for warning signs, including worsening depression...talk of suicide...sleeplessness...agitation...and social withdrawal.

• ***Varenicline*** **(Chantix).** This prescription pill can help some people quit smoking. But for years, the FDA has required this medication to be labeled with a black-box warning alerting users that the drug has been linked with serious mental health problems, including suicidal thinking and behavior.

In 2016, citing new data, the FDA removed the strong warning, saying that the benefits of using Chantix to quit smoking outweighed the possible mental health risks and that those risks appear to be lower than previously suspected.

However, the risk for suicidal thinking continues to be mentioned on the manufacturer's website.

What may not be brought to your attention: Some of the best smoking-cessation tools, including nicotine-replacement products such as gums and patches, are available without a prescription and have not been linked to suicidal thinking. In-person and telephone counseling (call 800-QUIT-NOW) also can help some smokers.

My advice: If you're uneasy about taking Chantix, try one of the other approaches mentioned above. But do stay resolved to quit smoking!

Other Drugs

The list of widely used medications linked to suicidal thoughts or actions also includes the OTC allergy drugs *cetirizine* (Zyrtec) and *levocetirizine* (Xyzal)...the acne drug *isotretinoin* (Accutane)...the nerve pain drug *pregabalin* (Lyrica)...and a variety of medications, including *carbamazepine* (Tegretol) and *divalproex* (Depakote), that are used to treat seizures. Studies differ on which seizure medications are associated with the risk, so the FDA requires warnings on all of them.

Good rule of thumb: If you don't feel "right" when starting any new medication or a new dose of a medication, talk to your pharmacist, physician or other health-care provider. You also can read about the possible side effects of any medication at FDA.gov—search "Index to Drug-Specific Information."

Critically important: If you or someone you know is having suicidal thoughts, immediately call your doctor...go to a hospital emergency room...or call the confidential and toll-free National Suicide Prevention Lifeline at 800-273-TALK (8255). Help is available!

In Case of an Emergency ...Always Carry This Health Info

David Sherer, MD, is an American physician, author and inventor. He is the lead author of *Dr. David Sherer's Hospital Survival Guide: 100+ Ways to Make Your Hospital Stay Safe and Comfortable.*

Those of us of a certain age will remember a radio (and later television show) called *Dragnet*, where the hard-boiled detective Joe Friday would tell witnesses to alleged crimes, "All we want are the facts, ma'am..." The detective, played by Jack Webb, was often short on time and full of questions, so he needed to get to the point.

When you as a patient need to go to the emergency room, and time counts, the doctors and nurses need "just the facts" to get a rapid and accurate assessment of your medical history and condition. Recently, a financial services adviser I know wanted to make a service available for his clients. The service would provide essential medical information in just such a scenario so that medical personnel can quickly assess what's important in one's medical history. I thought that was a great idea.

In light of that, I'd like to share the kind of information you need to share quickly and accurately, whether on a 5" x 8" card, a piece of paper or some electronic device, in case of a medical emergency.

Roughly, the information falls into five basic categories: drug and food allergies, medication list, ongoing medical conditions, prior surgeries and medical directives. Most are self-explanatory, but let's talk about each.

- **Drug and food allergies** (and sensitivities) are essential to communicate to medical people. An allergy is where you get a true anaphylactic reaction to a drug or food—where you may break out in hives, you have difficulty breathing and your windpipe swells. This is not to be confused with a sensitivity or adverse reaction, where an antibiotic might cause stomach upset. Also, food allergies, such as to shellfish, are important to know about because some intravenous contrast dyes might cause an anaphylactic reaction when given to such patients.

- **Your medication list is an important part of your medical history.** You should include all prescriptions, over-the-counter medications and supplements on this list. This ensures that medical folks know what you are taking and what drug choices to make when treating you while you are under their care. It's also helpful to reduce the incidence of adverse drug interactions or overdose.

• **Medical conditions.** The importance of divulging your ongoing medical conditions is self-explanatory. Doctors and nurses need to know your major medical conditions, such as hypertension, diabetes, thyroid problems, cancers, autoimmune diseases and the like. Use common sense when compiling this list; it's not essential that personnel know you once had poison ivy or an ear infection years ago.

• **Prior surgeries.** Again, use common sense. The fact that you had your appendix out is very important if you have abdominal pain. The fact that you had a small non-cancerous skin lesion removed 10 years ago is not important. When in doubt, ask your doctor what to put down on your list.

• **Medical directives.** Finally, your directives regarding your "code" status (relating to heroic, life-saving measures), your religious preferences (e.g., Jehovah's witnesses do not accept blood transfusions), whether you have a living will, your organ donor status, and the contact numbers for your primary doctor, family and friends who are responsible for you go a long way in reducing ambiguity and confusion.

So be smart and take time to fill out these items. Carry it with you...give copies to key loved ones...and remember to review it periodically for updates. That way, when you are asked to present "just the facts," you'll be ready.

Getting Hospital Care—at Home

Linda DeCherrie, MD, associate professor at Icahn School of Medicine at Mount Sinai, New York City, and director of Mount Sinai Hospital's Mobile Acute Care Team. Her clinical and research interests include the care of complex frail patients and innovative models of care.

Your chest hurts, you are short of breath and you're shaky from fever and chills. The ER doctors diagnose pneumonia. Since you also have a heart condition, they decide that you qualify for immediate hospital admission.

But you're not admitted. Instead, you're sent home to recuperate. A brush-off? Bad medicine? Not at all! You'll be getting intensive hospital-quality care in your own home. Within two hours, you have the medications and equipment you need to get well, plus a team of health pros to check on you daily.

What sounds like a health-care fantasy may one day be routine. "Hospital-at-home" programs are increasingly the norm in England and Australia and gaining traction in the US, too. For good reason—people who recuperate at home have better outcomes than those who stay in hospitals.

Hospitals—despite the full medical staff, fully equipped labs and stocked pharmacies—are dangerous. Patients can suffer sleep interruption, exposure to superbug bacteria and risk "sundowner syndrome" (delirium that often happens during a hospital stay). Hospital care at home helps you avoid these risks—and get better faster.

Your Bed Is Better Than a Hospital Bed

Seniors are more likely to be admitted to the hospital than younger people. The hospital-at-home movement is seeking to change that. *Technological advances that make that possible include...*

• **Home infusion**—medication that must be delivered by needle or catheter, such as antibiotics, can now be safely administered at home by a health-care professional or, in some cases, you can do this yourself.

• **Point-of-care testing**—simple "lab" medical tests can now be done at the bedside.

• **Telehealth technologies allow doctors to diagnose, treat and monitor patients from afar.**

Even such conditions as severe urinary tract infections, pneumonia, emphysema and deep vein thrombosis, which normally keep older patients in the hospital, can be safely treated at home under the right conditions.

Who Can Be Treated?

Only certain patients, with certain conditions, qualify for this kind of care. Doctors apply strict criteria, only accepting people who aren't likely to require constant oversight, technical hospital-based procedures (such as endoscopy) or the kind of intravenous medication that can be done safely only in a hospital (such as intravenous cardiac medications or intravenous blood thinners). Research shows that about 30% of older patients are eligible for at-home hospitalization. *Besides clinical qualifications specific to his/her medical condition, a patient is a good candidate if...*

- **She can get to the bathroom,** prepare meals and answer the door or telephone.
- **She has a caregiver** (a family member or an aide) who can help out.
- **It's safe for the medical staff to go to the home** (no unattended pets, not too much clutter, etc.).
- **She lives within the area that the program serves.**

How Hospital-at-Home Works

If the patient is offered at-home hospitalization and accepts, as about 80% do, a hospital-at-home team—including a doctor who oversees care, an administrative assistant who checks insurance and arranges transportation and a nurse manager who schedules nurses—takes over.

Pharmacy and laboratory services are arranged, and medical equipment, if needed, is procured—all within two hours. If it takes longer and it's after 8 pm, the patient is sent to a bed in the hospital for one night and hospital-at-home starts the next morning.

Here's what we require in our program at Mount Sinai Hospital, where we are studying hospital-at-home under a federal grant...

- **A nurse visits once or twice a day.**
- **A doctor or nurse practitioner visits once a day.**
- **A social worker or physical therapist visits at least once.**
- **Lab services are performed in the patient's home.**
- **If a patient needs an extra visit with the doctor,** the nurse will conduct a video visit with the doctor back at the hospital.
- **Paramedics can also be dispatched,** if needed, to evaluate the patient's condition.

The Rewards

At Mount Sinai, patients in the hospital-at-home program remain under care for less time than those who are admitted to the "real" hospital for the same condition. Costs are substantially lower. Not surprisingly, patient satisfaction is higher, too. Complications and mortality are also reduced.

Despite these beneficial outcomes, there are only a handful of full-fledged programs in the country. Besides the Mount Sinai program, there's one at the Presbyterian Hospital in Albuquerque, New Mexico (for Medicare Advantage patients), one at the Cedars-Sinai Medical Center in Los Angeles and one at Brigham and Women's Hospital in Boston. The Veterans Affairs (VA) hospital system has programs at several locations, including Boise, Idaho...Honolulu...New Orleans... Philadelphia...Portland, Oregon...and Bend, Oregon.

A key reason why so few such programs are offered in the US is the way we pay for health care. Most hospitals get paid for every service they provide, but hospital-at-home often requires fewer services at less cost, so it's less financially attractive for the hospital. On the other hand, "capitated" insurance plans (VA, some managed-care plans, Medicare) pay a fixed amount to the hospital to cover each patient based on the diagnosis. So if hospital-at-home care saves money, it benefits the plan. Capitated plans are gaining in popularity, but it will be several years before hospital-at-home programs are widely available.

In the meantime, if you are admitted to the hospital, ask whether you can arrange for the kinds of services that might allow for an early discharge—such as home visits by a skilled nurse or hospital treatments that can be provided at home.

No one should be discharged from the hospital too early, but if you can safely shave off a day or two (for instance, by finishing the last few days of an infusion for antibiotics at home), it will help you avoid some of the downsides of traditional hospitalization—and might give you some of the better outcomes of healing at home.

Doctor Loyalty Has Perks

Patients who regularly see the same primary care physician over time are less likely to be unnecessarily hospitalized.

Details: Among more than 230,000 patients ages 62 to 82, those with the highest continuity of care had 12% fewer hospitalizations for conditions that are considered preventable with good quality primary care (such as asthma and pneumonia) than those with the lowest continuity.

Why: Regular visits to a trusted health-care provider may lead to greater understanding of health issues and more appropriate treatments.

Isaac Barker, MSc, data analyst, The Health Foundation, London.

Is That Medical Test Really Necessary?

Dennis Gottfried, MD, an associate professor of medicine at University of Connecticut School of Medicine, Farmington, and a general internist with a private practice in Torrington, Connecticut. He is the author of *Too Much Medicine: A Doctor's Prescription for Better and More Affordable Health Care.*

Getting all the health screening tests possible sounds like a great idea. After all, frequent screening tests help detect diseases early and help you live longer, right? Not always...

Do You Need That Test?

People who are sick obviously need medical attention and appropriate tests. So do those at high risk for certain diseases. If you have a family history of melanoma, for example, I believe an annual skin check is wise. But many tests administered to millions of healthy people every year have no clear benefits. So why, then, do doctors order unnecessary tests? According to a 2014 physician survey, more than half admitted that they do it to protect themselves from malpractice lawsuits...36% said they recommend these tests "just to be safe"...and 28% said they do it because patients insist.

My advice: Before getting any medical test, ask your doctor why he/she is recommending it and what he will do with the information. Will the test reveal a problem that needs to be fixed? Is it likely that you will live longer if your doctor confirms a tiny thyroid nodule? If the answer is no, the test might be unnecessary—and needlessly risky.

Common tests you may not need...

Late-Life Colonoscopy

Most people are advised to have a colonoscopy every 10 years, starting at age 50. The benefits seem obvious. Colonoscopy allows doctors to detect early-stage cancers and remove precancerous growths. Overall, the test has reduced the risk for death from colorectal cancer by about 40%.

Exception: For those who are age 75 or older, the risks of colonoscopies usually outweigh their benefits. A Harvard study looked at data from more than 1.3 million Medicare patients between the ages of 70 and 79. The researchers found that while colonoscopy slightly reduced cancer death rates in those who were under age 75, the test made little to no difference in those who were older.

Why: Between 30% and 50% of Americans will eventually develop polyps in the colon, but the vast majority of polyps will never turn into cancer. This is particularly true in the elderly because cancers take a long time to develop. Someone who's age 75 or older probably won't live long enough for the polyps to become cancerous.

Routine colonoscopies are generally safe but not totally risk-free. Bleeding and perforations can occur, and in rare cases, there have been deaths as a result of complications of colonoscopy. Plus, the test is expensive, and the "bowel prep" can be very unpleasant.

My advice: Get a colonoscopy every 10 years starting at age 50 (or as directed by your doctor), but if nothing serious is ever found, you can skip the test after age 75.

Skin Exams

Millions of Americans ask their dermatologists to perform an annual head-to-toe skin exam. The early detection and removal of melanoma skin cancers is critical. More than 80,000 cases are diagnosed annually, and almost 10,000 people will die from melanoma. But only about 1% of all skin cancers are melanomas. The vast majority of skin cancers are basal and squamous cell carcinomas, which are slow-growing and present little health risk.

The US Preventive Services Task Force (USPSTF), an independent group of national experts that makes evidence-based recommendations about tests and other medical services, concludes that the evidence is insufficient to recommend for or against annual dermatological screening for melanomas. According to the group, the downsides of screening include overdiagnosis (the detection of diseases that are unlikely to ever be a threat) and the possibility of disfigurement caused by needless biopsies. There is also the expense of procedures and visits to the dermatologist. The USPSTF consciously did not address screening for basal and squamous cell carcinomas because of their relative medical insignificance.

My advice: An annual skin screening by a dermatologist doesn't make sense for everyone—particularly individuals who don't have a personal or family history of melanoma or those who are not severely immune impaired, such as people who have HIV. However, do be sure to see a dermatologist if you notice a mole, growth or "spot" that meets the ABCDE criteria—Asymmetrical...Border irregularity...Color that is not uniform (often with shades of black, brown or tan)...Diameter greater than 6 mm (which is about the size of a pencil eraser)...and Evolving size, shape or color, or new symptoms such as bleeding or itching. These are the changes that are most likely to signal melanoma.

Thyroid Screening

Ultrasound technology has made it easier to find and evaluate growths in the thyroid gland. As a result, there has been a threefold increase in the diagnosis of thyroid cancers, but there hasn't been any change in the thyroid cancer death rate.

A study from the Department of Veterans Affairs Medical Center and Dartmouth Geisel School of Medicine concluded that the apparent increase in thyroid cancer was mainly due to improved detection. About 87% of the cancers measured were just 2 cm or smaller and were unlikely to ever pose a threat. Yet patients were treated surgically with the risk for bleeding, vocal cord paralysis and disfigurement. They also had to deal with the psychological trauma of being told they had cancer. Radiation is also standard treatment for thyroid cancer and can cause side effects. Additionally, radiation exposure presents a cumulative lifetime risk of developing cancer.

My advice: Don't get routinely screened for thyroid cancer. However, if you have a neck mass or lump...you notice changes in your voice...or have a family history of medullary thyroid cancer, an ultrasound of your thyroid may be advised.

Remember: At the proper age and appropriate intervals, screening tests, such as colonoscopy, mammograms and Pap smears, are necessary. Also be sure to get a cholesterol test every five years and blood pressure checks annually...and regular dental and eye exams.

How to Check Out a Doctor

Charles B. Inlander, consumer advocate and health-care consultant based in Fogelsville, Pennsylvania.

Most of us assume that if a doctor loses his/her license to practice in one state, that same doctor couldn't retain or get a new license to practice in a different state. But that's not necessarily true. A recent investigation conducted by the *Milwaukee Journal Sentinel* newspaper and website MedPage Today uncovered laxity on the parts of the federal government, state medical licensing boards, hospitals and other organizations that are responsible for keeping patients safe from incompetent and/or dishonest physicians. For example, several doctors who had been sanctioned in one state for sexually assaulting patients were practicing without restrictions in another state.

Each state licensing board is required to review the entire National Practitioner Data Bank annually to make sure a doctor who was sanctioned in one state is not practicing unnoticed in another. Hospitals are required to check on new hires and existing practitioners. Sounds good, but studies have found poor compliance with those requirements. Fortunately, you can check out any doctor you use or are considering. *Here's how...*

• **Check the state licensing board.** Every state must publicly disclose any action it takes against a physician. Most state boards put it on their websites. To find contact information for all state licensing boards, go to FSMB.org/contact-a-state-medical-board. You do not have to be a resident of that state to gather the information. For clues on which states to search, ask your doctor (or the practice he is associated with) for the other states where he has formerly practiced or currently practices. If you live in an area where residents frequently cross state lines for services, check all those states.

• **Look for board certification.** While it's no guarantee of character, board certification ensures that a doctor meets nationally recognized standards for education, experience and skills in a specific medical specialty. To be sure your doctor is certified by a legitimate and highly regarded board, consult the American Board of Medical Specialties (ABMS). Its specialty boards are considered the best in each specialty, and they will verify that your doctor is in good standing. Go to ABMS.org and click on "Is Your Physician Certified?" or call 866-ASK-ABMS (866-275-2267). *Note*: The certifying board looks at its own criteria for competence and not necessarily any license revocations.

• **Ask a nurse.** Nurses are great sources of information about doctors. If you know a nurse, ask about the doctor in question. You can find out about the doctor's reputation or learn about the nurse's direct experience with him.

Also ask the nurse: "Would you use this doctor for yourself or for a family member?"

• **Be direct.** It's perfectly reasonable to ask any doctor you currently use or are considering whether he has been sanctioned by any state licensing board...or ever had his hospital privileges suspended or revoked. If so, ask why. Doctors are required to answer honestly. If a doctor resists, look for another one.

Genetic Testing Could Torpedo Your Insurance

Lee J. Slavutin, MD, CLU, principal of Stern Slavutin-2 Inc., an insurance and estate-planning firm in New York City. SternSlavutin.com

If you expect to apply for life insurance, disability insurance or long-term-care insurance, think twice about getting a DNA test.

DNA testing has become so inexpensive in recent years that many people are having it done as a precaution—or simply out of curiosity. For $250 or less, companies such as 23AndMe (23AndMe.com) will analyze a sample of your saliva and tell you about your heritage and/or your health.

Example: Some people learn that they have inherited genes that put them at high risk for breast, ovarian, colorectal or prostate cancer. If knowing this inspires them to make anticancer lifestyle changes or to be checked for cancer more frequently, it could help them stay healthier.

But if a DNA test reveals that you have a genetic predisposition to a serious health problem, you may be required to inform life, disability and long-term-care insurers of this when you apply for coverage. (Genetic testing that explores only your ancestry and not your health should not create this problem.) And insurance companies may respond by imposing higher premiums or declining to cover you at all. The federal Genetic Information Nondiscrimination Act bars health insurers from requesting the results of genetic tests or discriminating against applicants based on such tests, but this law does not apply to other forms of insurance.

What to do: If your doctor advises you to get a genetic test because of a specific, pressing medical concern, do so. But if there is no pressing health concern and you intend to apply for life, disability or long-term-care insurance in the future, delay DNA testing until after you have been approved...or choose a test that reports on your ancestry only and not on your health.

Skimping on Rehab Can Lead to Arthritis

Joseph M. Hart, PhD, associate professor of kinesiology at University of Virginia Curry School of Education in Charlottesville.

If you suffer a serious injury to a joint, there's a good chance that more bad news lies ahead—but you can avoid that if you know what researchers recently discovered about joint injuries.

Not only are joints that have been injured often later reinjured—these joints also face substantially increased risk for painful and potentially debilitating osteoarthritis. The new research found, for example, that people with a history of knee injuries are three to six times more likely to develop osteoarthritis in the injured knee than people with no history of knee problems. Osteoarthritis is especially likely if you rush back to your previous level of activity after an injury, short-circuiting the rehabilitation needed to allow the joint to heal fully. The knee is not the only trouble spot—injuries to hips, shoulders and ankles also have been linked to significantly increased risk for osteoarthritis.

Sustaining a serious injury to a joint can destabilize the joint...weaken the muscles surrounding it...and/or alter the way you use the joint during activity, leading to greatly accelerated cartilage wear. That's why adequate recovery, including a rehabilitation program to strengthen the muscles that support the injured joint, is crucial.

What to do: If you sustain an injury to a joint, ask your doctor about a physical therapy program and then stick with this physical therapy program for its entire recommended duration even if the joint has stopped hurting.

Ask your doctor or physical therapist what types of exercise are safe for the joint while it still is recovering, prior to returning to unrestricted physical activity.

Finally, if you have suffered a major knee-joint injury, have the joint and surrounding muscles reevaluated by a physical therapist, athletic trainer or sports medicine professional prior to returning to full activity levels and periodically in the years following your injury—even if it feels as good as new. There might be lingering issues such as muscle weakness or altered movement patterns that are too subtle for you to notice but that could increase your risk for osteoarthritis.

When Your Doctors Disagree

Charles B. Inlander, a consumer advocate and health-care consultant based in Fogelsville, Pennsylvania. He was the founding president of the nonprofit People's Medical Society, a consumer advocacy organization credited with key improvements in the quality of US health care, and is the author or coauthor of more than 20 consumer-health books.

If you've got a medical problem, you need to feel certain that your doctor knows what's wrong with you and is recommending the best treatment. That's why second medical opinions are so important—they give you a greater level of confidence that the diagnosis is accurate and/or the treatment is appropriate. If the second opinion confirms that of your original doctor, then you've got a green light. But what happens when your second-opinion doctor disagrees? Studies going back more than 40 years show that roughly 20% of diagnostic second opinions do not confirm the original doctor's diagnosis. Meanwhile, when Mayo Clinic conducted a recent study focusing on second opinions sought from them, researchers found that the original diagnosis was confirmed in only 12% of the cases, and it was better defined/refined in 66% of cases.

If you're dealing with a major diagnosis such as cancer or a complex heart problem...or have to decide between getting a risky surgery or taking a medication with potentially serious side effects, this puts a lot of pressure on you. *My advice for making the right choice when medical opinions conflict...*

- **Find out what led to each opinion.** Ask the physicians you've consulted to give you the reasons—including specific scientific evidence—that each doctor used to arrive at his/her opinion. The doctors should be reviewing the same evidence. If it's a diagnostic conflict, how many other patients with similar symptoms or test results has each doctor successfully diagnosed? Unless it's a rare disorder, the doctor should have treated at least 50 cases such as yours. If it's a treatment conflict, what experience does each doctor have with each of the proposed treatments? I'd look for a doctor who has treated at least 100 cases such as mine...or at least 10 cases for a rare problem.

- **Get a third or fourth opinion.** Getting a third or maybe even more opinions may be a good idea, especially if there seems to be real conflict between the first and second opinions. Most insurance plans pay for these follow-ups. At this point, you are seeking a consensus among as many doctors as possible. When looking for other opinions, consider contacting major medical schools or hospitals with national reputations for specific conditions—for example, you can check *US News & World Report's Best Hospitals* ratings.

Insider tip: Many hospitals and well-known institutions, including Mayo Clinic, Cleveland Clinic, Massachusetts General Hospital and others, have highly regarded online second-opinion programs. Do an online search for such services to find out details.

Note: Most insurers won't pay for online second opinions. Prices typically range from $500 to $800.

- **Ask each of the doctors providing opinions to review the other doctors' opinions.** Whenever possible, using this approach may lead to quicker agreement about what is wrong or should be done. One doctor may raise an issue the other(s) didn't consider, such as another condition that's mentioned in your medical history.

- **Review the recommendations.** Take the time to carefully go over each of the opinions. When doing this, you may want to enlist the help of your primary care doctor.

Remember: The final decision is yours! But having all the relevant information will definitely make it easier for you to make the right choice.

Hospice Helps You Live Better

John Mastrojohn III, RN, MSN, MBA, executive vice president and chief operating officer of the National Hospice and Palliative Care Organization (NHPCO), NHPCO.org. To learn more about hospice, consult CaringInfo.org.

Everyone's life ends. But not everyone has the same quality of life at the end of life. Many are in pain or not comforted physically, emotionally or spiritually. Others die in a hospital when they would have wanted to die at home, surrounded by loved ones in a beloved place.

Yet sadly, countless individuals who could receive hospice care don't get it. Many don't even know it's an option. And among those who do use hospice, many take advantage of it only in the last week or two of life. But research shows that hospice can provide important benefits—and for a much longer period of time than just the final few days.

Scientific evidence: In a study published in *Journal of Clinical Oncology*, researchers from Harvard Medical School and two cancer centers talked with 2,307 family members of individuals who had died.

Results: When hospice was used, patients had more appropriate relief from pain, better symptom relief and higher-quality end-of-life care...they received care that was more in accordance with their wishes...and they were more likely to have died in a preferred place (usually at home, rather than in the hospital).

What you and your loved ones need to know about hospice care...

The Facets of Hospice Care

Even though most people assume that they know what hospice is, few can explain exactly when it's used in the course of an illness or how it works. Medicare, the main payer of hospice care, defines hospice as a system of care for people who have approximately six months or less to live if the disease runs its normal course. In order for a patient to elect hospice care, he/she must be certified as meeting the criteria described above by an attending physician and the hospice medical director. Over 90% of people in hospice receive care at home or in the place they reside.

Hospice care is delivered by a team of doctors, nurses, home-health aides, social workers, therapists, chaplains, counselors and trained volunteers. The care plan varies according to the patient's needs, but it is not around-the-clock care (except for in the rare cases when continuous home care is needed for a brief period of crisis, such as uncontrolled pain). For that reason, family caregivers are an integral part of the care team.

Managing the patient's pain and/or controlling symptoms is a priority, and hospice provides medication and medical equipment and supplies (such as a hospital bed and/or oxygen) for these purposes. During hospice care, curative treatment for the illness itself is discontinued. *In addition, hospice care...*

- **Provides emotional support to address the myriad of feelings and issues affecting hospice patients and their families.** Spiritual support is also offered for those patients who choose it and can be delivered by the hospice and/or the patient's clergy or other faith leader.
- **Offers the surviving family bereavement care and counseling,** typically for 13 months following the death of a patient. These services include written materials, phone calls, visitation and support groups.

Important: Though the Medicare hospice benefit is the predominate payer of hospice services, managed care and private insurers will often cover hospice services.

Debunking Myths

Common myths about hospice stop many people from getting the end-of-life care they need. *For example...*

MYTH #1: **Hospice mainly serves terminal cancer patients.** Only 37% of hospice patients have cancer. Other terminal diagnoses include dementia, heart disease, lung disease, stroke, kidney disease, liver disease, HIV/AIDS and others.

***MYTH #2:* The doctor must bring up hospice.** Anybody can inquire about and refer to hospice—the patient, a family member, a counselor or the doctor. But only a physician can certify that a patient is eligible for hospice care.

***MYTH #3:* The hospice patient can't keep his/her own doctor.** Hospice encourages a patient to keep his primary physician. The primary physician typically knows the patient best and can consult with the hospice medical director and other hospice team members to provide the best care. Patients may still visit their primary care physician if they choose.

***MYTH #4:* Hospice care hastens death.** Hospice neither hastens nor postpones dying. Just as doctors and midwives lend support and expertise during the time of childbirth, hospice provides specialized knowledge and skill for patients and families at the end of life.

***MYTH #5:* Hospice means giving up.** Hospice is not about hopelessness or giving up. For example, if a patient decides to seek curative care for any disease, he can revoke the hospice benefit at any time and return to curative therapy or even try a new therapy.

Finding Hospice Care

All hospices are licensed by the state in which they operate and certified by Medicare. But not all hospices are alike. In the US, 60% are independent...20% are part of a hospital system...16% are part of a home-health agency...and 4% are part of a nursing home. Hospices are both large and small, rural and urban, and range from for-profit national chains to local nonprofits.

To find a hospice program anywhere in the US: Use the National Hospice and Palliative Care Organization's "Find a Provider Tool" at: Moments.nhpco.org/find-a-hospice. Once you (or the certifying doctor) contact the hospice, enrollment should happen quickly.

Helpful: Look for a hospice that is accredited by an independent accrediting organization, such as the Accreditation Commission for Health Care...the Community Health Accreditation Program...or The Joint Commission.

My advice: Have the conversation about end-of-life care with your loved ones early so you understand their wishes. If you decide that you want hospice care, once you've chosen the program, you'll have an initial consultation to develop a plan of care, typically with a hospice nurse.

If the patient is comfortable with the idea, I encourage not only the family caregiver (such as a spouse) but other family members (such as adult children) to attend the initial consultation. In that way, all those involved with the patient's care will hear the same information regarding hospice care and will have the opportunity to get their questions answered. This approach also helps the hospice nurse understand the patient's needs and develop a personalized plan of care.

Your Biopsy Results Might Not Actually Be Yours

John D. Pfeifer, MD, PhD, professor and vice chair for clinical affairs in the pathology and immunology department at Washington University School of Medicine in St. Louis. WUSTL.edu

It's no secret that biopsies occasionally produce inaccurate results. But what if the biopsy result you get is accurate—but the tissue sample came from someone else's body?

Yes, it happens. A study of more than 13,000 prostate biopsies found that switched or contaminated samples caused the wrong patient to be told he had cancer approximately three times in 1,000. Additionally, three times in 1,000, a patient is told he doesn't have cancer when in fact he does. And there's no reason to assume that such mix-ups are limited to prostate biopsies.

Lab mix-ups such as these can have catastrophic consequences. A healthy person might be subjected to life-altering treatments, including surgery, chemotherapy and/or radiation, for someone else's medical problem. Meanwhile, the person who actually has this major medical problem might be told that he is fine, delaying potentially lifesaving treatments.

What to do: When the stakes of a biopsy are high, ask your doctor, "Does it make sense to do a DNA test to confirm that the tissue that was tested originated from me?" Some private labs that do DNA testing for criminal investigations also test to make sure that biopsied tissue samples truly came from the patients who received the results. This type of DNA test typically is covered by health insurance—contact your insurance provider for details. If not, expect it to cost several hundred dollars.

Example: Strand Diagnostics, a reputable DNA-testing lab that is accredited by the FBI and CLIA, charges $295 (KnowError.com).

Get Your Money's Worth at the Doctor

Get more value when seeing your doctor. Write down your concerns, and refer to your notes during the visit. Prioritize—decide on your main concerns and discuss the most important one first. Bring a list of all your medicines, prescription and over-the-counter, so your doctor can look for interactions and no-longer-needed drugs. Take notes during the visit. You might not remember everything your doctor says, especially if you're not feeling well. Take advantage of available help. The office may have specialists who can help with your specific issues—a dietitian for weight-loss concerns, for example. Expect some face-to-face quality time with your doctor—doctors must enter data during a visit for electronic recordkeeping, but if your doctor focuses only on the screen and not on you, consider finding another doctor

Roundup of experts on health care, reported at *Consumer Reports.*

Chapter 16

VERY PERSONAL

To Enhance Sexual Desire, Women Need "Just Right" Testosterone

When it comes to testosterone, women share a few things with men. Like men, they produce the hormone, although in much smaller amounts. Like men, they make less as they get older. And like men, women with low libidos who get testosterone treatments often experience a boost in sexual desire and enjoyment. No wonder millions of American women turn to their doctors to get testosterone prescriptions to enhance their sex lives—even though it's not FDA-approved for women.

Yet, when it comes to testosterone and libido, women aren't really like men—at all. For women, unlike men, just a little extra "T" can backfire in the bedroom.

Background: "Hypoactive sexual desire disorder" (HSDD)—the medical term for low libido—affects both men and women, but it's particularly common in postmenopausal women. While there are many factors, including vaginal dryness, that can affect sexual comfort, low levels of testosterone may play a role, too.

Women make small amounts of testosterone in their adrenal glands, ovaries (even after menopause) and in cells with testosterone receptors, but levels start declining in their 20s and are often quite low by their 50s and beyond.

In women with HSDD, testosterone treatment can be an effective treatment, studies show. But there are sometimes side effects, including hair growth, acne and even mood changes.

Study: My colleague and I reviewed existing studies, including animal research, to identify whether women respond to testosterone treatment for HSDD differently from men—and why. One reason the FDA has approved dozens of testosterone products for men but none for women, they suggest, is that the proper dose for each individual woman isn't understood yet.

Results: Men taking testosterone have a linear dose-related response when it comes

James A. Simon, MD, professor of obstetrics and gynecology, George Washington University School of Medicine, Washington, DC, and coauthor with Jill M. Krapf, MD, of an article titled "A sex-specific dose-response curve for testosterone: could excessive testosterone limit sexual interaction in women?" published in *Menopause.*

to libido. At higher doses of testosterone, men have a bigger increase in libido than they do when taking a smaller dose.

In women, more testosterone may actually mean less desire.

Example: 318 postmenopausal women with HSDD were treated with different doses of testosterone or a placebo for 24 weeks. Those who got the lowest daily doses—150 micrograms (mcg)—didn't have any sexual benefit. Those who got 300 mcg had more sexual desire and more frequent "sexually satisfying" events. But increasing doses up to 450 mcg not only didn't increase those benefits, it was actually associated with lower levels of desire. Plus, unpleasant side effects were a little higher in these women.

Women, it appears, don't have a linear response to testosterone treatment—their response is more like a bell curve. You might call it the "Goldilocks effect"—the amount of testosterone that is just right for them.

Surprising finding: To dig deeper into what's behind this phenomenon, we reviewed animal as well as human studies. One possible reason for the bell curve—while increasing concentrations of testosterone in women increase sexual function, at a certain point the "masculine" effects get in the way. These physical effects include deepening of the voice, hair loss where there should be hair, excessive hair where there shouldn't be and acne. Not exactly turn-ons. Psychological effects of too much testosterone treatment may also include aggression, anxiety and depression.

Any of these features may affect a woman's sexual desire and function—and she may become less sexually attractive to her partner. That's true in animals. Human sexuality is a lot harder to study, we admit, so it's just a thought experiment for now.

Bottom line: Discuss with your doctor whether this is the best approach for you—depending on your issues, there are many libido-boosting options.

Because there is no FDA-approved testosterone treatment for women, there is no approved dosage, either. If you do decide to be treated using testosterone, work with your doctor, who should be a hormone expert, to determine the dose that seems best for you…and then pay close attention to how the dose you're taking is affecting you—body and mind. Just a little too much might actually dampen desire. In women, testosterone appears to work best in moderation.

Sex Gets Better in Menopause...Believe It!

Lynnette Leidy Sievert, BSN, PhD, professor of anthropology at University of Massachusetts Amherst and author of *Menopause: A Biocultural Perspective*.

Say the word "menopause," and chances are you'll instantly come up with a list of negatives, from hot flashes and chin hairs to a thicker waistline and nonexistent libido. So naturally, most American women view this stage of life with dread and trepidation.

As an anthropologist who's traveled the globe studying this topic for the past 30 years, I've discovered that many women in other parts of the world actually welcome menopause. And one of the reasons is…sex gets better.

Gynecologists will tell you that sex becomes problematic during menopause, but that's partly because the women they see are the ones who are having problems. In my first study in upstate New York, half of women said their sex life had gotten *better* after menopause. No more birth control! No more periods! More spontaneity!

The ones who thought their sex lives were going downhill said it was because their husbands had back problems or they weren't having sex because they were widowed. These are the same reasons that women in other countries give for not having sex.

Of course, vaginal dryness is a common complaint, but instead of viewing this condition as the inevitable end to their sex life, women all over the world use their ingenuity to find ways to make sex more comfortable.

When I was in Puebla, Mexico, for instance, I found that pharmacies didn't sell lubricants. Women used a little olive oil instead. Now, that's creative problem-solving that comes with maturity.

Keep Your Love Life Alive!

Barry McCarthy, PhD, a psychologist, sex therapist and marital therapist who is a professor of psychology at American University in Washington, DC. He is coauthor, with Michael Metz, PhD, of *Enduring Desire: Your Guide to Lifelong Intimacy.*

There are a multitude of reasons why some couples stop having sex as they age. But a chronic health problem is definitely a big one. Fortunately, it doesn't have to be that way.

Sexual satisfaction remains within reach for just about everyone who wants it...and most people still do want it. Not only that, sexual activity has its own health benefits—for example, it helps lower blood pressure, improves sleep and relieves pain.

Adopting a New Mind-Set

If you're depriving yourself of sexual intimacy because of a health problem, the key is to start thinking about sex in a new way. Instead of viewing a sexual encounter as a pass/fail test that involves intercourse and mutual orgasm, it's time to think of it as an opportunity for sharing pleasure. How you achieve this is largely up to you. *To get started, you'll want to talk to...*

- **Your doctor.** Schedule a single consultation for you and your partner to meet with your internist, cardiologist, oncologist or other physician who is treating your health problem. Ask him/her to explain how your condition might affect your sexual intimacy and to give you any advice on what you can do medically to minimize those issues.
- **Your partner.** It's crucial for you to be able to talk about sex with your partner. Don't wait until you're in bed...or after a negative experience. Instead, bring up the subject (ideally on the day before a sexual encounter) while you're on a walk or having a glass of wine together. Avoid any blaming, and be clear that you're simply making sexual requests so that the experience is more comfortable and pleasurable.

In addition to what you learn by talking to your doctor and your partner, consider these specific steps to get your sex life back on track if you are affected by...

Back Pain

Take a man with low-back pain and have him engage in intercourse the way 70% of Americans do—with the man on top of his partner performing short, rapid thrusts—and you've got a perfect recipe for uncomfortable sex.

A better approach: The man with the bad back can invite his partner to go on top, and they can try a circular, thrusting motion. If a woman has back pain, the couple might try the side rear-entry position and long, slow thrusts. If your partner also has back problems, take lovemaking to the shower, where the warm water can loosen sore muscles.

Also helpful: If you're in chronic pain, such as that caused by arthritis, your doctor can refer you to a physical therapist, who can give you additional positioning tips.

Taking your favorite over-the-counter pain-reliever or using a heating pad about 30 minutes before sex also helps. This approach often reduces back and joint pain for an hour or more.

Even if your pain is not entirely eliminated, you may get enough relief to enjoy yourself. And after orgasm, your pain will likely be less intense for a period of time.

Cancer

Cancer treatment, such as surgery, radiation and medication, can create pain, fatigue and all kinds of psychological and physical fallout.

With breast cancer, it's common for a woman to worry about her partner's reaction to her altered body and how her breasts will respond to touch, particularly if she has had reconstructive surgery, which reduces sensitivity.

What helps: When talking about these issues, don't be afraid to get specific. Some women will not want to be touched on the affected breast or breasts, at least for a while. Others will crave that touch. Some might feel uncomfortable about nipple stimulation but fine about touching on the underside of the breast.

Cancers that affect other parts of the body, such as cervical or testicular malignancies or even mouth cancer, can also interfere with intimacy. If a man has been treated for prostate cancer, for example, he may want to focus more on pleasure-oriented sexuality rather than the traditional approach of intercourse and orgasm. Whatever the situation, talk about these vulnerable feelings and enlist your partner's help as a sexual ally.

Excess Body Weight

Too much body weight can get in the way—both psychologically and physically.

It's common for a person who is overweight to think: I don't feel sexy now, but I will when I lose some weight. While weight loss is a healthy idea, putting your sexuality on ice until you reach some ideal state is not. Learn to love and care for the body you have.

What helps in bed: Think beyond the missionary position, which can get pretty awkward and uncomfortable if one or both parties carry a lot of weight around the middle. Try lying on your sides instead. Or try a sitting and kneeling combination—a woman might sit on the edge of a sofa, supported by pillows behind her back, while her partner kneels before her.

Heart and Lung Problems

The fatigue often associated with heart and lung disease can douse your sexual flames. But a bigger issue is often the fear that a bit of sexually induced heavy breathing will prove dangerous or even fatal.

If this is a concern, ask your doctor whether you are healthy enough for sex. A good rule of thumb is to see if you can comfortably climb two flights of stairs. If the answer is yes, then almost certainly you're healthy enough to have sex.

What helps: If you still feel nervous, you can gain some reassurance by pleasuring yourself. A bout of masturbation produces the same physiological arousal as partnered sex. And it gives you a no-pressure chance to see how that arousal affects your breathing and heart rate.

Parkinson's and Related Conditions

People with frequent tremors, muscle spasms and other conditions in which a loss of control over the body occurs can still enjoy sex.

What helps: When talking to your partner about sex, decide between the two of you, in advance, on what you will say if, during lovemaking, your body becomes too uncooperative. It might be just a single word—"spasm," for instance—that tells your partner you need to pause.

Then agree on a "trust position" you will assume as you take a break to see if you want to return to sexual activity. For example, some people will cuddle or lie side by side.

Bad Hot Flashes? Watch Out for Pelvic Organ Prolapse

Angelo Cagnacci, MD, professor of gynecology and obstetrics, University of Udine, Italy, and lead author of the study "Association Between Pelvic Organ Prolapse and Climacteric Symptoms in Postmenopausal Women," published in *Maturitas, the European Menopause Journal.*

If you've ever talked to a woman who's had pelvic organ prolapse, you'll be motivated to prevent it. It's an uncomfortable condition in which one or more of the pelvic organs—the bladder, uterus, vagina and rectum—can bulge toward or out of the vaginal opening. It's a common problem in women, especially as they age.

Now there's a new way to know you're at risk—the severity of menopausal symptoms. If you're a postmenopausal woman and you've been experiencing severe hot flashes and other menopausal symptoms, it's a wake-up call to take steps to help prevent this condition. Fortunately, there's a lot that you can do.

Background: The "pelvic floor" is a network of muscles, ligaments and other tissue that acts like a sling to support a woman's pelvic organs. The bowel and bladder are controlled by contracting and relaxing these muscles and tissues. When the pelvic floor becomes weak, the organs above it can bulge toward your vaginal opening and even push out of it. The medical name for this hernia of the pelvic organs is pelvic organ prolapse.

Risk factors for it include menopause, age, obesity, repeated heavy lifting and traumatic injury—as may happen during childbirth, for example, or from a hip or back injury. But there's been little research into whether menopausal symptoms themselves are linked to prolapse risk.

Recent study: Italian researchers analyzed data on 1,382 postmenopausal women attending an outpatient service for menopause at a university hospital. The women were asked 21 questions to rate the severity of menopausal symptoms such as hot flashes, night sweats, fast heartbeats and sleep problems. The incidence of prolapse was also tracked.

Results: Women with a higher degree of menopausal symptoms were more likely to suffer pelvic organ prolapse—specifically, a prolapsed bladder. This study wasn't designed to show how it might happen, but the researchers note that high levels of the stress hormone cortisol—which often rise in the menopausal transition—can impair collagen tissue that's a key component of the pelvic floor.

Bottom line: If you have severe menopausal symptoms, explore ways to ease them—including mind-body approaches. But now is also a good time to check with your doctor to see whether you also have pelvic floor weakness that may lead to prolapse. You may be able to prevent this condition by losing weight and practicing Kegel exercises, which strengthen the pelvic floor muscles. Even if you already have prolapse but it's not causing significant symptoms, such lifestyle approaches may be enough to keep it from getting worse. Treatment options include the use of a pessary—a medical device that provides structural support—or surgery.

A Fountain of Youth for Your Vagina?

Lauren F. Streicher, MD, medical director, Center for Sexual Health and Center for Menopause, and associate professor of clinical obstetrics and gynecology, The Feinberg School of Medicine, Northwestern University, Chicago. She is author of *Sex Rx: Hormones, Health, and Your Best Sex Ever.* DrStreicher.com

---

Better living through lasers? That's the promise of a new treatment for postmenopausal women experiencing vaginal changes that make having sex difficult (or nearly impossible).

It's not a pill. You may remember the buzz over Addyi, the "female Viagra" for premenopausal women experiencing low sex drive. It turned out to be somewhat of a disappointment.

The new laser therapy doesn't claim to boost your desire...but it may help you enjoy sex again. It aims to treat vaginal dryness—and other changes that occur with menopause that can make sex uncomfortable—by promoting tissue healing, restoring the vagina to a more "youthful" state.

Does it work? Is it better than more low-tech alternatives? Is it safe? To find out, we spoke with Lauren F. Streicher, MD, medical director of the Center for Sexual Health and the Center for Menopause at Northwestern University's Feinberg School of Medicine in Chicago and author of *Sex Rx: Hormones, Health, and Your Best Sex Ever*. She has been offering the procedure in her practice for a year.

If you've been experiencing painful sex—or avoiding sex altogether because it hurts—here's what you need to know.

The technology itself isn't new. This particular treatment uses the same kind of laser technology that's used in skin "resurfacing" to improve the appearance of skin marked by acne, scars and other blemishes. A few years ago, Italian researchers had the bright idea to see whether it could help restore the health of the skin in and around the vagina.

The treatment uses concentrated ultraviolet light to create tiny "microwounds" in the skin of the vagina and vulva (the area outside the vagina). It may seem counterintuitive, but creating these small wounds activates the body's repair mechanism and stimulates regrowth of healthy skin. A doctor uses a wand-type device to deliver the laser pulses inside and outside the vagina.

Don't call it "vaginal rejuvenation." Some doctors—often dermatologists or plastic surgeons—are marketing the procedure to patients as "vaginal rejuvenation," a way to make your vagina look younger or tighter. But while there may be noticeable physical changes, this treatment isn't cosmetic and shouldn't be pitched as such. Instead, it aims to treat a medical condition called vulvovaginal atrophy, aka "genitourinary syndrome of menopause," that is caused by the dip in estrogen levels after menopause. As many as 70% of postmenopausal women experience this condition. The vaginal lining becomes thinner, less elastic and less lubricated, causing symptoms such as itching, burning, dryness, irritation and pain. The vagina also tends to become more prone to infections. These symptoms together take a toll on a woman's sex life.

Treatments are quick. You can literally have the treatment—comprised of three sessions over 12 weeks—on your lunch hour. Each treatment takes less than five minutes and involves no preparation, anesthetic or need for pain relief. Most women see an improvement in their symptoms after the first session.

It's backed up by (early) research. There are many European studies that confirm the safety and efficacy of this treatment. The initial US study—funded by the manufacturer but conducted and interpreted by researchers at Stanford University and a Cincinnati hospital and published in the peer-reviewed journal *Menopause*—found significant improvements in vaginal health and sexual function in women who tried MonaLisa Touch, the first such system that received FDA clearance. Almost all of the women in the trial—26 out of 27—said they were satisfied or extremely satisfied with the therapy three months after their last treatments.

It's not cheap—and no one knows how long its effects will last. The cost ranges from around $1,800 to $3,000 for the full course of therapy—and it's not covered by insurance. It's also unknown how long the benefits will last and whether women will need "maintenance" treatments after a year.

Women's health groups urge caution. While the results in this study were positive—and were enough, along with other data, to get the technology cleared by the FDA—it's not conclusive. That's why major women's health organizations, including the American College of Obstetricians and Gynecologists and the North American Menopause Society, have taken a cautious stance. They advise waiting until larger, long-term, randomized placebo-controlled studies—now underway—are completed.

Should You Try It?

If you're considering this approach, here's what Dr. Streicher wants you to know...

- **My patients swear by it.** While I agree on the need for more studies, in my own clinical experience, vulvar vaginal laser therapy has often been a game changer for my patients. Not only does the health of their vaginal lining improve, but they also appear to experience fewer urinary symptoms such as recurrent urinary tract infections, burning and urgency. Many report being able to have sex comfortably for the first time in years. The procedure is also showing promise for treating an itchy, painful condition called lichen sclerosus that affects the skin of the vulva outside the vagina.

• **It is not the only treatment.** For many women, more low-tech, and certainly less expensive, options may work just fine. Some women find relief by using a silicone vaginal lubricant and/or a long-acting moisturizer. Many women need more help than a lubricant or moisturizer can provide and benefit from a prescription option such as a low-dose estrogen delivered in a suppository, pill, cream, or ring placed in the vagina. Local vaginal estrogen is safe for virtually every woman. There also is an oral medication (*ospemifene*) that works similarly to estrogen to reduce vaginal symptoms and pain with sex. Another option is a new FDA-approved vaginal insert that uses the estrogen-precursor hormone DHEA to help you make your own vaginal estrogen—Prasterone.

But if these don't work for you or you simply prefer to not use medication, you may want to ask your ob-gyn about laser therapy. It's also an option for cancer patients with estrogen-receptive tumors, who are advised not to use hormone therapies.

• **Beware other products.** While there are other lasers on the market for gynecological use, I recommend the MonaLisa Touch because it is the device that has the most published scientific studies.

I do not recommend treatments using radiofrequency devices, even though they are a lot cheaper than laser therapy, because I do not believe there is enough scientific proof to support the claims being made for them.

• **It should be done by a gynecologist.** While other doctors, such as plastic surgeons or dermatologists, may offer MonaLisa Touch, it's best to see your gynecologist. Painful intercourse can be caused by many other gynecologic problems that will not be alleviated by a laser treatment (some of which mimic menopausal changes). Only a gynecologist is trained to diagnose these problems. Your gynecologist can also spot and address related gynecological issues that might need to be treated along with vulvovaginal atrophy, such as pelvic floor muscle issues.

The Sex-Starved Marriage

Michele Weiner-Davis, LCSW, founder of The Divorce Busting Center in Boulder, Colorado, which helps on-the-brink couples save their marriages. She is the best-selling author of eight books including *Healing from Infidelity*, *The Sex-Starved Marriage* and *Divorce Busting*. DivorceBusting.com

It has been two months since Janet and Mark have had sex. They're hardly speaking to each other. If you asked Janet about this, she would say that their home has become a battle zone—they fight about every little thing. Janet goes out of her way to avoid Mark to protect herself from his wrath.

Mark tells a different story. His anger, he believes, is justified. He is fed up with Janet's lack of interest in their sexual relationship. "She never initiates sex. She recoils when I try to kiss or hug her. I'm tired of being rejected." To cope with his unhappiness, Mark spends longer hours at work and busies himself on his computer at night, deepening the chasm between them.

Both Mark and Janet think that the other one is to blame for the problems between them. They have hit an impasse.

The result: A sex-starved marriage. And sex-starved marriages are surprisingly common. In fact, in about one in three marriages, one spouse has a considerably larger sexual appetite than the other. This in and of itself is not a problem—it's how couples handle their differences that matters.

Here's what you need to know to fix a sex-starved marriage and make you both happier…

Yearning for Contact

In a sex-starved marriage, one partner is longing for more touch—both sexual and nonsexual—and the other spouse isn't interested and doesn't understand why such a fuss is being made about sex. The less interested spouse thinks, *Is this just about having an orgasm? That's not such a big deal.* But the spouse yearning for more physical contact sees it differently. Being close physically is more than a physical release—it's about feeling wanted and connected emotionally.

When a misunderstanding of this magnitude happens and the less interested spouse continues to avoid sex, marriages start to unravel. Couples stop spending time together. They quit putting effort into the relationship. They become more like two distant roommates. Intimacy on all levels ends, which puts the marriage at risk for infidelity or divorce.

Typically, the spouse with the smaller sexual appetite controls the frequency of sex. If she/he (contrary to popular belief, men also can have low sexual desire) doesn't want it, it generally doesn't happen. This is not due to a desire to control the relationship—it just seems unthinkable to be sexual if one is not in the mood.

Furthermore, the lower-desire spouse has the expectation that the higher-desire spouse must accept the no-sex verdict and remain monogamous. The higher-desire spouse feels rejected, resentful and miserable.

How do two people with differing sexual appetites begin to bridge the desire gap? Regardless of where you stand on the sexual-desire spectrum, it's important to keep in mind that loving marriages are built on mutual care-taking. Don't wait for your spouse to change first. Be the catalyst for change in your marriage. *Here's how...*

If You Are the Lower-Desire Spouse

Just do it—and you may be surprised. Over the years, countless clients in my counseling practice have said, "I wasn't in the mood to have sex when my spouse approached me, but once we got going, it felt really good. I had an orgasm, and my spouse's mood really improved afterward."

Why would that be? For many people, the human sexual response cycle consists of four stages that occur in a certain order—desire (out of the blue, you have a sexy thought)... arousal (you and your partner touch, and your body becomes aroused)...orgasm...and resolution (your body returns to its normal resting state).

But for millions of people, stages one and two actually are reversed. In other words, desire doesn't come until after arousal. These people must feel turned on physically before they realize that they actually desire sex. Therefore, being receptive to your partner's advances even from a neutral starting place—when you do not feel desire—makes sense because chances are that sex will be enjoyable for both of you.

Give a "gift." Let's face it, there are times when people—even people with the typical desire/arousal pattern—simply don't feel like having sex. It's perfectly acceptable to decline your partner's offer from time to time. But when "no" substantially outweighs "yes," you are creating deep feelings of frustration and rejection—guaranteed.

What's the solution to an "I'm not really in the mood for sex" moment? Give a gift—a sexual gift—or to be more blunt about it, pleasure your spouse to orgasm if that's what he/she wants, even if you're not in the mood for the same. This is an act of love and caring and completely appropriate within a marriage.

If You Are the Higher-Desire Spouse

Speak from your heart. If you're feeling frustrated that your spouse hasn't understood your need to be close physically, chances are you've been irritable and angry. Anger is not an aphrodisiac—it pushes your spouse further away. Press your mental-reset button, and approach your spouse differently. Speak from your heart—express your vulnerability (yes, you are vulnerable, no matter how "tough" you are!) and your hurt.

Example: Instead of saying, "I'm angry that we haven't had sex in so long," it's better to say, "When we don't have sex for this long, I miss being close to you. I feel disconnected. It hurts my feelings that you don't seem interested in me sexually."

Rather than complain, ask for what you want. Complaining, even when it's justified, leads to defensiveness. Instead, ask for what you want in a positive way.

Example: Instead of saying, "You never initiate sex," say, "I'd really love it if once in a while, you threw your arms around me and said, 'Do you want to make love?' That would make me feel great."

Figure out what turns your spouse on. If buying sex toys or downloading X-rated videos has failed to entice your spouse to nurture your sexual relationship, there's probably a reason. Your spouse might need to feel courted by you first. You might be married to someone who feels more connected to you when you have meaningful conversations... spend enjoyable, uninterrupted time together other than having sex...are more affirming and complimentary...or when you participate in family activities together. This is how your partner feels loved—and the truth is, there are many people who want sexual intimacy only when they feel loved first.

If you're uncertain about your spouse's way of feeling cherished by you, ask. Say, "What can I do to make you feel loved?" Believe it or not, meeting your partner's needs, though different from your own, may be a turn-on for him/her. Try it.

Ovarian Tissue Freezing vs. Egg Freezing

Ovarian tissue freezing could be a fertility alternative to egg freezing. Nearly 40% of women who had the procedure to preserve fertility gave birth later in life, a new study reports.

Reproductive Sciences.

Can You Be Allergic to Estrogen Cream?

Mache Seibel, MD, professor of gynecology and obstetrics, University of Massachusetts Medical School, Worcester, a leading expert on women's health and menopause, and author of *The Estrogen Window: The Breakthrough Guide to Being Healthy, Energized, and Hormonally Balanced—through Perimenopause, Menopause, and Beyond.* DrMache.com

For most women, estradiol and other hormone creams don't burn, and it's pretty rare to be allergic to estrogen. If estrogen cream is causing discomfort, it's more likely that you have some other condition that's not related to perimenopause or low estrogen.

For example, you may have something called vulvar dystrophy, in which an area of thickened skin and gray or white plaque develops on the vulva. It itches like crazy. A lot of women will scratch the spot, sometimes at night when they're asleep, which can lead to cracks and abrasions. And then when you apply estrogen cream, the medium it's mixed in may get into the tiny cracks and make things worse. (For estrogen to be absorbable, it has to be whipped into a gel or cream that you then apply to your skin.)

If you are experiencing pain and itching after using hormone creams, I suggest you do two things...

- **First, try an over-the-counter topical product called Replens.** It doesn't have any hormones in it...it is less likely to burn or irritate your skin...and it will bring moisture to your vaginal tissues. This will give you some relief from itching and also be a clue as to whether the creams you've been using are causing the burning.
- **Make an appointment as soon as you can to see a doctor familiar with vulvar conditions** such as a gynecologist who treats vulvar conditions, or a dermatologist who treats the skin of the vulva.

Here's why: Few medical schools provide much training in vulvar problems, so it's a good idea to check with a specialist. If you have vulvar dystrophy, you might be prescribed short-term use of a topical steroid. Your doctor will also evaluate you to figure out if it is a different problem, such as an allergic reaction, a yeast infection, psoriasis—or, more rarely, a potentially precancerous condition of the skin.

Bottom line: Topical estrogen is highly unlikely to cause vaginal burning. If you have persistent vaginal itching, see your doctor to get to the root cause—and the right treatment.

Solving the Mystery Behind Breast Tenderness

Laurie Steelsmith, ND, naturopathic physician who writes the blog "Natural Healing Secrets for Women" at BottomLineInc.com. She is coauthor of three books—*Natural Choices for Women's Health*, the critically acclaimed *Great Sex, Naturally* and her latest, *Growing Younger Every Day.*

Susan, a 42-year old engineer and mother of two, came to me complaining of acute breast tenderness before her periods. While Susan was no stranger to changes in her breasts—she had breastfed both of her children—she was experiencing significant sensitivity in them before her periods. The tenderness would get so intense she could not hug her partner or children, and found that any jarring movement—including the jogging she loved—caused discomfort. She also complained of feeling short-tempered and "generally blue" before her periods.

Over the course of a thorough discussion, it became clear that Susan's symptoms had started slowly but had gradually grown worse. A breast exam revealed she had neither cysts nor lesions and, after learning that her symptoms were cyclical—they came and went with menstruation—I suspected hormonal imbalances. I ordered a 24-hour urine test on the 21st day of her cycle, which would allow me to assess her levels of estrogen, progesterone and testosterone, as well as her levels of the stress hormones cortisol and DHEA. Further, I requested a blood test and a basal body temperature test to examine her thyroid hormone levels, which are essential to healthy ovulation (and manifest in healthy levels of progesterone).

What my evaluation revealed: Susan's results were classic. She had an overabundance of estrogen but a shortage of progesterone, which was not a surprise given Susan's age. Women tend to have less-robust ovulation as they mature, and ovulation helps trigger production of progesterone. Susan's test results, as well as her symptoms, pointed toward "estrogen dominance"—a condition in which a woman has more estrogen than progesterone in the second half of her cycle. In addition to breast tenderness, women with estrogen dominance may also experience irritability, weepiness, frustration, moodiness, bloating and fatigue—exactly the sort of things Susan endured every month. Additionally, she had signs of low thyroid function, which can also affect progesterone production (among other things).

More Progesterone, Less Estrogen

To help Susan's body get back on track, I pinpointed three primary goals—lower her estrogen...boost her progesterone...and improve her thyroid function.

To tackle the first, we examined Susan's diet and exercise regimen. While she was an avid jogger—generally hitting the pavement two to three times a week—she admitted to "slacking off" the week before her period and not getting much other exercise besides her running. She agreed to move in some way every day—a vital component to striking hormonal balance, as working out helps one's liver to do its job of detoxifying the body (including removing excess estrogen).

I also advised Susan to step away from processed foods and instead reach for foods that aid the liver in breaking down estrogen, such as cruciferous vegetables (broccoli, cauliflower, Brussel sprouts), which contain compounds that convert unfriendly estrogen into friendly estrogen. What this means is that our bodies are constantly breaking down hormones, including estrogen. We can break down estrogen into compounds that are "anti-proliferative," which means anti-cancer, or those that could promote proliferation of estrogen-sensitive cells, thus becoming more pro-cancerous.

The great news is that you can impact which kind of estrogen dominates with your diet! Additionally, I suggested adding beets to her plate (beets are an excellent source of betaine, which promotes hormonal balance) and sipping on dandelion tea—an herb well-reputed for its ability to diminish bloating.

I further proposed that Susan take 100 milligrams of Vitamin B6 per day. A water-soluble vitamin that's found in turkey breast and chickpeas (among other foods), Vitamin B6 can bolster mood by activating "feel-good" hormones like dopamine and serotonin.

To boost Susan's progesterone, I recommended balancing her estrogen and progesterone with 175 milligrams of my all-time favorite herb, chaste tree berry. It contains compounds that lower the release of luteinizing hormone from the pituitary and that, in turn, decreases the breast tenderness. Chaste tree berry also heightens progesterone production in the ovaries.

Winning Formulas

Stanford University tested a formula containing chaste tree berry, called FertilityBlend for Women, and found that the herbal combination boosted progesterone by 150%. Not only did the formula help women conceive, but it also helped them with their premenstrual symptoms. In fact, the company repackaged the product for women with PMS and hormone imbalance and called it Asensia. I've been using this product in my practice and it has been effective.

Hearing this, Susan was immediately on board.

Finally, I recommended a thyroid-supportive product packed with nutrients to help the conversion of the inactive thyroid hormone T4 to the active form, T3. Not only does this support progesterone production, but it also upregulates the production of energy in every cell in the body—including the ovaries. The specific supplement I proposed contained a combination of iodine, gugulipid, ashwagandha and amino acids—all of which encourage this thyroid hormone conversion. By improving her thyroid function, we would also be promoting healthier ovulation and, thus, more progesterone to balance her estrogen—which would hopefully decrease her breast tenderness.

The patient's progress: Susan noticed an immediate improvement in her energy with the protocol I gave her.

Even more exciting: The tenderness in her breasts was virtually nonexistent when her next cycle arrived. Susan remained my patient for several years, and the support I offered her in her early 40s helped her through perimenopause and later as her body transitioned at menopause. With less dramatic symptoms, she was able to not only hug her children and partner and jog...she was also able to thrive.

Five Embarrassing Health Problems with Shamelessly Easy Solutions...

Bill Gottlieb, CHC, a health coach certified by the American Association of Drugless Practitioners and former editor in chief of Rodale Books and Prevention Magazine Health Books. He is author of 16 health books including *Speed Healing* (Bottom Line Books). BillGottliebHealth.com

Do you have an embarrassing health problem? Unfortunately, embarrassment can keep people from seeking solutions to their problems. And that's a shame because there are simple, fast, natural solutions for most embarrassing health problems.

Caution: If nondrug remedies don't work after a week or two, see your doctor—your health problem may have a serious cause that requires medical attention.

Bad Breath

Sulfur-generating bacteria in the mouth cause most cases of bad breath. And those bacteria usually are on your tongue.

Solution: Use a tongue scraper.

Scientific evidence: A study in *Journal of Periodontology* showed that tongue scraping reduced "volatile sulfur compounds" by 75%, while cleaning with a toothbrush reduced them by 45%.

What to do: First, buy a tongue scraper, available for less than $10 online and in drugstores.

Your goal is to remove the creamy-looking white, brown or orange layer of gunk on your tongue with the scraper. Gently but firmly scrape both the top and the sides of your tongue (but not the underside) from back to front. Start scraping as far back on the tongue as you can without gagging. If the gunk isn't completely gone, go over the same area until it is removed. After you are done, rinse the scraper.

Also helpful: In a scientific study published in *The Journal of Clinical Dentistry*, chewing gum with cinnamon essential oils reduced sulfur compounds in the mouth by more than 50%. And in a new study on bad breath, published in *Archives of Oral Biology*, scientists tested 10 essential oils and found that cinnamon oil was the most effective in reducing sulfur in the mouth.

Good product: Cinnamon-flavored, sugarless Spry gum, which contains bacteria-reducing xylitol. Chew it after every meal.

Passing Gas

You need to pass gas—it's a natural part of digestion, and the average person does it anywhere from six to 21 times a day. But passing it excessively is uncomfortable and embarrassing.

Most excessive passing of gas is caused by dysbiosis—an imbalance in intestinal bacteria, with "bad" bacteria such as Clostridium difficile outnumbering "friendly" bacteria such as *Lactobacillus acidophilus*.

Solution: Take a daily probiotic, a supplement containing friendly bacteria.

Scientific evidence: Researchers from the Mayo Clinic and other institutions analyzed the results of six studies on probiotics involving more than 560 people—and found that the supplement "significantly improved" flatulence.

Also helpful: If you're about to be in a social situation where gas is a no-no, take a preventive dose of activated charcoal, which works by binding with toxins (including unhealthful bacteria) and ushering them out of the body. Follow the dosage recommendations on the label.

Anal Itching

There are many possible causes of anal itching including diarrhea, incontinence, psoriasis, genital warts or a yeast infection. But one common cause is hemorrhoids, the swollen and inflamed anal veins that affect half of Americans over age 50. (If you have pain and bleeding with the itching, a hemorrhoid is the likely cause. But confirm the cause of anal itching with your doctor.)

Solution: To ease itching from hemorrhoids, one vein-strengthening food factor works particularly well—hesperidin, a flavonoid (plant pigment) found in citrus fruits.

Scientific evidence: A study in *British Journal of Surgery* analyzed 14 other studies on flavonoids and hemorrhoids, involving more than 1,500 people. The scientists found that consuming flavonoids cut the risk of itching from hemorrhoids by 35%—and also significantly reduced bleeding and pain.

What to do: Look for a supplement containing diosmin, a specially processed form of hesperidin. Take 500 milligrams (mg), twice daily. Diosmin is very safe, but a few people may experience intestinal discomfort—if that happens, stop taking the supplement.

Also helpful: Other ways to help prevent and heal hemorrhoids include drinking more water (60 ounces a day is a good goal)...increasing your intake of fiber-rich foods such as fruits, vegetables and whole grains...and regular exercise, such as brisk walking.

Dandruff

The flaking and itchiness of dandruff are caused by overproduction of a substance called sebum from glands in the scalp. These glands typically are hyperactive when the scalp is excessively dry. While dandruff shampoos control symptoms, they don't address the underlying problem. In fact, they often contain harsh cleansers that destroy the scalp's delicate balance of water and oil, further irritating the scalp and perpetuating the problem.

Solution: I often recommend a simple, natural, homemade antidandruff lotion, developed by aromatherapist Roberta Wilson. It normalizes the water- and oil-secreting glands of the scalp, helping to eliminate dandruff.

How to make it: To eight ounces of unscented, mild shampoo, add 10 drops of tea tree oil, eight drops of cedarwood oil, six drops of pine oil, six drops of rosemary oil, four drops of clary sage oil and four drops of lemon oil. Use the shampoo two or three times weekly, leaving it on for a minute or two each time. You should see results within a week or two.

Caution: If you have very sensitive skin, test each essential oil first. Put a dab on the inside of your wrist. If there is any redness or irritation after a few minutes, don't use it.

Award-Winning, Noninvasive Answer to Hair Loss

Lorraine Dahlinger, founder and CEO of From the Lab, a revolutionary beauty company giving women exclusive access to next-generation luxury products at an affordable price. Lorraine is passionately committed to helping women cut through a cluttered and often confusing beauty landscape to discover the joy of finding effective products that feature safe, sustainable and ethical ingredients.

Approximately 80 million people in the US experience hereditary hair loss, also known as androgenic alopecia, and 40% of those people are women. While male-pattern baldness generally manifests as a receding hairline and thinning crown, female-pattern baldness is characterized by a widening of the center part as the hair on top of the head thins and becomes brittle. For both men and women, however, the emotional side effects of hair loss can be devastating, leading to extreme treatments, which can include anything from painful surgeries to harsh prescription drugs.

Introduced in 2014, the active ingredient Redensyl became the first cosmetic alternative to hair transplantation surgery. A powerhouse combination of two patented molecules designed to stimulate stem cell proliferation and neutralize scalp inflammation, Redensyl dramatically reverses the effects of alopecia, demonstrating a 214% increase in hair growth. That's almost double the results of Minoxidil!

To better understand hair loss—and how Redensyl works—it's important to understand the normal growth cycle of your hair. Hair follicles cycle through three distinct phases of growth and rest stages. The Anagen phase is the growth phase. This period, which lasts for approximately three years, is then followed by the Catagen, or transition, phase, a period of about three weeks. Finally, the Telogen phase, during which the hair dies and falls out, lasts around three months before the entire cycle repeats.

Hair loss occurs when the follicle's stem cells become sluggish and less capable of supporting hair follicle growth, and become less efficient in communicating with the stem cells. Instead of continuing to cycle through the three normal stages of growth, your hair's Telogen phase lasts longer and longer while its transition to the Anagen phase becomes increasingly difficult. Your hair thins, dies, and falls out without being replaced efficiently.

Redensyl reactivates hair growth by triggering a new hair cycle. This increased nourishment allows the stem cells to switch on the Anagen phase faster, resulting in dramatically visible hair growth. *In just three months, clinical tests indicate that Redensyl...*

- **Increases the percentage of hair in the Anagen phase by 9%**
- **Decreases the percentage of hair in the Telogen phase by 17%**

In recognition of its efficacy and scientific innovation, Redensyl was awarded the Silver by In-Cosmetics Group for their Innovation Zone Best Ingredient Award in 2014.

It's important to remember that hair loss can be caused by any number of factors, including diet, medication, or even hair-care techniques, but sudden hair loss can be an early indicator of illness. If you experience any significant, unexplained changes in your hair, consult with your doctor before pursuing treatment.

Solving the Mystery of Thinning Hair…

Francesca J. Fusco, MD, assistant clinical professor, dermatology, Mount Sinai Hospital, New York City.

Hair loss can have many causes. Stress, thyroid disease, anemia and hormonal imbalances all can cause or worsen hair loss. Speak with your doctor about doing a panel of blood tests to identify whether any of these conditions—or a vitamin deficiency, such as low levels of vitamin D—are causing your hair to thin. Medications, such as beta-blockers, antidepressants and high-dose vitamin A, also can be culprits.

Psoriasis, persistent and chronic dandruff, eczema and allergic reactions to hair dyes all can cause inflammation of the scalp and subsequent thinning. You might also have androgenetic alopecia, a common genetic condition that makes you predisposed to hair loss. This condition can gradually result in a widening part and hair loss all over the scalp or just at the crown.

With any of these conditions, identifying and treating the cause of your hair loss can make a big difference in slowing it down or stopping it altogether. Medications to treat underlying disease…supplements to make up for vitamin deficiencies…and medicated shampoos and topical scalp treatments for inflammatory conditions (such as shampoos with coal tar or zinc pyrithione for psoriasis or dandruff, or a topical corticosteroid cream) can all stem hair loss and allow hair to gradually grow back.

Up to half of women with androgenetic alopecia notice some hair regrowth and/or slowdown of thinning after several months of using *minoxidil* (Rogaine), an over-the-counter, FDA-approved topical treatment. If the cause of your hair loss is your medication, your doctor may be able to switch you to a different drug.

You Have a Skin Microbiome—Here's How to Protect It

Kara Fitzgerald, ND, clinical director of the Sandy Hook Clinic, a practice devoted to functional medicine in Sandy Hook, Connecticut. DrKaraFitzgerald.com

Your skin is alive with visitors. Each square inch hosts millions of microbes…and that's a good thing. Like the "good bugs" in your gut, the skin's microbiome protects your health in many ways.

Consider skin bacteria. Some hold in water, helping to moisturize. Others protect you from ultraviolet light. But the most amazing benefit is the ability to help protect skin from infection by communicating with immune cells. A microbiome imbalance has been linked with eczema, psoriasis, rosacea, acne, poor wound healing, fungal infections—even plain old dandruff.

On the horizon: Topical live "probiotics" that treat eczema and other skin conditions.

But there's something we all can do now—protect this beautiful, elegant system. A healthy diet (fruits and veggies, little sugar, few refined carbs) and staying hydrated are essential but only the start…

- **Shower less often.** You're stripping your skin of natural moisturizers, literally washing away beneficial bacteria. If you now shower or bathe daily, try doing so every other day, even every third day.

Tip: If you're not particularly dirty or stinky, skip washing areas exposed to light and air such as your arms and neck.

• **Swear off antimicrobial soap.** The FDA has banned triclosan, an antimicrobial compound, from soaps and cleansers. It kills "good" bugs and may promote antibiotic-resistance in "bad" bugs. But now some soap manufacturers have switched to other antimicrobials, and there's no evidence that they are safer.

What to buy: Soap that doesn't mention killing microbes/bacteria on the label.

• **Wash lightly.** Regular soap often is alkaline and can interfere with the natural acidity of skin, which is key to preventing the growth of harmful organisms. Even gentle soap can wash away beneficial bacteria if you use it too frequently. One product that won't disturb skin microflora is Face & Body Cleanser from MotherDirt, which costs $15. *(Disclosure:* the company is a sponsor of my blog).

• **Do wash your hands.** Here's an exception to the "wash less" idea—to prevent the spread of infection, wash your hands with soap and water, especially if you're sick, you sneezed, you used the bathroom or you are going to handle food.

Tip: If you're not near soap and water, an alcohol-based hand sanitizer is a good idea. Still, don't overdo it—do you really need to squeeze that bottle 10 times a day?

• **Lotion up.** I like lotions that contain ceramides, fats that are a natural constituent of skin cells and help repair the skin's protective barrier. They help treat eczema and psoriasis (ask your doctor if you have one of those conditions).

• **Work up a sweat.** Perspiration is good for your skin microflora. It is believed to act as a prebiotic—food that these critters feed on. Working up a sweat two or three times a week should help keep your skin happy.

Excess Weight May Raise Rosacea Risk

Wen-Qing Li, PhD, assistant professor, dermatology and epidemiology, Brown University, Providence, Rhode Island.

Ross Levy, MD, chief, dermatology, Northern Westchester Hospital, Mount Kisco, New York, and clinical associate professor, dermatology, Albert Einstein College of Medicine, New York City.

Journal of the American Academy of Dermatology.

The skin disorder rosacea should be added to the list of chronic diseases linked to obesity, researchers report.

Their large new study found that the risk for rosacea increases among women as weight rises.

The researchers reviewed the records of nearly 90,000 US women, tracked over 14 years. They found a 48% higher likelihood of rosacea among those with a body mass index (BMI) greater than 35 than among women of normal weight.

A BMI of 30 or higher is considered obese. For example, a 5-foot-5-inch woman weighing 180 pounds has a BMI of 30. At the same height, someone who weighs 211 pounds has a BMI of 35.

"Particularly considering the chronic, low-grade inflammatory state associated with obesity, and also the [blood vessel] changes caused by obesity, it is not surprising obesity may increase the risk of rosacea," said study author Wen-Qing Li, PhD. He's an assistant professor of dermatology and epidemiology at Brown University in Providence, Rhode Island.

"Our study holds general public health significance, [adding] rosacea to the list of chronic diseases associated with obesity," Dr. Li said. "A healthier weight should definitely be encouraged for general health and well-being."

About Rosacea

Rosacea is characterized by facial redness and flushing, bumps and pimples, skin thickening and eye irritation, according to the National Rosacea Society. It's estimated to affect 16 million Americans.

The condition typically develops after age 30. Symptoms can wax and wane, varying by patient. There's no cure for rosacea, which is managed with oral and topical medications, antibiotics and laser treatments, among other therapies.

Study Details

Dr. Li and his team identified more than 5,200 cases of rosacea among tens of thousands of participants in the national Nurses' Health Study. They were tracked from 1991 to 2005. Not only was the risk of rosacea markedly higher among those with BMIs above 35, but there was a trend toward higher risk for rosacea among those who had gained weight after age 18.

What's more, the likelihood of developing rosacea increased by 4% for every 10-pound weight gain in study participants. The researchers also noted significantly higher odds of rosacea as girth—waist and hip measurements—rose.

The study was published in the *Journal of the American Academy of Dermatology*.

Implications

Dr. Li said the findings may prompt dermatologists to advise their patients with rosacea to reach a normal weight to "relieve their disease," though further clinical evidence is still needed.

About a third of US adults are classified as obese. Obesity has been linked to an increased risk for many health problems, including diabetes, cancer and early death, as well as inflammatory skin conditions such as psoriasis and acne.

Dr. Li also noted that his research didn't delve into the various subtypes of rosacea, which can be triggered by different factors. Also, the study only found an association between obesity and rosacea, rather than a cause-and-effect link.

"It is warranted to examine the effect of obesity on each type separately," Dr. Li said. "A large-scale clinical study would also be required to confirm that losing weight helps the relief of rosacea severity."

Expert Commentary

Ross Levy, MD, chief of dermatology at Northern Westchester Hospital in Mount Kisco, New York, said he wasn't surprised by the study's findings. He agreed with Dr. Li that obesity-driven inflammation could account for the increased risk for rosacea with weight gain.

"I would never tell somebody that if you lose weight your rosacea will get better, but I would probably hint to them that it might," said Dr. Levy, who wasn't involved in the new study. "Obesity is probably the No. 1 killer in the US. No one thinks of it that way, but it has such a great impact on everything."

The National Rosacea Society has answers to common questions about rosacea at Rosacea.org/patients/faq.php

---

Surprising Causes of Skin Rashes

Amy Chen, MD, assistant professor of dermatology, University of Connecticut School of Medicine, Farmington.

Julian Trevino, MD, professor of dermatology, Wright State University School of Medicine, Dayton, Ohio.

When it comes to avoiding painful, itchy rashes, everyone knows to steer clear of the Big Three—poison ivy, poison oak and poison sumac. But you should watch out for more than just the usual suspects, because something as simple as enjoying a poolside margarita or doing a little gardening can lead to skin irritation, rashes or worse.

Did you know...if the lemon or lime juice in that refreshing drink comes in contact with your skin, it can cause a chemical re-

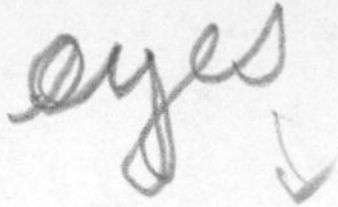

action that makes skin ultrasensitive to the sun (a condition called *phytophotodermatitis*), leading to burning, itching, stinging and even large blisters on areas of contact?

Allergic reactions can occur in some people when touching common houseplants such as chrysanthemums and Peruvian lilies, or plant bulbs such as daffodils or hyacinths. The bristly spines and small nettles or hairs on plants like cacti and thistles also contain chemicals that can irritate some people.

Foods such as chili powder and horseradish contain irritating chemicals that can cause burning, redness and hives when they touch a person's skin.

Note: The chemicals in these foods can irritate the skin in some people, but consuming them will not necessarily cause a reaction.

Self-defense: The American Academy of Dermatology (AAD) says the best defense is to avoid touching these irritants, but suggests some common-sense precautions as well, including wearing protective clothing (such as long pants, long-sleeved shirts and gloves) when working in the garden or taking a hike, and washing thoroughly after you come inside. Applying sunscreen can protect skin from the chemical reaction caused by the combination of citrus juices and the sun, as can rinsing the skin after contact.

If you do get a rash: Fortunately, most plant-related rashes can be treated with an over-the-counter or prescription antihistamine or topical steroid. However, the AAD does urge individuals to seek medical attention for a rash that doesn't fade, that spreads near your eyes or becomes infected (it might feel warm, ooze green or yellow fluid, swell or develop red streaks), if you develop a fever or body aches or if you have any difficulty breathing.

What to Do About Dark Circles and Puffiness Under Your Eyes

Ginger Hodulik Downey holds a BS in foods and nutrition, an MS degree in nutrition and a CNS (Certified Nutrition Specialist). She is currently the co-owner and vice president of R&D for DermaMed Solutions.

Dark circles don't discriminate. They affect people old and young, male and female and from all types of backgrounds. And they are one of the most frequent complaints I hear in my work in the skincare industry because they are so difficult to remedy. Even the best eye creams can only offer a small improvement in the dark appearance.

To me, the best approach is to figure out if there is some sort of health or lifestyle issue causing the problem and address the raccoon eyes from the inside out.

- **Not enough sleep.** Most people associate dark circles with lack of sleep, which certainly is a valid cause. When our bodies don't get enough rest, the blood vessels dilate (expand), and that's what creates the dark tint under the eyes. It's sort of like pressing a blue balloon under a thin white sheet; the closer it is to the surface, the more you see it under the sheet.

Poor sleep can also cause puffiness from the same blood vessels that bring fluid to the skin under the eyes. Like dark circles, the puffiness leaves us looking ragged and tired.

Rx: Get eight to 10 hours of quality sleep per night. To prevent puffiness, try elevating your head slightly with a pillow or two while sleeping. Also, drink plenty of water and watch your sodium intake. We tend to retain water when we are dehydrated or have too much salt in our diets.

- **Allergies and skin conditions** like eczema and dermatitis are an often-overlooked cause of dark circles. The issue here

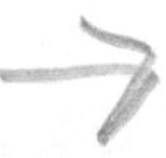

stems from the nasal-swelling congestion that comes with these conditions. The sinuses are located all around the eye area. When there's swelling on the inside you will see more circles under the eyes as all these tiny blood vessels expand. Additionally, sneezing and watery, itchy eyes will cause you to rub at the already-irritated area, increasing the redness and swelling.

Rx: Work with your doctor to manage skin conditions with proper diet and medications or supplements. In addition to taking an antihistamine to reduce swelling, many people benefit from daily sinus cleaning with a neti pot or nasal saline rinse. For "emergencies," like before a special event, try topical and oral arnica to relieve the swelling.

• **Your genes** cause the toughest cases, which frankly is completely out of your control. Certain ethnicities tend to have more melanin (pigment that makes our skin dark) under the eye area than others—namely people from Greece, the Middle East, Italy and India.

Rx: These folks can try using a skincare product with ingredients proven to lighten excess melanin.

My favorite ingredients are: Haloxy, a powerful peptide for dark circles and puffiness...kojic acid...azelaic acid...alpha arbutin...mandelic acid...and vitamin C. The acids can be a little strong for daily use under the eye area. My top pick is Haloxyl, which is found in high-end eye creams like our eyeradiance K'reme. It is also critically important to wear sunscreen every day, rain or shine, and to wear sunglasses.

• **Your age.** An equally difficult challenge is battling dark circles brought on by the aging process. As we age, our skin becomes thinner, increasing the appearance of the vessels under the skin. Also, over time our vessels get leaky and do not do their job as well as before. Blood vessels transport fluids and nutrients to the cells, as well as remove toxins from them. Age-related impairments in these processes cause more puffiness and pigment.

Rx: The fix here includes the Rx from the genetic approach above. This group can also benefit from practicing excellent hydration and by eating a variety of fresh plant foods, rich in vitamins and minerals, every day to support good vascular health. An omega 3 supplement can also help support vessels and lower inflammation to keep the blood flowing properly.

As you can see, there are many causes of dark circles and puffiness under the eyes, and plenty of lifestyle interventions to help you keep them under control. When all else fails and you just can't seem to get rid of those pesky circles, use a good moisturizing eye cream, a light reflecting concealer and a big bright smile...and no one will even notice those dark circles.

What Are Those Mysterious Little Bumps?

Jeffrey Callen, MD, chief of dermatology, University of Louisville School of Medicine, Louisville, Kentucky.

They can suddenly appear on your thighs... arms...bottom. These are areas you don't normally shave, so what's going on? Several common skin conditions can cause these occasionally reddish bumps, so it's important for you to get it checked out by your physician or dermatologist.

• **Keratosis pilaris,** commonly known as KP or "chicken skin" (because it resembles the skin of plucked chickens), often develops on the arms, thighs or buttocks. It occurs when hair follicles get clogged with dead skin cells. The clogged follicles form tiny, harmless red or tan bumps and often resemble goose bumps. To improve KP, use a moisturizer that contains lactic acid or urea within a few minutes after getting out of your bath or shower. Both of these ingredients help dissolve the dead skin cells plugging the follicles. (See next article for more remedies.)

• **Molluscum contagiosum** is a common, generally harmless skin condition characterized by waxy-looking bumps that result from a skin infection caused by a virus. They usually clear up by themselves within 12 to 18 months but may keep reappearing if the infection spreads to adjacent areas. A dermatologist can remove molluscum bumps (and the virus) with liquid nitrogen or by scraping them off. Both methods are somewhat uncomfortable. A prescription cream containing *tretinoin* or salicylic acid can also help clear them up.

• **Folliculitis** is caused by a bacterial infection of the hair follicles. Tight clothing can rub against the skin and irritate follicles. Folliculitis often goes away in a couple of weeks if you wear loose clothing that allows air to circulate. To speed healing, use a warm compress once or twice a day for about three minutes. To make a compress, soak a washcloth in warm water and wring it out. If this doesn't help, see a dermatologist who may prescribe a topical antibiotic.

Stop Hiding Your Chicken Skin Arms! Help for Keratosis Pilaris

Ginger Hodulik Downey, CNS, co-owner and vice president of R&D for DermaMed Solutions. She writes the blog "Beyond Beauty" for BottomLineInc.com.

"Chicken skin" is an embarrassing and sometimes uncomfortable condition that may prevent you from feeling your most confident...that cute spaghetti-strap dress stays on the hanger! If you are embarrassed by little pink- or flesh-colored bumps on your arms, read on.

Keratosis pilaris, the technical name for these unwelcome bumps, is a very common and medically harmless genetic condition that affects an estimated 30% to 50% of the adult population and approximately 50% to 80% of all adolescents. It is more common in women than in men, and is often present in otherwise healthy individuals.

Keratosis pilaris is caused by a buildup of keratin, which clogs the opening of the hair follicle and forms hard little plugs. Keratin, by the way, is a protein in our skin that protects us from infections and bacteria. We need keratin to maintain our immunity, so it serves an important function.

This annoying skin condition, which typically begins during childhood, can also show up on the tops of the thighs and on the buttocks. Many people grow out of it, but those who continue with it during adulthood may notice that it is worse during the winter, when the air is drier, and that it can completely clear up during the humid summer months. This condition is also more common in those with eczema and other atopic (allergy-related) skin conditions.

There's no magic cure for keratosis pilaris, but there are many ways you can help reduce the visual and physical symptoms with a treatment regimen that includes proper skin hydration, exfoliation, and good nutrition to support healthy skin from the inside out...

• **Bathe with warm water rather than hot and limit your time in the water to maintain your natural skin oils.**

• **Use cleansers and soaps that contain added lipids.** Look for coconut oil, shea butter, jojoba and/or squalene in product ingredient lists.

• **Apply a thick shea-butter- or coconut-oil-based moisturizer to the skin immediately after bathing and repeatedly during the day, as needed.**

• **Run a humidifier in your home to add moisture to the air.**

• **Remove dead skin cells from the surface of your skin by exfoliating with keratoytic (keratin removing) agents.** Choose creams and serums that contain acids such as glycolic, lactic acid and/or salicylic acid. For additional exfoliation, apply topical retinoids. These products will help to prevent the hair follicles from getting plugged up. (With this condition, a chemical exfoliation is preferred over a mechanical one like salt or sugar scrubs.) Women who are pregnant, nursing or may become pregnant should avoid topical retinoids.

• **Include ample omega-3 fatty acids in your diet.** They provide the skin cells with the lipids they require to maintain moisture and also reduce inflammation. Aim for two servings of fatty fish per week. You can also get omega-3s from plant sources like walnuts, flax and chia seeds.

• **Feed your skin the right minerals.** Magnesium and zinc support skin integrity. Spinach, nuts and seeds are good sources.

For those who have exhausted all of these healthy lifestyle approaches and still suffer, consider laser treatments. Hair removal using Intense Pulsed Light (IPL) is an excellent choice because it targets the hair follicle, shutting it down so no clogging can occur. Our hair follicles each grow in different phases, so it may take several sessions before you see results. Four treatments are typically recommended. (These treatments would not be covered by insurance since there is no medical reason for them.)

What to Do About Sweaty Palms

Jenny Murase, MD, associate clinical professor of dermatology, University of California, San Francisco Medical Center.

Sweat is a natural response to prevent the body from overheating during hot weather, vigorous exercise or in situations that trigger anxiety or anger. But sweat that's uncontrollable and excessive (your palms may be so sweaty that you have difficulty typing on your keyboard, for example, or you leave moisture stains on paper) could be a sign of a condition called *hyperhidrosis*.

People with hyperhidrosis sweat excessively for no apparent reason—often from the palms, feet, underarms or head. It can run in families or result from another medical condition, such as a thyroid problem or diabetes—or even menopause.

Powder or a bit of antiperspirant containing aluminum chlorohydrate (which plugs sweat glands) may help. (Apply antiperspirants at night to completely dry skin. But don't cover your hands once you have antiperspirant on them or you risk irritating the skin.) But if your palms still drip with sweat, consult a dermatologist, who can prescribe a more potent antiperspirant, such as Drysol, or *glycopyrrolate* (Robinul), an oral medication that reduces sweat and other secretions.

Botox can be injected to block nerves that stimulate sweating, but it is very painful when done on the palms. Other options include *iontophoresis*, a procedure that uses electricity to shut down the sweat glands. The procedure is usually done several times a week until sweating lessens, then treatments are continued on a regular basis (typically once a week) to maintain results. Insurers may cover these treatments.

Severe cases of hyperhidrosis may require surgery to cut nerves in the chest that send signals to sweat glands. The surgery usually has good outcomes, but there are potential risks, such as infection and bleeding.

INDEX

Eyes

61 allergies ✓
63
281 282 287 ✓
109, 283, 284, 286

327-328 ✓

131, 286, 287 ✓

58 ✓
284-286 ✓
286 ✓
281, 287 ✓
284-287 ✓
282, 287 ✓

58
89

F

P

Q

R

S